THE PIPER PROTOCOL

THE PIPER PROTOCOL

The Insider's Secret to
Weight Loss and Internal Fitness

TRACY PIPER

WITH EVE ADAMSON

WM

WILLIAM MORROW

An Imprint of HarperCollins *Publishers*

This book is written as a source of information only. The information contained in this book should by no means be considered a substitute for the advice of a qualified medical professional, who should always be consulted before beginning any new diet, exercise, or other health program.

All efforts have been made to ensure the accuracy of the information contained in this book as of the date published. The author and the publisher expressly disclaim responsibility for any adverse effects arising from the use or application of the information contained herein.

THE PIPER PROTOCOL. Copyright © 2014 by Tracy Piper. All rights reserved. Printed in the United States of America. No part of this book may be used or reproduced in any manner whatsoever without written permission except in the case of brief quotations embodied in critical articles and reviews. For information address HarperCollins Publishers, 195 Broadway, New York, NY 10007.

HarperCollins books may be purchased for educational, business, or sales promotional use. For information please e-mail the Special Markets Department at SPsales@harpercollins.com.

FIRST EDITION

Designed by Lisa Stokes
Photography by Jeff Skeirik, a.k.a. Rawtographer, www.rawtographer.com

Library of Congress Cataloging-in-Publication Data has been applied for.

ISBN 978-0-06-231705-6

14 15 16 17 18 OV/RRD 10 9 8 7 6 5 4 3 2

To my grandmother, Ellen, to Tucan and Niko, and to all my beloved clients, who have inspired my passion for this work.

Contents

Preface

MANY YEARS AGO, AS I was finishing my training as a cardiologist in New York, I became very sick. I visited three specialists, got tons of medical tests, and was given three different diagnoses, followed by seven prescriptions for medication. I was told I would need them all in order to function. But the drugs did not take care of the underlying problem. Their only purpose was to silence my symptoms.

Even though I had been trained to treat my patients in exactly this way, being on the patient side of things changed my perspective, and all those prescriptions didn't make sense to me. I decided to find a different solution—a drug-free solution. I found my way back, not only to vibrant health but also to looking and feeling ten years younger, through cleansing and detoxification.

During this journey, I met some remarkable people who taught me a lot. Tracy Piper is up there with the best of my newfound friends. Her vast knowledge, experience, and compassionate bedside manner, along with her hurricane-strong shamanic spirit, helped me to heal. I wish someone had given me her book back in the days when I was so sick. It would have saved me a lot of time and money as I searched desperately for a solution to my health issues. Because the truth is that the path to health is much simpler than many doctors will lead you to believe.

I highly recommend her book to anyone who wants to get and stay healthy, or help others do the same.

With much love and respect,

—*Alejandro Junger, M.D.*, New York Times *bestselling author of* Clean, Clean Gut, *and* Clean Eats

Foreword

NO PHYSICIAN CAN "HEAL thyself." It is hard to admit we as doctors need help sometimes. As someone who is both a doctor and a person who suffers from celiac disease, hypothyroidism, and other immune disorders, I was one of those doctor-patients who needed help from other healthcare practitioners, because despite the fact that I knew a lot about disease and its conventional and integrative treatments, I needed someone to step in and help me heal.

During my leadership at the Atkins Center for Complementary Medicine in early 1999, I became familiar with colon hydrotherapy. I was intrigued by this procedure and its reported effectiveness in the treatment of many bowel conditions. Some of these bowel conditions are associated with systemic disease, and I thought this therapy might help me. I inquired within my network of colleagues, and that's when I found Tracy Piper.

After visiting her and then referring patients to her, it was my turn to try the process for myself, to see if it could do something for my "sick" colon. I completed a series of colonics with great ease and no distress, and for the first time in decades, my colon began to heal. I was impressed. Tracy and I began to work together. Combining our knowledge, we have been able to increase and restore internal fitness, not just to me but to countless others. Of course, a new dietary and exercise lifestyle has been of great importance, as well. Tracy and I spent countless hours at conferences discussing different remedies and approaches, and it is with great admiration that I recommend this book, as a handbook for the future of internal fitness. I believe her approach will soon become an integral part of mainstream medicine.

But it can become a handbook for you *today*. Internal fitness is essential for everyone. You cannot be externally fit unless you are internally fit. The gut, or the digestive system, is the gateway to all disease, so you must take good care of it. More than 70 percent of Americans are affected with diseases of the digestive system, such as colitis, constipation, irritable bowel disease, candida, and unexplained weight gain or weight loss, not to mention autoimmune conditions like celiac disease and the epidemic of obesity in our culture. As Tracy so clearly states, without internal fitness, we would not be healthy. There are some of you that suffer from eczema, brain fog, decreased glandular function, urinary tract infections, and thin, weak hair. All of these are directly caused by an ineffective cleansing of your colon. A toxic environment, a Westernized diet (with too many processed foods), daily stress, and poor lifestyle choices are the major causes of the digestive disease epidemic.

Since our patients seek our guidance and expertise in overseeing their healthcare, this book is long overdue. In fact, it is one of the best cleansing books ever written that frankly and directly addresses colon cleansing with candor and honesty. It also clearly explains and helps the reader to implement many other health strategies that I myself recommend and utilize. These practices are no longer "fringe." There is a body of experiential strategies and evidence-based literature to support the utilization of these integrative strategies in healthcare.

Although I was not born in St. Thomas nor have I lived in Tortola and although I have never met Tracy's "Granny," I can relate to her personal journey. As her Granny gave her cod liver oil every day, my Nanny made sure I, too, had my daily spoonful of cod liver oil before I left for school. Different cultures and different people share one common denominator: Earth Mother's many remedies for sickness and tools for healing. Let Tracy Piper be your translator.

The Piper Protocol will take you on a journey. It might well be a journey you never thought you would venture into, but it is a journey that will change you for the better. I ask you to challenge yourself with this educational, inspirational, and compelling book about self healing and internal fitness. I feel privileged to have been part of Tracy's journey, and I know how privileged she feels to be part of yours.

—*Patrick Fratellone, M.D., R.H. (AHG), F.I.M., F.A.C.C., integrative cardiologist, Fellow of Integrative Medicine, director of Fratellone Medical Associates in New York City, president of the New York City chapter of the American Herbalists Guild, nationwide lecturer, and host of the show "The Integrated Physician" on BlogTalkRadio. Dr. Fratellone was also recognized by The National Academy of Medicine for his outstanding excellence in humanitarianism. Follow his daily dispatches at www.fratellonemedical.com.*

Who I Am and Why
I Can Help You

THIS BOOK WILL TAKE you on a journey. It will take you from wherever you are now to a cleaner, purer, more vibrant, and more alive place, where you will feel better than you do right now. It is about cleansing your inside and your outside—your body, mind, and spirit. But it is also about more than cleansing. It is about *living* by freeing yourself from the behaviors and influences that keep you from being as healthy, radiant, and fit as you can possibly be.

There's no more important or basic level of fitness than what is inside you, at your very center. All other fitness and all health begin with digestion; without regular maintenance, your body won't work as well as it could and should. No matter how experienced or inexperienced you are at cleansing, there's always more to do, as the body constantly transforms food into flesh and processes the detritus of living so it doesn't harm you.

In this book, I'll take you through your own body and show you exactly what's happening, where things can go wrong, and what you can do about it. We'll begin by covering the mechanisms of the body, how your body cleanses naturally, and how you can help this process, and then I'll show you what I show my celebrity clients every day: How to make your body, your mind, and your spirit feel better, look better, and behave better on every level. I'll show you how to be not just more beautiful on the outside but, much more important, more internally fit—because that is where beauty begins.

I have a lot of information for you, and I hope you will absorb it and let it change you. Each chapter in the first two parts of this book will tackle a topic you need to understand in order to become internally fit, and at the end of each chapter, I'll give you an Internal Fitness Prep Step to help you develop some great internal fitness habits. These will build upon each other, stepping you up to a place where you will be ready for the Piper Protocol, given in Part Three.

Then we'll jump into the serious business of cleansing. I'll introduce you to the Piper Protocol, the program I use with my clients in my clinic in SoHo, and with my many actor and model clients who hire me to get them ready for film shoots, photography sessions, and awards ceremonies. However, I've modified the program just for you—I believe cleansing is individual and must be flexible if it's going to help you. I've created varying levels of intensity, and you can jump in where you want to and whenever you're ready to begin. You can also jump off when you need to, or stay where you are for as long as you need to; only when you are ready do you increase the intensity. The Piper Protocol is built to adapt to *your* needs and to progress only when your body is ready to move forward.

WHAT YOU SHOULD KNOW ABOUT CLEANSING

In the United States, we take cleanliness for granted. We assume things are generally safe, if not sterile, and as long as we take showers and eat vegetables once in a while, our bodies will self-clean. People seem to have this idea that their insides are clean, too—a clean-as-a-whistle tube from mouth to rear, where the food slides through and the walls remain smooth and slick as glass. Or we don't really know, or care to know, what happens in our insides—what it looks like in there, what else lives in there, how well things are moving along, how effectively our organs are functioning. Until something hurts, most people don't tend to pay too much attention. Until something goes wrong, we may not even consider the idea of "doing a cleanse."

In recent years, however, I've seen the beginnings of a curiosity about cleansing—people are wondering about it, asking about it, trying cleanses they hear about or find here and there. My clients ask me about cleanses all the time, and they have a lot of very specific questions, many of which they are embarrassed to ask. There's definitely a buzz out there about cleansing, but it's hardly a mainstream topic yet; and compared to diet books, there aren't a lot of books on cleansing that go into the details or give people the answers they seek.

A few years ago, I was one of those people seeking answers, and this is the book I wish had been there for me when I first began my cleansing journey. It answers all the questions people have about cleansing, even the embarrassing ones nobody wants to talk about. It answers the questions you may not even know you had until you read the answers. It's a book without fear or shame, a book that delves deep into what's happening inside your body and how you can optimize that process. It's the book you didn't know you needed, but that you *do* need—I would even venture to say *need urgently*. You need this book because practically everyone could improve his or her internal hygiene for more vibrant health; and from what I see in my practice, most people's internal hygiene isn't nearly as good as they think it is. And that leads to bad health news down the road, including obesity, chronic pain, and disease.

But cleansing can turn all that around, changing your future prospects from grim to great and your future silhouette from stout to slim. It can restore your energy and may even help your body gain control over chronic conditions.

I believe that everyone needs to cleanse periodically, and that cleansing should be both safe and effective. Whether you're new to cleansing or are a cleansing veteran, you can find a place within the Piper Protocol, and you can make progress toward a cleaner, fresher, stronger, more energetic and vibrant body. You can become internally fit—a literal embodiment of health.

But who am I to tell you how to cleanse? Let me introduce myself.

MY CLEANSING JOURNEY

Cleansing has always been a part of my life, long before I became a cleansing specialist, long before I even realized "cleansing" was a "thing." Where I come from, cleansing is just what people do. I was born in St. Thomas, in the U.S. Virgin Islands, but I moved to Tortola, in the British Virgin Islands, when I was just three years old to live with my grandmother. With four children, my parents were overwhelmed, and my grandmother needed company, but we didn't have an easy life in Tortola. Our home was modest, and although it was always clean, luxuries like indoor plumbing were beyond our reach. I grew up using a latrine. Sometimes I had to use an enamel pail and carry my "belonging" to the latrine to dump it. I was tiny and my grandmother didn't want me sitting up there—she was afraid I would fall in!

My grandmother led a simple life and so, by necessity, did I. I didn't have computers or video games or designer clothes, and when someone got sick, it wasn't a matter of traipsing off to the nearest world-class surgeon at a major medical center, or driving past the pharmacy pick-up window for a fully-covered-by-insurance bottle of $500 medicine. The Caribbean is beautiful, but life is hard. People practiced prevention seriously in those days because it was much easier to stay healthy than to be sick. Of course, that's true for everyone, but back then, it was more obvious; the consequences of *not* doing everything you could do to prevent illness were dire—even a matter of bankruptcy . . . or life and death!

My granny was a woman of great wisdom, generous with her laughter and her herbal remedies, and knowledgeable about what nature had to offer us. I grew up eating natural foods. Nothing was processed. I never ate anything from a package. My grandmother cooked daily. We ate fruit and vegetables picked from the neighbors' trees and purchased from the local market, where on Saturdays everyone sold their crops in the market square. Much of what we ate was raw, rich with minerals from the soil: sugar apple, pomegranate, cane, soursop, genips, limes, mangoes, bananas, spinach, pumpkin, cherry tomatoes, pigeon peas (gandules), avocados, aloe, hibiscus flowers, papaya, and coconuts. My grandmother would carry me down to the bay to the fishermen's spot to get our fresh fish. I always got the best doctor fish and yellowtail because one of the fishermen was our neighbor.

My grandmother also had her own particular cleansing rituals. Every Friday night before bed, she gave me a spoonful of castor oil and steaming cups of foul-tasting bush tea to drink, to help move my bowels. I hated those tastes—I can still taste them today!—but in the Caribbean, it was a common thing to do. Still, I would whine, "Why do I have to take this?" My grandmother always answered in the same way: "To keep your insides clean." I couldn't exactly argue with that. I couldn't prove they were already clean, the way I could hold up my fingernails or feet for inspection. I had to trust that my granny knew what she was doing.

I learned a lot about herbal medicine from my granny. She took me with her on her outings to collect botanicals. We picked the plants and then went home to make tea or other remedies. Crab bush tea was for colds and flus, soursop leaves were for insomnia and cancer, and there was an orange vine that strangled the life out of other plants if it wrapped around them. We called it "orange spaghetti," because that's what it looked like. It was known in Tortola as the only cure for jaundice, and it worked.

I had my own personal interactions with the Caribbean plant life. My grandmother worked as a housekeeper for a neighbor. Every Saturday, she took me with her. While she worked indoors washing, folding, and ironing the clothes, I had to stay outside and be quiet so as not to disturb Mr. and Mrs. Smith. They had lots of flowers on their grounds and I made "perfume" from them:

alamanda, night-blooming cactus flower, hibiscus, and white ginger. I would mix some flowers in a bowl and grind them to make my perfume from their oils. Little did I know I was studying aromatherapy.

My granny believed that nature's gifts, its plants and herbs, would keep us healthy. She prayed a lot, and she believed that everything lived and worked according to the cycles of the moon and stars. These were my first lessons in raw food, aromatherapy, herbology, and cleansing—and I was a good student and obedient cleanser. The more I learned, especially later in my training, the more I saw this reflected also in many other cultures—every organ has its natural timing and its natural cycle. I also saw my granny's ways reflected in my own. I live in New York City now, but I maintain that same respect and reverence for what nature has to offer us, including how a natural, internal balance and cleanliness, along with a healthy respect for spirit, can heal people.

But I also developed some unusual health problems—things even my granny wasn't sure how to handle. I didn't eat very much. In fact, I was so skinny that people made fun of me. The problem was, every time I ate more than just a tiny bit, I would throw up.

My weight got so low that, at one point, my teacher called the police, suspecting my grandmother wasn't feeding me. They came to the house and made me eat food in front of them, to prove that my grandmother was telling the truth when she said that she did indeed feed me, but that I couldn't keep anything down. Dutifully, I ate the food in front of me—then promptly threw it all back up again.

The doctors said I had something called involuntary bulimia, due to an overactive vagus nerve. Now I know all about the vagus nerve, but at the time, neither my grandmother nor I understood what this meant. The prescription was steroids, which would increase my appetite and dampen the regurgitation response; but when the steroids didn't work within a few days, they increased the dosage, and then increased it again. Finally, the steroids kicked me into overdrive. I started eating and stopped throwing up, and I started gaining weight . . . and more weight, and more weight, and more. Steroids often have this effect, swelling the body and encouraging the body to retain water, as well as hang on to fat. When I became quite overweight, I tried to lose weight, but when my weight began to drop again, they gave me more medicine. For the next few years, my weight went up and down, up and down. I became obsessed with losing weight and I started dieting at a very young age, all in a desperate attempt not to be fat. I'm sure this situation did some terrible damage to my body, which wouldn't show up until I was an adult.

But my grandmother needed me, and I was there for her, despite my own troubles. When she developed terrible arthritis and could not use her hands for a while, I was able to return all the care she had given me by taking care of her. She taught me to cook by telling me what to do. When we moved to St. Thomas after she took sick, a nurse came to show me how to give my grandmother her daily injections. I became so good at giving injections that I was told I had the hands to become a surgeon. That stayed in my mind. I began to believe I had a gift for healing.

When I was eleven, my grandmother passed away and I moved back with my parents, but my motivation to heal others only grew stronger. At fifteen, I volunteered as a candy striper at a local hospital, and I loved it. It was the proudest moment in my life thus far, when I put on that uniform (which my mother sewed for me) and went to the hospital to *work*.

Then one day I got run over by a bicycle on the street. (I'm still frightened of bicycles and never learned to ride one—don't laugh!) I lost all my teeth and so I ate nothing but ice cream for nine months. That sounds like every kid's dream, but believe me, on about day three, pistachio ice cream loses its charm. I also began to have chronic congestion. All through junior high and high school, I always had a runny nose and felt stuffed up. I would keep a roll of paper towels with me and go through a whole roll in two days, just blowing my nose—and I would use every inch of that tissue. My mom wanted to know why I was always blowing my nose, but of course, I didn't know any more than she did.

Then I developed a cyst on the side of my chin, which I had to have removed. Then I developed another cyst on one of my ovaries, and I had to have that removed, too. That was two surgeries, and I was still in high school. I couldn't understand why I would have developed cysts.

I remember asking the doctor why I was having this problem. Now, if you are aware of the Caribbean rule of elders, you know that you never look your elder in the eyes, you don't ask questions, and you don't talk back. I was going against everything I had learned, but I reasoned that this was a doctor and he must have answers, and I needed those answers because this was about my body! He was annoyed, as would be expected in our culture, but he answered me anyway, and the answer surprised me.

"Too much mucus. Too much dairy. Milk, cheese, that kind of thing." And then he left the room.

I thought back to those nine months of ice cream. I thought about the thick canned milk I poured on my cream of wheat or oatmeal every morning—a typical Caribbean breakfast. I thought about the cheese I liked to snack on. I still didn't realize I was severely allergic to dairy products and that it was all related to why I was always blowing my nose, and I didn't yet know I had set up my body for chronic inflammation I would fight for years to come, but I decided that I had no interest in returning to that doctor or that hospital again.

I vowed to quit drinking milk and eating ice cream or cheese. I ate my cream of wheat or oatmeal without milk thereafter—not yet knowing I was also very reactive to gluten. Even after I gave up dairy, I continued to suffer from chronic congestion, as well as brain fog, fatigue, and mild depression, but I got good grades so nobody thought anything was wrong. And me? I just thought this was how everybody must feel all the time.

AS I GREW OLDER, the healing arts came naturally to me. Maybe it was because of my own health challenges, or maybe it was because of my grandmother—or both. I was still working at the hospital, and taking care of the patients became a passion. I decided to become a doctor and make my grandmother proud. As I watched sick people get better, I knew I wanted to be a part of that.

I worked in that hospital for many years, completely focused on my budding career. I didn't care about parties with my friends or hanging out. I spent all my free time studying and working. My hard work paid off when I was promoted to a position working for a physical therapist in the hospital. Then I took a job in a private physical therapy office while working on my biology/ pre-med degree at the University of the Virgin Islands (UVI). While I was there, I would sometimes do massages on people, and I noticed that the people who got the massages along with their physical therapy responded much faster than the people who got only the physical therapy. This fascinated me, and I began to wonder about getting certified as a massage therapist.

After I graduated, I moved to New York City with $100 to my name and big plans to eventually attend medical school at Boston University. But first, I wanted to learn more about massage therapy. I attended the Swedish Institute, where I became a licensed massage therapist, all the while fully intending to enter medical school. My friends were already there, and they considered American medical school easy compared to the grueling schedule and teachings at UVI, so I knew I could handle it.

Then, something shocking happened that changed my life forever. My roommate's boyfriend became sick quite suddenly, and then he was dead. The reason? Severe constipation. He had one regular bowel movement a day, like most people, so we were all stunned to hear that his colon had burst and poisoned him. He died from a massive infection that resulted from a burst diverticulum. One moment he was a young, seemingly healthy man. The next moment he was gone. My roommate was devastated and I was in shock. I couldn't help thinking back to my childhood, with those spoons of castor oil and that horrible-tasting bush tea. Maybe my grandmother was wiser than I knew.

I had heard about colon hydrotherapy before, but I couldn't imagine ever actually getting something so extreme as a colonic. Still, I couldn't stop thinking about what had happened to my friend. Almost on a whim, I looked up colon hydrotherapy in the yellow pages and made an appointment. I went in for my first session, thinking once would be enough to reassure me that my body was fine.

I was nervous, but the colon therapist reassured me that the procedure was safe and would make me feel great. It was a bit startling at first, but I did feel good afterward—until she showed me what had come out of me. I didn't want to look, but yet I couldn't help doing that. I couldn't believe my eyes when I saw what had, just moments before, been inside my body.

She told me I needed to come back the day after tomorrow. I was emphatic: It wasn't necessary! Why would I have to come back? I remember saying, "I'm sorry, but I just shit for forty-five minutes. There is nothing left." She told me to humor her and come back that Wednesday.

So I did. I figured that maybe, just maybe, there might be a little residue left. To my surprise, I released more on Wednesday than I did on Monday.

"See?" she said.

However, I was stubborn. I refused to believe that what came out was older than two days. Surely it was from whatever I had eaten between Monday and Tuesday. The colon therapist told me that we can hold twelve or more meals inside of our colon at one time, depending on how often we go to the bathroom, so she said I should get a package of three colonics. I was skeptical.

"Fine," I said. I figured as long as I'd done two already, I might as well get the third one. But I'm a Scorpio, you see, and I wanted to show her that she was full of it (and that I wasn't!). I decided to drink nothing but unrefined apple juice until my next colonic that Friday.

When I came in on Friday, I was pretty proud of myself, and a little bit excited to prove her wrong. I told her about my devious apple juice agenda, and she just smiled and said, "Good. Now we can really get down to business."

Once the colonic started, I looked around to see that nothing was coming out, and to my surprise, my body released more than on Monday and Wednesday combined! How could this be? I didn't eat. Seriously, I did not cheat one bit. This was mindboggling to me. (Never let your ego get the best of you—it's quite humbling!)

When I saw the results, I was sold. I wanted it all out of me. I decided to do the little dietary changes she asked me to do: drink more water, stop eating sugar, and have a salad every day. I lost 5 pounds by the end of the week, and two and a half months later, I was 55 pounds lighter and felt as if I'd begun a whole new life.

I bought a series of fifteen colonics and put it on my credit card. I had just moved to New York, so I didn't have a lot of money. Because I was so serious about my health after that, the colon therapist put me on a payment plan and let me pay what I could because she wanted me to heal. I was impressed with her dedication, patience, and honest caring. It made me realize that I wanted to do what she did—to help people on a deeper level (literally!).

The more I learned, the more I continued to refine my own diet and lifestyle. I still had occasional symptoms of bloating and inflammation, which I hadn't noticed until I lost weight. I yearned for more knowledge and truth, so I immersed myself in the science of digestion. While I worked part time at Barnes & Noble, I came across Dr. Peter D'Adamo's book *Eat Right 4 Your Type*. I was fascinated by that book! It totally resonated with me. After two weeks of following the Blood Type O diet, I had no more gas. I tried to find some inside me. I would strain and test myself—but there was nothing. I was gas-free, bloat-free, for the first time in years. As a further test, I ate a few of the "forbidden" foods, and sure enough, the gas came back. I began putting two and two together, and before I knew it, I had a whole new plan for my life.

I decided medical school wasn't for me after all. Instead, I enrolled in the Pacific College of Oriental Medicine. In 2001, I received a master's degree in acupuncture and Chinese herbology. And the more I learned, the more I wanted to know. I was hungry for truth.

I remember the moment when I first thought of going to school to study colon therapy. I was in Manhattan, on the F train heading home from acupuncture school, and it came into my mind: I would open my own cleansing center. I couldn't stop thinking about it and planning it. I didn't sleep that night. Instead, I envisioned my entire life forward: my own business, what it would look like, what type of disciplines I would have in it, everything.

After that epiphany, I went to Toronto and enrolled in the Canadian Natural Health and Healing Centre, where I studied to become a certified colon hydrotherapist. After I received my certification, I returned to New York and studied iridology (a technique for diagnosing health issues by studying the iris of the eye) with Judy Vedder, a former student of Bernard Jensen and the owner of the New York Center for Iridology.

Armed with knowledge and ready to start my own business, I opened the M.A.R.C. Holistic

Center, which is now called The Piper Center for Internal Wellness, in New York City. My first celebrity clients were a supermodel and her A-list movie director husband, who came in for massages. This opened the door for other celebrities to find out about me. People tell other people when something works. When your life changes, you want to talk about it. You want to help other people. It was all the advertising I needed.

Life was looking great—until in 2010 I was diagnosed with a serious health challenge. My thyroid, which could have been damaged as far back as those early days when I was given high doses of steroids for years, developed hypothyroidism and then Hashimoto's thyroiditis. My voice grew hoarse and I had trouble swallowing because of the swollen lymph nodes in my neck and a nodule on the right side that kept getting bigger and harder.

I had to do something. By this time, I had so much health training that I knew just what I still needed to learn. I went to the Ann Wigmore Natural Health Institute in Puerto Rico, where they taught a living food curriculum, and I embarked on a new raw-food lifestyle. When I returned, I had blood work done, and all my abnormalities were down 50 percent, in just two weeks! I couldn't believe the stunning results. I realized I had been cleansing others while not exactly practicing what I preached.

My recovery inspired me further. If raw and living foods could work this quickly on me, what could they do for others? I studied at many different schools, including the Cayce/Reilly School of Massotherapy in Virginia Beach, the school founded by Edgar Cayce, the American mysticist who is credited with being the father of holistic medicine. I learned even more about detoxification and the effects of chemical exposure from the Dr. Robert Morse International School of Detoxification in Florida. I learned more about inflammation, and the effects of acidity in the body, as well as how to make the body more alkaline. I learned about water and juicing and raw food preparation, and even how to teach colon hydrotherapy. Everything I learned I then proceeded to apply to myself—and to offer to my clients.

Today, I have hundreds of high-profile and celebrity clients who fly me all over the country to get them ready for whatever they need to do. They have to look good, but more important, they have to feel good from the inside out. I am constantly advising, massaging, counseling, and cleansing people ages eighteen to eighty-five, ranging from models to doctors, to Wall Street power brokers, and from raw-food devotees to magazine editors, to personal trainers, and to the group I affectionately call the "Tribeca Moms"—the women who got me on my feet when my clinic first opened by spreading the word about what I could do.

However, there's only so much I can do in person. I decided that I want to help more people than just those who come into my clinic or who can afford to fly me to a movie set. I want to help you.

You see, I know what it's like to feel poorly. I know what it's like to suffer a health crisis. I still struggle with health issues. Every time I let my diet slip and start eating more cooked food, every time I'm under a lot of stress, every time I get lax in maintaining my healthy lifestyle, the inflammation increases and I feel my energy waning. My body becomes more acidic, and problems resurface.

I also know what it's like to pinch pennies and not be able to afford the healing you need. I've been there, for most of my life. I also know what it's like to get by, thinking that the fatigue, excess weight, low energy, dull skin, and that feeling that you won't quite ever be able to do what you want to do in life are all *just the way it is*.

You shouldn't have to settle for mediocre health, for feeling "okay" or as if you're "just getting by." You can feel clearer, stronger, and more energetic. Your skin can firm up and take on a healthy glow. Your hair and nails can be strong and shiny. Your stomach can revert to its natural size, and you can feel better—so much better that you'll be able to break out of that malaise and start making real, positive changes in your life.

It all starts with cleansing. You can get your body back to its healthiest, most vibrant state— a state in which it can cure its own imbalances and thrive. You can look better than you look today, feel better than you feel right now, and manifest the life you only imagined you could have if only you had the energy. You can have the energy because that energy comes from internal fitness. It isn't difficult. You just need to know how to do it. Cleansing and living a healthy life, and improving your internal fitness is a process, and nobody's ever perfect, but we can do better together, with a system in place and the knowledge of why cleansing and caring for the body you've been given is so crucial for a thriving life.

Come with me on this journey, and *let's remake you.*

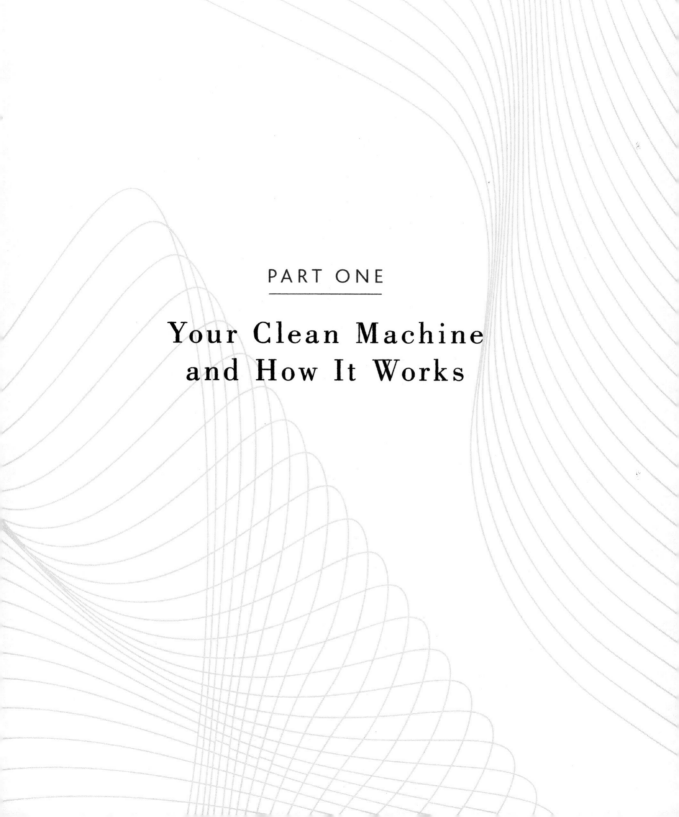

PART ONE

Your Clean Machine
and How It Works

CHAPTER 1

Are You F.O.S.?

CLEANSE. IT'S SUCH A nice word. It sounds so . . . well, clean. Hygienic. Refreshing. It's also a trendy word. You've probably heard about cleanses, and maybe you've even tried one or two of them. Or maybe you're just cleanse-curious. You want to know what a cleanse is, and you especially want to know whether you actually need one or not.

The short answer? *You need one*. How do I know this, even though we've never met? I'll tell you the same thing I tell my clients (even the celebrities): You need to cleanse because you are F.O.S.

(That's "Full of Sh*t," in case you weren't sure what I meant.)

Now, don't be insulted! It's not just you. It's everybody. We're all F.O.S., and without a healthy, well-toned digestive system—without good internal fitness—we're all going to stay that way. You can take three showers a day, but unless you clean your insides as well as you clean your outsides, you could be suffering from any number of chronic uncomfortable, even health-destroying conditions. Internal toxicity can be at the root of, or at least contribute to, the severity of those conditions:

Acidity in the body	Bloating
Acne	Body odor
Bad breath	Brain fog

Calcifications in the joints (as with arthritis and gout)

Candida

Chronic fatigue

Circulation problems

Colitis

Concentration and thinking problems

Congestion of the liver and gallbladder

Constipation

Decreased glandular function

Decreased organ function

Eczema

Endometriosis

Flatulence

Gastritis

Generalized aches and pains

Impaired vision

Irritable bowel syndrome (IBS)

Knots in the muscles

Lupus

Multiple sclerosis

Parasitic infestation

Premenstrual syndrome (PMS)

Psoriasis

Rashes

Thin, weak hair

Unexplained weight loss

Urinary tract infections

Weight gain

When your body isn't cleansing effectively, nothing will work as well as it should—not your organs, not digestion, not even sleeping. Poor internal fitness impedes the healthy, functional processes your body is meant to undergo as it takes nutrients out of the food, turns the remainder into waste, and shuttles it out the back door. But poor internal fitness impedes even more than that. Your kidneys, liver, lungs, heart, even the blood flow throughout your body can all suffer from the drag caused by a compromised internal cleansing system.

You see, your body has many built-in mechanisms for cleansing itself, but because of the way we live, we make that difficult. We get in the way. Imagine filling up your house with moving boxes packed with junk and old furniture, then trying to vacuum around it all. Most people in the developed world make poor food choices and combine foods in a way that impedes digestion. They lead sedentary lives, under crushing stress, and they breathe in, drink in, and have constant contact with environmental pollutants. These in particular are a significant reason you need to cleanse. So many of the foods we eat today contain preservatives, chemicals, artificial colors, flavors, and fillers—things our bodies have a hard time recognizing as nutrition.

These chemicals do some pretty nasty things to our bodies. For one, they make us fatter, pure and simple. One of the body's most efficient ways to protect its vital organs from toxins is to surround and isolate those toxins in fat cells. That means you need to make more fat cells, and the ones you have are going to get bigger. Yikes!

But our bodies can store only so much in the fat cells. When toxins circulate freely through our bodies and get into our organs, they can do all kinds of damage. They can trigger organ dysfunction, weird immune system reactions, and even cell changes. They can mess with hormones and blood sugar levels, causing metabolic disorders and diabetes, and perhaps most frightening of all, some of them can cross the blood-brain barrier and start affecting our nervous systems and brains, triggering problems from ADHD to Alzheimer's.

Just what are these chemicals that are so harmful, and that we're so constantly exposed to in our food and environment? Here's a roundup of some of the worst offenders:

Artificial flavoring, including MSG: Chemical mixtures that mimic the real flavors of food, these flavorings have side effects including skin disorders like eczema and dermatitis, allergic reactions, thyroid dysfunction, and inhibited enzyme activity.

Artificial food coloring: Derived from coal tars and sometimes tainted with heavy metals, artificial food colorings have been linked to cancer, headaches, allergic reactions, skin rashes, asthma, hyperactivity, an over-stimulated appetite, swelling, and neurological issues. That pretty color doesn't seem so pretty anymore!

Azodicarbonamide: This common bleaching agent and chemical found in packaged processed foods and in foamed plastics is linked to higher cancer risks but yet is found in frozen dinners, flour mixes for baking, boxed noodle mixes, and bread. It is also used to make yoga mats and sneakers. Why are we eating it?

Benzoate: If it has any benzoate or any derivative of it, avoid it. That includes things like BHA, BHT, TBHQ, benzoic acid, sodium/calcium/potassium benzoate, and ethyl 4-hydroxybenzoate. These chemicals are food preservatives that keep fat from going rancid so processed food stays "edible" longer. Read the labels to check for these preservatives, which have been linked to tumors, hyperactivity, rashes, hormonal imbalance, and more.

Bisphenol A (BPA): This is a chemical found in canned foods (especially canned tomatoes) and plastic containers. It leaches into foods and drinks, especially when in contact with acidic substances or heat. It's a man-made chemical that acts like estrogen in the body, and it has been linked to obesity, increased cancer risk, diabetes, metabolic disorders, heart problems, ADHD and other behavioral patterns, and obesity—in everyone, but especially in infants and young children. I'll pass, thanks.

Bromated vegetable oil (BVO): This flame retardant has been approved for food use, even though it's banned in Europe and Japan. It's a vegetable oil made from corn and/or soy that's bound with bromine; it gives bottled beverages like sodas, sports drinks, and "fruit" drinks their bright colors. It's a well-known endocrine inhibitor, attaching to iodine receptors so real iodine can't attach. This is a recipe for thyroid problems, and sure enough, BVO has been linked to hypothyroidism. BVO has also been linked to heart, liver, kidney, and testicular damage, as well as increased cholesterol and triglyceride levels. Just one more reason to skip the sodas and sports drinks!

Olestra: This is an indigestible fat used as a fat substitute in baked and fried foods. It stops the absorption of nutrients from the food and causes various types of gastrointestinal problems: bloating, gas, diarrhea.

Perfluorooctanoic acid (PFOA): This chemical is found in the lining of the bags and containers we use to microwave our TV dinners and that Friday night popcorn. When the heat from the microwave cooks this chemical, it falls right into our food, in the same way aluminum leaches into our food when we bake or grill on aluminum foil. PFOA is also in the steam that comes out when we pull the lid back or open the popcorn bag, and then breathe it in. PFOA has been linked to thyroid cancer. It's so toxic that it's on the list to be banned here in the United States, even though it has been banned in Europe for some time.

Polysorbate 60: This emulsifier is made from corn, petroleum, and palm oil. Because it doesn't oxidize and thus won't spoil, it's used as a replacement for dairy products in packaged food. It's also in pickles, coffee creamer, whipped cream, and frozen desserts. It has been linked to reproductive issues, organ toxicity, and cancer. Who wants a little polysorbate 60 in their coffee?

Propylene glycol: This is a stabilizer, emulsifier, and food thickener that is also used in the cosmetic industry and the auto industry in anti-freeze and de-icers. Although there are different grades of propylene glycol, and studies show it "probably" doesn't cause cancer, it does cause skin reactions and allergic reactions in many people, and has also been linked to liver and kidney damage.

Refined sugar, artificial sweeteners, high-fructose corn syrup: All these sweeteners, whether "real" or artificial, are highly processed and come with a laundry list of health issues, from obesity and tissue damage, heart disease and cancer and diabetes, to neurological impairment. Whether artificial sweetener gives you a headache or you can't stop eating sugar, this category is a huge challenge in internal fitness efforts.

Sodium hydroxide: This potent chemical, also known as lye, is extremely corrosive and can dissolve glass, metal, and living tissue. Yet, it is contained in many food and household products, from soap to toothpaste to drain cleaner and oven cleaner, as well as in many processed foods. Solutions are extremely caustic and a known health hazard, but very low doses in household chemicals and food-grade sodium hydroxide in food products are supposedly safe. However, I've seen evidence of serious health issues due to exposure, including infertility. Unfortunately, you will even find sodium hydroxide in many supposed "health foods." Read the label and don't ingest this or use it on your skin!

Sodium nitrite/nitrate: Preservatives that prevent botulism in preserved meat, these substances have been linked to cancer. There are many nitrite- and nitrate-free preserved foods available now. They might cost a little more, but they certainly cost less than one visit to the doctor.

Pretty disgusting, right? The worst part is that you already have a lot of this stuff *inside you*. This is just a partial list of the environmental chemicals to which we are all exposed on a daily basis. They come from everywhere—not just our food and drinks but also in the form of air pollution, water pollution, and soil pollution. Our carpets and furniture emit toxic gases, our microwaves warp the structure of our foods, and even the constant bombardment of radio waves and electricity may be damaging to us. The products we put on our skin and hair contain chemicals that were never meant to enter our bodies, and yet, there they are. Yes, even that sweet-smelling perfume you love to wear—it's *toxic*!

So what can we do? How do we manage? Fortunately, the human body is extremely resilient, but at this point in history, it really does need a little bit of help. Doing a cleanse can reboot your system, optimizing your body's natural elimination processes so it can get ahead of the mess again.

This is why you need a cleanse. Your environment and your lifestyle are stacked against you when it comes to your chances of achieving internal fitness. A cleanse can tip the odds back in your favor again, building and strengthening your internal fitness so your body's natural detoxification system can work the way it's supposed to work. It's body maintenance, and it's *important*.

INTERNAL VS. EXTERNAL FITNESS

In my work with celebrities, I hear a lot about how everybody wants to be fit, toned, and beautiful, but I know that when people say this, they mean they want to be *externally* fit, toned, and beautiful. External fitness is the condition of having an outward appearance that's appealing to the eye. It means having muscle definition and not too much body fat, clear skin, bright eyes, and shiny hair. Some people are genetically predisposed to a fit-looking body, and some people work very hard to get and maintain one through calorie restriction and exercise, because our culture values external fitness.

My focus, however, is on *internal fitness*. Internal fitness is the condition of having healthy, efficient, functional organs, tissues, and cells. It is being free of disease, with a strong immune system. It is having the digestive system toned and in good working order. It is the body in balance, as nature intended. Although calorie restriction and exercise can have certain benefits for internal fitness, my program is more directly related to eating in balance, eliminating foods that gum up the works, effectively detoxifying the body on a regular basis, and continually rejuvenating the body with a lifestyle that builds the body up rather than tears it down.

Of course, internal fitness leads to external beauty, and that's one of the great perks of being internally fit. Not everyone who is externally fit is also internally fit. You can be a supermodel with terrible digestive issues, or a glamorous movie star with an autoimmune disease. You can look fantastic in the mirror and be on the brink of a major health crisis. In these cases (which are many in "the industry"), external beauty is fleeting. It's temporary, and when things go wrong inside, eventually they will show on the outside.

But when you're internally fit, external beauty is part of the package. You have glowing skin, shiny hair, high energy, and a body that works, doing what you need it to do. Internal fitness promotes the development, strength, endurance, and health of all organs, tissues, and cells. It promotes a positive bacterial balance in the gut, good muscle tone in the digestive system, the most beneficial pH inside the body, and the proper handling of food as it moves through the body, including the most efficient uptake of nutrients and the most effective processing and elimination of waste. It goes above and beyond external beauty, creating a body that can live long, feel good, and do what you need it to do for the rest of your life. That's what I want for you, and that's the direction we'll be going in this book.

Internal fitness isn't as sexy as external fitness, and it's not as obvious, either, at least not from the outside. You can see a six-pack or firm upper arms, but you can't see the inside of your colon. However, internal fitness *feels fantastic*. Better yet, internal fitness is the key to health and beauty. When your organs, tissues, and cells are strong and healthy, then you will be, too.

CLEANSING: THE PATH TO INTERNAL FITNESS

Cleansing efforts are natural and normal. Cleansing, in its ideal form, is a dance of natural processes and lifestyle behaviors entwined to produce vibrant health. It's not weird or New Age or "fringe." It's a natural part of having a body. Every living thing has a detoxification process. Even animals fast when they need to heal. Nature encourages cleansing by changing what foods are available in each season, limiting variety.

Cleansing may be trendy, but it's nothing new. Humans have been doing it for thousands of years, and every culture worldwide has its own versions or methods for cleansing. For some, it's fasting, or drastically limiting what foods should be eaten, or by ingesting certain herbs or teas or tinctures, or sitting in saunas, or using some ancient version of colon irrigation. As far back as 3000 B.C., the Chinese were concocting herbal formulas for cleansing. Saunas cleanse the body through sweating, and those date back to about 1100 B.C. Cleansing the colon with water goes back to the time of Cleopatra.

Today, in our culture of information and health obsession, we've taken these concepts and made them high tech—or taken them even further. Sometimes, this works. But sometimes people go too far and do things that aren't safe, like drastic fasting without medical consultation, or taking herbs without understanding what they do, or using sweat lodges without safe supervision, or getting colonics by someone who isn't experienced. But what this really means is that humans have a natural impulse to help their bodies cleanse; and the more you know about how to do this effectively and safely, the more you'll be able to maximize your own health, increase your energy and vibrancy, and even look more beautiful. I want to show you how to do this the right way, the safe way, and the natural way.

THE SEVEN PATHWAYS OF ELIMINATION

Let's consider some of the ways the body detoxes naturally, so you can be better aware of what you'll be supporting in your own body when you cleanse. The body eliminates toxins, including the ones our bodies naturally produce, as by-products of metabolism. Also, the external toxins we're exposed to make their way inside of us. In response, the body contains seven different detoxifying systems. The seven pathways of elimination are:

1. BLOOD

Blood circulates and permeates every part of you. It's the highway through which nutrients are delivered to every part of the body, and by which waste and other toxic materials are funneled into the liver for processing. Because blood flows through every part of your body, it should be as clean as possible. Ideally, your body cleans the blood, but when your body is overwhelmed with toxins, this can become more difficult.

2. COLON

This is the tail end of the digestive tube, where the body absorbs any last water, vitamins, minerals, and electrolytes from the indigestible food matter, and then eliminates the remaining waste. The colon begins with the cecum, which leads to the ascending colon, then the hepatic flexure (named for its position next to the liver), then it goes across the abdominal cavity where it is called the transverse colon, makes a turn on the left side called the splenic flexure (named for its position next to the spleen), then turns down into the descending colon with another turn toward midline to the sigmoid. Finally it empties into the rectum and out the anus. The colon contains 400 to 500 different species of bacteria—about 100 trillion total bacteria—that feed on the fiber of the indigestible food, breaking it down. Because so much waste is processed through the colon, it's vital to keep things moving along.

3. KIDNEYS

The kidneys are a pair of bean-shaped organs the size of an adult's closed fist. They are located in the back of the abdominal cavity and are responsible for filtering the blood to get rid of excess fluid, as well as water-soluble toxins. This makes urine. The metabolism of vitamin D is one of the functions of the kidneys. They also control blood pressure and help to regulate the body's electrolyte balance. The kidneys are very important, so fortunately you have two of them. If one fails, you can live on the other one; but if both fail, as in end-stage renal failure, the body completely shuts down. In order for the kidneys to be in tip-top shape, they need to be well hydrated at all times or else these toxins can build up and injure them. Poor nutrition, stress, and too much salt can harm the kidneys.

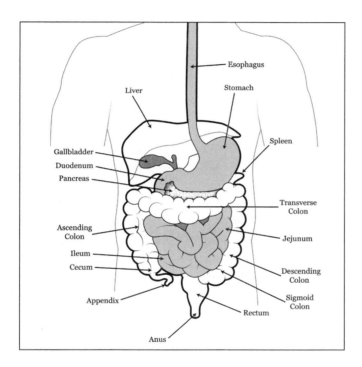

4. LIVER

The liver is located in the upper right quadrant of the abdominal cavity. It's shaped like a cone and it's the largest internal organ you have. The average, normal size of a liver is about the size of a football, but tends to be a little smaller in women and a little larger in men. Much bigger or smaller is a sign that something is wrong. The liver can store one pint of blood at any given time, and it's the only organ that can regenerate itself.

The liver is tough and resilient—your liver can lose up to 75 percent of its cells before it ceases to function. It's no coincidence that the word *liver* contains the word *live*! However, the liver can be damaged by alcohol, drugs, insecticides, pesticides, heavy metals, and overeating carbohydrates and proteins. It's the major organ of elimination, as it processes toxins out of the body, including chemicals, drugs, poisons, bacteria, and waste products. It also produces immune factors to help the body eliminate infection. Waste broken down by the liver is excreted into the blood or bile, which goes through the gallbladder and is stored until the small intestine signals the body to release it into the intestines. Bile is eliminated through the feces. (Toxins released to the blood travel to the kidneys for processing.) I think of the liver as the chief executive officer of elimination, working in conjunction with its board of directors: the gallbladder, kidneys, and pancreas. These in turn work with the colon (chief operating officer of the digestive system) to get everything out of the body.

When the liver is working optimally, it is able to reduce cholesterol, release excess estrogen in the body, and perform many other important functions.

....

ABOUT THE GALLBLADDER

The gallbladder is a small organ that sits just under your liver, and it helps you to digest fat and concentrate bile. It also initiates peristalsis of the colon. The liver dumps its waste into the gallbladder, where it is stored in bile until your body gives the signal to release it into the intestines for elimination. Many people develop gallstones, and when these become painful, a doctor may want to remove your gallbladder. This isn't usually a problem, but on the other hand, why remove the poor gallbladder when the stones are really the fault of the liver? Keeping the liver cleansed and strong can reduce or eliminate the buildup of gallstones.

....

5. LUNGS

A beautiful pair of spongy, air-filled organs that are located in the chest area (thorax), the lungs connect to the trachea or windpipe, which directs inhaled air into the bronchi, which branch into smaller and smaller structures called bronchioles and alveoli. This is where the oxygen from the air you inhale is absorbed into the blood, and carbon dioxide, the waste product of respiration, travels from the blood into the alveoli to be exhaled. Lung cleansing starts with deep breathing, which will increase oxygen absorption. I recommend deep breathing for a few minutes every single day. This also strengthens the lung muscles, so they can contract more forcefully, allowing deeper cleansing of the bronchioles. Any cardiovascular exercise will also strengthen and cleanse the lungs.

6. LYMPHATIC SYSTEM

Lymph is a clear fluid filled with immune cells called lymphocytes that are crucial for immune function. Lymph travels through the bloodstream and then moves through capillary walls that are too small for red blood cells to penetrate. It flows through your body all around your blood vessels, picking up waste products and delivering white blood cells for infection control and general immune system work. Then it flows into the vessels and capillaries of the lymphatic system, which direct it to the lymph nodes to be filtered and cleansed of any toxins and debris. The clean lymph then flows back into the bloodstream and the process starts all over again. The lymphatic system does not have valves, so its fluid moves only by our movement. If we are sedentary, then so is our lymph, and when the lymph gets sluggish, the result can be swollen ankles, hands, or a generalized puffiness all over the body. Exercise and deep breathing are crucial for a healthy lymphatic system. They keep lymph moving. Dry brushing and lymphatic massage also stimulate lymphatic flow, leading to more efficient toxin removal.

7. SKIN

The skin is our protective covering. It keeps things in (like blood and water) and keeps things out (like bacteria and ultraviolet rays), but it also lets things in (like compounds in skin lotion) and lets things out (like sweat). The skin is the largest eliminatory organ, which means it releases more waste than any of the other six channels of elimination. Your skin is also your ambassador to the world. It allows you to feel touch, pressure, pain, and temperature. It regulates your body temperature by retaining or releasing heat (sweating via the eccrine glands helps with this process), and it also regulates blood flow to the skin (which is why you sometimes blush or go pale).

Because the pores in your skin are the outlets for sweat, which can carry some toxins from the inside to the outside, skin problems are often the first sign of a health issue. When I see serious skin issues, I liken this to "pooping through the skin." When your body is overburdened, all that toxic waste has to come out somewhere, and releasing it through the skin is one way your body tries to preserve organ function. A plain and simple hot shower is an excellent skin cleanser that opens pores and helps wash away what the body releases. Sweating is great for helping the skin with its elimination duties—try a sauna or steam room periodically. In cases of serious skin problems, however, more internal detoxification is often required.

THESE ARE THE SYSTEMS you need to support, the systems that so easily get bogged down by life in the modern world. Let's begin with our very first Internal Fitness Prep Step. I call them IFs, my acronym for Internal Fitness, but also the word *if* to remind you of the possibilities internal fitness offers you. I'll give you one at the end of each chapter leading up to the Piper Protocol, so that when we get ready to begin the business of real cleansing, your body, mind, and spirit will be ready. Each Prep Step is meant to be repeated daily, but move through them at a rate that makes you comfortable.

Some people will take on one more each day, or one more each week. As you take on these healthy habits, you'll feel your body changing and working better, little by little. Starting today, you're already cleansing.

Here's the first one. IF you are ready, here we go!

....

INTERNAL FITNESS PREP STEP #1

IF you want change, you have to prepare your body and mind to receive new information and discard old habits that aren't serving you. Starting today, take just a few minutes to sit in a quiet place, relax, and then take five slow, deep breaths, inhaling to a count of five and exhaling to a count of five. Repeat five times. Why all the fives? In numerology, five is the number of change, and I want you to feel empowered to make positive changes in your life. It may not seem as if you're doing much, but trust me: This is a profound habit that will help you stick with what's to come. Five minutes, five breaths, five seconds in, five seconds out, repeat five times. Do this every day, and you will be laying the groundwork for change.

....

CHAPTER 2

Digestion 101

ONCE UPON A TIME you had a thought about food. Maybe you thought about it because you hadn't eaten in a while and you felt hungry. Maybe you thought about it because you saw a billboard displaying food or a commercial showing food at a restaurant, and that set the wheels turning. Maybe somebody mentioned sugar cookies or prime rib or a steaming hot slice of pizza. Whatever the trigger, the *thought* of food is actually the moment when digestion begins. Just reading these words might have triggered digestion in *your* body, right now, because digestion begins not in your stomach, not even in your mouth, but in your head.

But what is it exactly, this powerful process that is so instrumental in building your body, maintaining your energy, lifting your mood, and keeping your whole system working smoothly? Healthy digestion is the basis for health and poor digestion is the root of disease. Digestion can impact nearly everything about your health—not just the effectiveness of your waste removal system, but also the robustness of your immune system and even your mental state. Poor digestion can destroy health, and robust digestion can restore it. It's *essential* to maximize strong, healthy digestion, but if you don't understand what it is—if you don't know what happens to your food from entrance to exit—you won't prioritize it or do what you need to do for maximum digestive vitality.

Every time you make a decision about what to put into your mouth, and every time you chew too little or eat too fast, and every time you experience indigestion or intestinal gas, and every time you have a lot of stress while you're eating (or in your life in general), and every time you stay up too late and sacrifice hours of sleep for something that doesn't matter that much to you, and every time you decide not to take that walk because you're too comfortable on the couch, and every single time you use the bathroom, you have an opportunity to either facilitate this process or notice when it isn't going as well as it should and do something about it.

I'm always amazed to discover how little most people know about what happens to food between the moment it goes into the mouth and the moment its remnants come out the other end. What kind of magical processes are going on inside your body that transform a perfectly lovely apple or delicious bowl of soup into *you,* and then how do the parts of that apple or bowl of soup your body can't use get to the exit? It's a pretty amazing journey, and it's happening inside your very own body every time you eat. You should know what's going on in there because it couldn't be more personal. But your torso isn't fitted with a window, so instead, I'm going to tell you a story. The Story of Digestion. Like all stories, this one has a beginning, a middle, and an end.

THE STORY OF DIGESTION

Once upon a time there was a slice of chocolate cake. It sat on a plate looking delicious, and when you saw it, the process of digestion began in your body. As you considered savoring it, your stomach began to contract, knowing in its body-wise way that it would soon be receiving that cake. As you looked at it, your small intestine began to secrete enzymes to digest it, and as you smelled it, your olfactory nerves triggered your salivary glands to release saliva, which is full of enzymes for digesting starch.

When you finally took a luscious bite of that chocolate cake, two things happened in your mouth. First, you began to chew. This is one of the primary modes of *mechanical digestion.* Your teeth ground up that cake, aided by your tongue, into a mush. As this happened, all the taste buds on your tongue got to savor the chocolate flavor (this is the part that makes eating so enjoyable).

As you chewed, that cake was getting mixed with your saliva. Saliva is the first step in *chemical digestion,* converting the starches in the cake into sugar, so your body can more easily utilize the energy that lives inside that cake. Chewing also releases the enzymes that might exist in the food you eat (especially fruits, vegetables, and meat). As you chew, your tongue helps out by rolling the cake around in your mouth, and then in a bittersweet moment, your taste buds say good-bye to the bite of cake as it hits the back of your throat and launches into your esophagus.

As soon as you swallow, your *autonomic nervous system* takes over. It's like that moment at the airport when you push your shoes and laptop computer onto the conveyor belt, which then takes over and carries them into the X-ray machine. You don't have to think about it anymore (because you're probably thinking about the *next* bite of chocolate cake). Now, that bite of cake doesn't much resemble cake anymore. It is more of an egg-shaped pellet, which is called a *bolus*. It moves quickly down the *esophagus*, the tube from throat to stomach, thanks to a series of wave-like muscle motions called *peristalsis*.

At the bottom of the esophagus, the lower esophageal sphincter opens up to let the food pass into the stomach, then snaps shut again to prevent any stomach acid from splashing back up into the esophagus. (When this mechanism doesn't work correctly, food and acid can back up into the esophagus, causing acid reflux. If this becomes a chronic condition, it can damage the esophagus. This is called gastrointestinal esophageal reflux disease, or GERD.)

....

GHRELIN AND LEPTIN, AND LOSING WEIGHT

Your body is a complex chemical factory, and many chemicals interact to make digestion happen, but two chemicals in particular are important for getting you started eating in the first place. Ghrelin is the hormone that increases appetite. It's manufactured in the stomach when your stomach is empty, and ghrelin signals your brain that you need to eat. It's your body's way of saying, "Feed me!"

As you eat, another hormone monitors the situation. It's called leptin, and it is produced by your fat cells. If you have a lot of fat cells, you have a lot of leptin, and it's telling your body, "Okay, that's enough. We're good." Leptin helps regulate fat metabolism; ideally, if you have a lot of fat, you won't need to eat very much because your leptin will keep things in check, knowing it has plenty of energy in storage.

The system should work, but some things can happen to cause trouble. In people who are overweight and especially obese, the body gets resistant to leptin. It stops paying attention to the signal. It's good with ghrelin—they're best buddies. Ghrelin says, "Eat!" and the body says, "One step ahead of you, big guy!" Meanwhile, poor leptin is shouting, "Stop! Stop! You don't need all that food, look at all this great fat we can burn for energy!" And your body is refusing to listen, metaphorically covering its ears and saying, "La la la la, I can't hear you!" It's not your willpower that's ignoring the cues to stop eating. It's your chemistry.

Another thing that can go wrong is that ghrelin can get a little too easily activated. Fatty foods, sugar, and lack of sleep all get the ghrelin revved up so your body is telling your brain that you're hungrier than you really are. "Eat now! It's an emergency!!" And you know what happens next.

To help get ghrelin and leptin back to working properly, you can do a few important things:

- **Eat more slowly.** Eat slowly, chew thoroughly, and take a good 20 minutes to eat your meal. That's how long it takes for leptin to kick in.

- **Eat more fiber.** Eat a diet high in fiber and protein, but low in fat and sugar. This will help to keep you more sensitive to leptin, and it's a good way to keep all your hormones happier and in good working order.

- **Get enough sleep!** People who chronically under-sleep (say, five hours a night versus eight) have both higher ghrelin levels and lower leptin levels.

- **Chill out**. Stress can mess with your hormones, and stress-reduction techniques such as meditation and yoga can even things out.

- **Move it**. Moderate exercise on most days may help your ghrelin levels stay within normal range, so you won't get unreasonably hungry.

- **Lose it.** Weight loss will help your body become more sensitive to leptin, so you get full faster and stop eating sooner.

OUT OF THE FRYING PAN, INTO THE FIRE

Now, digestion gets really serious. Your stomach is like a big high-speed blender—full of acid! Stomach acid is extremely potent and powerful. Even if you didn't chew very well, it can liquefy your food (well, maybe not corn . . .). Plus, the stomach releases digestive enzymes to break down food further (chemical digestion again), and the muscles around the stomach contract and expand so everything gets shaken up and broken down in there (more mechanical digestion). Pretty soon, there are no hard pieces left. It's all a kind of part-liquid, part-solid mass of stomach acid mixed with mushed-up food, called *chyme*.

Incidentally, it's pretty amazing that the stomach doesn't digest itself. That's because the stomach is lined with a thick, highly alkaline mucus coating that is impervious to acid and digestive enzymes. The stomach lining (made of epithelial cells) is also knitted together tightly to resist leaking, and these cells regenerate every few days to keep the stomach lining fresh, young, and strong. But get that stomach acid into your esophagus, and all bets are off. It can actually eat away at your flesh. It's that powerful.

THE LONG TRIP THROUGH THE SMALL INTESTINE

Next, the chyme has to enter the small intestine, but now that the food is all broken down, it doesn't leave the stomach all at the same time. Starches like bread and cake tend to move through the quickest because they don't need to spend as long in the stomach; they're easily broken down into energy-inducing sugars. Protein takes longer to digest, so it stays in the stomach longer. Fats take the longest to digest, so parts of that chocolate cake (like the carbohydrates from the flour and sugar) will be moving along more quickly than, say, that buttery chocolate frosting, which may spend a little more time in the "blender."

Chyme is still pretty acidic when it enters the first part of the small intestine, called the *duodenum*, which is kind of a holding tank or way station. This is where the chyme gets neutralized, so it doesn't burn your small intestine, and where everything gets further broken down to basic nutrient level for absorption in the lower parts of the small intestine. First, the gallbladder kicks in, delivering a dose of an alkaline liquid called bile, to bring down the acidity of the chyme. Along with the bile come a flood of digestive enzymes and bicarbonates from the pancreas, for further neutralization and for making all the sugars, amino acids, vitamins, minerals, and fatty acids available to your body. Once the acids are neutralized, the chyme enters the two remaining parts of the small intestine, the *jejunum* and *ileum*.

Now the work of absorption begins. This is an important part of digestion—everything up to this point has been for the purpose of breaking down the food so the nutrients can be absorbed. Mucus and more digestive juices mix with the chyme to dissolve it even further. Then, the small intestine, which is lined with tiny fingers of tissue called *villi* covered with even tinier hairs called *microvilli*, absorbs the broken-down sugars, proteins, fats, vitamins, and minerals, taking them in and releasing them to the bloodstream where they can be delivered to all the organs and muscles, wherever they are needed. The cool thing about all these tiny finger-like and hair-like projections is that they drastically increase the surface area for nutrient absorption. This primarily happens in the jejunum, but the ileum catches anything the jejunum missed. Body: officially nourished!

It's also important for you to know that the small intestine produces *most* of the body's serotonin. People think of serotonin as a brain chemical because it is a neurotransmitter, but there's actually a whole "brain" right there in your gut. I'll talk more about this later, but when the small intestine is malfunctioning, you may not produce enough serotonin, which could lead to depression, anxiety, and a host of other problems that *feel* mental but actually start right there in the middle of your body. (This is one reason cleansing is incredibly important for people who are experiencing emotional issues! You want your serotonin production to be working at maximum efficiency.)

A COLON CONVERSATION

So what's left? You've still got fiber, bile, and any other extras sitting there in the intestine, waiting to be dealt with. And don't you worry, your large intestine, also called your colon, knows just what to do with this stuff. It moves through the *ileocecal valve* into the first part of the colon, the *cecum*, and then the *ascending colon*, and this passage is all uphill! Fortunately, peristalsis (that wave-like muscle movement you first experienced in your esophagus) keeps that mass of fiber and waste products moving, even though it's going against gravity. After the ascending colon, it travels across the body in the *transverse colon*, then down the *descending colon* and into the *sigmoid colon*. Things can get stopped up anywhere along the way, but we're hoping they don't. (When they do, the colon can swell and bulge with the impaction—ouch!)

Now your colon has some serious work to do as the chyme passes through it. It absorbs water and electrolytes out of the chyme, compacting and solidifying it while sending the liquid off to the liver to be filtered and reused in the body. The colon also secretes mucus to lubricate the way and to help glue the remaining fibrous chyme into shape for easy passage. The colon also houses a whole lot of bacteria—about 3 to 5 pounds' worth in a healthy person! Most of this bacteria should be the good stuff (not the nasty stuff, *pathogenic* organisms like *E. coli, salmonella,* and cancer cells, although we all have a few of those). As long as this whole community of bacteria, or the *microbiome,* is mostly made up of the good guys that help ferment undigested food, manufacture B vitamins, and maintain the integrity of your intestinal walls, the bad bacteria won't be able to cause any trouble. Meanwhile, peristalsis keeps everything—all the fiber, bacteria, and waste—moving toward the rectum.

All that fiber acts like a broom, scrubbing the walls of the large intestine clean. Unfortunately, the system sometimes goes awry. I'll talk more about this later, but basically, if the large intestine absorbs all the water and the feces get too dried out, they can actually stick in the little pockets and folds of the large intestine walls that are meant for pushing the waste down the tube. These are called *haustra*, and they give the colon its segmented appearance. They are quite useful—as they fill up, they contract, propelling the waste material to the next pouch. It's this muscle action that keeps your bowels moving, but in the case of desiccated feces and dried-up mucus, things can get a bit stopped up. The haustrum may contract, but the feces don't move. This is called *colonic inertia*, and it's the failure of the muscles and/or nerves of the colon to move the bowels. This leads to constipation.

A sluggish colon can lead to disease, as well as bloating and discomfort. You can hold pounds of fecal material in the colon! It can stretch and become misshapen, and it can also form extra little pockets to hold more stool, called *diverticuli*. These can get infected, causing a painful condition called *diverticulitis*. Your colon shouldn't have to change and warp and develop these pockets, but depending on your lifestyle and what and how you eat, it could.

Now, you may have heard that all of this is untrue. Some people, even doctors, will tell you that the colon does not hold pockets of feces and that feces don't get backed up in there. Anyone who has been constipated, however, will likely disagree. I can attest, in my work as a colon hydrotherapist, that it's true because I've seen what comes out during a colonic. Trust me, I also have some personal experience with this. I lost 55 pounds in two and a half months for this very reason. I've seen pounds and pounds of old, dried-up material releasing from an impacted colon, and I've experienced it myself. It's much more preferable to maintain your internal fitness so this doesn't happen to you.

....

DESCENDING ENERGY

In Chinese medicine, an ancient, comprehensive system that I have studied for many years, energy (called *qi*) moves through the body in different directions. This energy doesn't correspond to the way conventional Western medicine looks at the body, but it is an ancient and still-practiced aspect of Eastern medicine. When the directions get reversed due to poor lifestyle habits or other environmental factors, that can cause discomfort and eventually disease.

The large intestine and the lungs are related, and should both contain descending energy, meaning the energy within these organs moves downward. (Never mind that you cough something "up." We're not talking about air; we are talking about *qi* and it should be moving downward.) If the energy doesn't descend in the lungs, they get clogged and we cough and get respiratory infections. If it doesn't descend in the colon, we get constipated. And guess what two of the most common cancers are in the United States, where internal fitness is such a problem? Lung and colon. I don't think this is a coincidence.

As long as we're in the colon, I want you to start thinking about this little nugget: According to Chinese medicine, the large intestine is an important center for emotion. This area is about letting go of old, toxic waste that no longer serves you, both physical and emotional. You won't get information like this from your primary care physician, but you can take it from me. According to one of the oldest texts in Chinese medicine, the *Huangdi Neijing,* the colon is (and this is a translation from the Chinese) "the official passage for the transmission of the way; change and energy emerge from it."

In other words, holding on to negative emotional thinking, past trauma, and blockages are like mental constipation; and just like physical constipation, these hold us back from living our best lives. This is also an old and dearly held belief in the Caribbean, where I grew up. We say that bottling up our emotions will cause emotional and physical harm. So it goes both ways: Gut dysfunction causes emotional dysfunction, and emotional dysfunction causes gut dysfunction. (Just in case you needed another good reason to try a cleanse!) I'll talk more about the connection between the gut and the emotions later. For now, let's get back to our story, which is nearing the end.

BON VOYAGE!

Now that your food has moved along through the sigmoid colon, it dumps (pardon the pun) into the *rectum,* which is like a holding tank. When the rectum gets full and the walls start to stretch a bit, your nervous system triggers your brain that it's time to poop. Remember the autonomic nervous system, which controlled all the aspects of your digestion without you having to think about it? Now you regain some control. The very beginning and the very end of the digestive process involve the voluntary nervous system.

If you decide to make your way to the bathroom, peristalsis kicks in again and the walls of the rectum contract, the anal sphincter releases, and all that waste material gets pushed out of your body. If you decide, however, that you do not want to go to the bathroom—maybe you're too busy or you're ignoring your body's signals—your body gets the message. If your rectum is too full, your colon can actually contract and pull the feces back up to relieve the pressure. That will work occasionally, but if you do this too often, the feces stay in the colon for too long and keep moving in the wrong direction. They can get hard and dry and resistant to coming out. You will be literally backed up. If you have to strain and push to accomplish this final step of digestion, then things aren't working as they should. Defecation should always be pretty easy.

Here's how it all works out, visually:

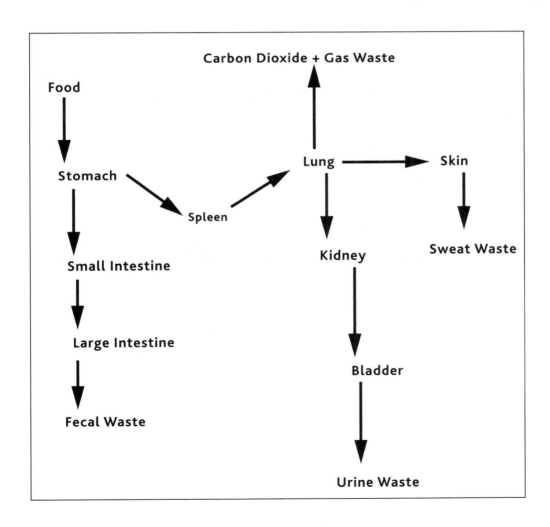

So there you have it—the story of digestion. A lot goes on between that first thought of food and that trip to the bathroom, and I've only scratched the surface. I could write a whole book about the complex chemical and mechanical processes that happen, but I don't want to bore you. This is Digestion 101—just the basics.

So what's it going to be? Bloated belly? Gas pain? Acid reflux? Constipation? Excessive weight gain? Depression? Low energy? Just feeling "blah" all the time? Or smooth sailing? Your internal fitness is up to you, and knowledge about what's going on in there is power—power to make the choices that will help you feel and look fantastic. Are you ready for your next Internal Fitness Prep Step? Keep doing your five minutes of deep breathing every day from the last chapter but now, add this one:

....

INTERNAL FITNESS PREP STEP #2

IF you want to make an active and powerful change to increase the efficiency and effectiveness of your digestion, do two things from your next meal forward:

- Take smaller bites.
- Chew your food thoroughly.

Use a small fork, such as a salad fork, to help you put less food in your mouth with each bite. Don't stuff the fork full. Food expands when you begin chewing and if you get too much in your mouth, you'll be more likely to swallow it prematurely. Take small bites and chew each bite 25 times or more, or until the food is completely dissolved and liquid in your mouth. This begins the process of mechanical digestion and chemical digestion, as the food morphs into smaller pieces and into mush and your body begins releasing digestive enzymes. The more you chew, the more flavor you'll extract (so you might eat less), and the less digestive work your stomach and pancreas have to do. Start today, and repeat with every meal and snack.

....

CHAPTER 3

The Rhythms of Life

THE EARTH GOES AROUND the sun once every 24 hours, and every living thing on this earth—from bacteria and plants to animals and people—has a rhythm that works in concert with the cycles of light and dark, sleeping and waking. As part of this earth, you have felt this, too, and these cycles are reflected inside you as well as all around you.

At the most basic level, you go to sleep at a certain time of day, and you wake up at a certain time of day. But your internal clock regulates much more than your sleep. You've probably noticed that sometimes you feel more energetic, or calmer. You feel mentally sharp during one hour, but you may feel as if your brain "turns off" at other times of the day. You may have noticed a pattern, or maybe these fluctuations in how you feel and what you do seem random to you.

You've probably also experienced what happens when this system goes awry. If you travel through several time zones (say, if you fly from the West Coast to the East Coast, or from the United States to Europe or Asia), you're likely to experience jet lag. Your internal clock gets confused because your body isn't adjusted to the new time zone. If you've ever pulled an all-nighter or slept for too long, you've also felt the mental confusion, physical exhaustion, and sluggish energy that occur when you get out of sync with your own clock. Or, you may notice a more subtle dysfunction in your rhythms—some days you just feel "off," never quite getting into sync or feeling like you're doing the right thing at the right time.

Your internal rhythms are more than just a curiosity. They affect your hormone regulating system, your sleep, your body temperature, your appetite, and your energy level. Did you ever wonder why one person is a morning person and another is a night owl? Personally, I'm a morning person, but my best friend claims to be a night owl. I could never stay up as late as he does. I think it would kill me! We each have our rhythms, and each individual is different, but in many cases, staying up too late, insomnia, and other rhythm issues are the result of bad habits or health issues.

There are patterns that apply to all humans, and knowing and understanding them can help you learn how your internal clock works, what can interrupt it, and how to get back in sync with yourself. Humans have noticed and studied this internal clock for centuries. In Western culture, we call these cycles *circadian rhythms,* and they set your internal pace. Light and dark influence this internal system, but so does everything else in our environments—what we eat, when we sleep, how we feel, and how we live. This system even alters according to daylight savings time, because we modify our environments and habits to match the changing clock.

Other systems, as in Asia, see the internal clock a little differently. In Chinese medicine, every hour of the day is associated with certain organs in the body, and every organ is associated with certain seasons, temperatures, elements, and energies. I see this system at work in my clients. When the internal clock is off, it can impact internal fitness by draining the energy from certain organs of the body or flooding them with too much energy. This in turn can further disrupt your internal clock; we've evolved to live in sync with the sunrise and sunset, but disharmony within the internal organs, either deficiency or excess, can manifest as an inability to sleep at night or to stay awake during the day. Night owls and early risers who get up before the sun may find that when they get internally fit, what they thought was just a personality trait corrects itself and gets them more in sync with the natural world.

GETTING OFF THE BEAT

You may be wondering whether your internal clock is off. If you're like most people, it's probably off at least a little, but let's look at some of the obvious symptoms that indicate your natural rhythms have gotten off beat. Check all that apply to you in the last month:

- Trouble falling asleep at night
- Trouble staying asleep—you wake up in the middle of the night and can't get back to sleep again

- Waking up too early, before you've gotten enough sleep, and are unable to fall asleep again
- Waking up every night at a particular time, like 3:20 A.M.
- Trouble getting a solid eight hours, no matter how hard you try
- Even when you get enough sleep, you wake up feeling tired
- Excessive fatigue during the day—all you want to do is put your head down and take a nap
- Irritability and/or mood swings with no apparent cause
- Inability to concentrate
- Depression for no apparent reason
- Excessive worry and anxiety for no apparent reason
- Brain fog that feels like jet lag—but you haven't gone anywhere!

If you checked *even one* of the items on the above list, something in your life or lifestyle is probably interfering with your natural rhythms. Let's get you back on track. You can feel a lot better than you're feeling right now.

If you went to a doctor for your sleep issues, she might tell you that you have a *circadian rhythm disorder*. This is the Western term for certain sleep disorders thought to be caused by a disruption in the sleep/wake cycle that is natural for humans. Various things can mess with these cycles—less daylight in the winter, shorter nights in the summer, getting in the habit of staying up too late or chronically getting too little sleep, working a night shift, or for those who are particularly sensitive, exposing yourself to too much light in the evening, such as from television or computer screens.

All these things can disrupt your natural rhythms, leaving you feeling tired, drained, and more vulnerable to picking up a virus or getting an infection, and causing even more serious, self-perpetuating issues, such as insomnia, anxiety, and depression.

Lifestyle habits of all kinds can mess with your internal rhythm and make you feel less energetic and healthy, even less happy than you could feel. Here are some common disruptors:

Travel.
I have to travel frequently for my work. Because I live in New York but am often called on to work on movies or before big events in California, it seems as if I'm always flying from coast to coast.

This can be a huge rhythm disruptor, and I've had to take extra good care of myself so I can recover quickly. Otherwise, it can take up to a week to adjust each time I travel across the country.

Light (including lighted screens).
The internal clock is controlled by something called the *suprachiasmatic nucleus,* which receives information from the optic nerve about how much light is present. When the brain gets the feedback that the light is going away (the sun is setting), it releases melatonin, which helps you to sleep soundly at night. If you leave lights on, watch TV, stare at a computer screen, or even spend the evening checking email and sending text messages on your phone, your optic nerve keeps seeing light, so it doesn't send your brain the signal to begin producing melatonin. Then you wonder why you can't sleep.

Habit changes.
When I lived in Tortola with my grandmother, we had no TV, we ate supper at 4:00 P.M., we went to evening mass between 5:30 and 6:00 P.M., we were home by 6:30, and I was in bed by 7:30 P.M. We got up in the morning with the crowing of the rooster at sunrise. By the time I moved to New York and lived in the big city with lots of light, late-night TV shows, and all the stimulation of the city, my internal clock was way off. I was eating late at night and going to bed late, but waking up early because my body was still trying to keep a natural rhythm. When I did wake up, I felt groggy and tired.

Late-night stimulation.
If you get excited, have arguments, go out dancing, drink alcohol, have caffeine, or otherwise stay stimulated in the evening, you may not release melatonin, and you may also find it hard to turn off your brain when you finally climb into bed and close your eyes. It's very important to begin calming yourself a few hours before bedtime, to send your brain the signal that you're getting ready to sleep.

You can't always do something about all of these disrupting factors, but whenever you can, adjust your schedule to the natural light. Turn off all screens and dim the lights in the evening. Try going to bed and getting up at about the same time each day, and keep calm, especially at night. When you have to travel, be out in the sun as much as you can, and then go to bed when it gets dark. Your jet lag will resolve more quickly.

THE CHINESE CLOCK

The Chinese clock attributes different times of day to the highest functioning times for different internal organs. I think this is fascinating—every season has its qualities, and is always moving toward the next season. Every hour has its properties, too—with a corresponding element, internal organ, and even feeling. You are more likely to laugh at certain hours of the day, and more likely to lose your temper during others.

Here is a chart that encompasses all the complex aspects of the Chinese clock. These are based on the meridians, or energy pathways, that run through the body (acupuncturists use these to guide where they put the needles, and massage therapists sometimes use these to determine where to apply pressure for various issues). As you can see, every season, every element, and every hour of the day moves through a cycle.

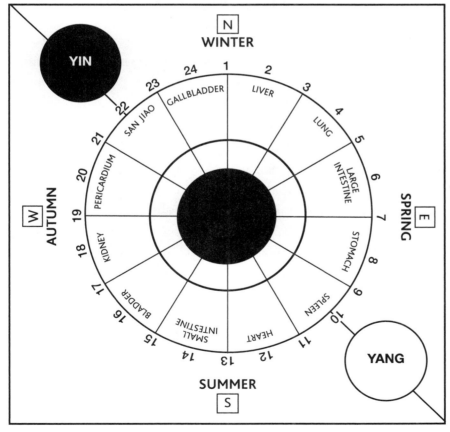

Follow the clock! The time of day on this chart, indicated by the numbers, coincides with the organs and systems in your body that are currently active and energized. Follow along to see when you should pay special attention to your stomach, when your liver is in peak detoxification mode, when your heart might need a little extra TLC, and when you're in particular need of more water and juice to help flush out your kidneys.

I know this chart contains a lot of information, but it's useful information, so let's break it down. At the most basic level, the rhythm of your days, weeks, months, and year can be considered in terms of *yin* and *yang*.

YIN, YANG, AND YOU

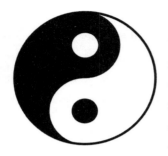

This is the yin-yang symbol, and although it may be familiar, it actually represents a concept that isn't that familiar to people in the Western world. We tend to think of things as either/or. It's day or it's night. It's dark or it's light. It's cold or it's hot. In Chinese medicine, however, practitioners think about things somewhat differently—day is always turning into night, and night is always turning into day. There is always some dark in the light, and some light in the dark; some cold in the hot, and some hot in the cold. Everything is a cycle, and everything is always turning into its opposite, and everything always contains a bit of its opposite. Pretty cool, right?

If you look at the Chinese clock on page 41, you will see that it is divided into many parts, but in the top left-hand corner, it says YIN, and in the bottom right-hand corner, it says YANG. Yin and yang are opposites, and everything in the universe is primarily either yin or yang, but also has a seed of the opposite in it. Here are some typical things that are primarily yin or yang:

YIN	YANG
Feminine	**Masculine**
Negative	Positive
Dark	Light
Silence	Sound
Unseen	Seen
Moon	Sun
Earth	Heaven
Night	Day
Passive	Active
Being	Doing
Soft	Hard
Cold	Hot
Intuition	Intellect
Emotion	Reason
Process	Goal
Nurturing	Assertive

Also notice that the chart has four seasons—winter, spring, summer, and autumn. Winter is the time of utmost yin, but as it moves into spring, the yang begins to grow in the yin. Summer is the time of utmost yang, and as time goes on, yin begins to grow again within yang until winter, when yin is again at its utmost. This happens within the day, too. Notice the ring of numbers—that's a clock. Every few hours the clock alternates to be more yin-dominant or yang-dominant, but whichever is dominant always contains a seed of the other, which is growing within it. That means you can always change—you can always improve and move toward health because you are not static.

So the first thing to think about in your daily rhythm is that you will be alternating between yin and yang throughout the day. You will have moments of dark and light, cold and hot, passive and active, intuition and intellect, even moments of feeling more feminine and moments of feeling more masculine. This is completely natural, and as it should be. The earth's environment is ever-changing and cyclical, and so are you.

Also notice that the Chinese clock is like a regular clock. It moves clockwise through 24 hours, and through different organs of the body. Each organ has a two-hour portion of this clock, and during those two hours, the energy of that organ is at its highest. This is based on something the Chinese call *qi*. (You may have also seen it spelled *chi* or *ch'i*.) *Qi* is life force energy that flows along meridians in the body that are like rivers of energy. Western medicine doesn't recognize these meridians, although some people believe they approximately coincide with certain aspects of the nervous system. Acupuncturists use the meridians to determine where to place their acupuncture needles, to stimulate different organ systems; the meridians are linked to both the organs and to the clock. You can learn a lot about which organs are out of balance by the interruptions in someone's daily routine. For example, if someone always wakes up between 2:00 and 3:00 in the morning and has insomnia, that is a sign that the liver is out of balance, either lacking energy or filled with too much energy. If someone is often nauseated from 11:00 P.M. to 1:00 A.M., he may have a problem with the gallbladder.

DANCE TO YOUR RHYTHM

So what do you do with all this information? Let's take a walk through your day. With each two-hour period, we'll look at what is going on within you, what organs are dominating, and exactly what you can do to maximize your rhythms and dance to your own beat. The middle of that two-hour period is your peak, when you will have the highest energy in that particular organ. So for example, between 5:00 and 7:00 A.M., which is the time of the large intestine, 6:00 A.M. will be your highest energy time, so it's a great time to hit the bathroom. Look back at the clock at any time to help remind you where it's all going.

Let's start in the morning:

LARGE INTESTINE TIME: 5 A.M. TO 7 A.M.

This is the optimal time to wake up, even on the weekends! If you're a night owl, you might not like the sound of this, and I'm not saying you always have to be up and out of bed before 7:00 A.M., but this is the ideal time your body wants to wake up. Give your body the chance to try it.

As soon as you get up, have a big glass of room-temperature or warm water (not cold; that's too much of a shock to a waking-up system) with half of a fresh organic lemon squeezed into it. This will help you to wake up and get your colon moving. Once you start the Piper Protocol, I'll have more things for you to do to get your body going in the morning, but if you can start with that lemon water, you'll be doing your body a favor. Don't have breakfast just yet. Give your body a few minutes to adjust and prepare for food.

After your system wakes up, this is the optimal time to hit the bathroom. Your body has been detoxing all night (you'll see exactly how when we get to the overnight hours), and now you want to get all that waste out so you can move on with your day feeling energized and clean, not to mention to make some room for breakfast. That lemon water will help wake things up in there. If you don't have the urge to move your bowels before breakfast, you probably need some internal toning. We'll get to that in time. For now, just give your body the space to use the bathroom. You might just be in a habit of forcing your body to wait.

By the way, if you've been using coffee to trigger your morning bathroom time, it's time to switch to lemon water and kick the caffeine habit. Coffee is acidic and an irritant to the colon, so it forces your body to evacuate in order to flush out the acid and mold and fungi and other chemicals and toxins common in conventional coffee. It also depletes the body of many minerals and vitamins, including calcium, vitamin D, iron, and the B vitamins, and it interferes with the absorption of magnesium, potassium, phosphate, and sodium. Lemon water, on the other hand, works with your body's natural processes, stimulating the liver to release bile, which causes the peristalsis action in the colon, causing a more natural bowel movement—all without depleting any nutrients. However, if you really want to keep your coffee, try one of the new clean, mold-free, fungus-free, alkaline coffees. I've listed brands in the Resources at the back of the book.

Here's an example of how you might spend Large Intestine Time. If your day doesn't go exactly like this, that's fine, but whenever you can, try to approximate this schedule:

Between 5:00 A.M. and 6:00 A.M.: Get up and have a glass of warm lemon water. While you are waiting for your body to respond, you can do some gentle stretching, start making breakfast for your family, or lay out your clothes.

6:30 A.M.: Toilet time. Let yourself relax and see what your body can do for you. If nothing happens, move on with your day. Your body is in training and will soon learn that this is what you want it to do at this time.

6:45 A.M.: Jump into the shower and get clean.

....

WHAT CAN GO WRONG DURING LARGE INTESTINE TIME

If you're not feeling it—if the bowels just aren't moving—then it might be your lungs, believe it or not. Yes, congested lungs can cause constipation! Weird but true. The reason is that the time right before waking, from 3:00 to 5:00 A.M., is Lung Time, and if you're having issues such as a sore throat, chest pressure, cough, or congestion in the lungs, or if you were out at the club smoking until 3:00 A.M. when Lung Time begins, you might not have had the energy to send the toxins down to the large intestine during the night, so your body might not be ready to expel them yet.

Remember, everything is always moving toward the next stage, so the lung energy should move into the large intestine at around 5:00 A.M. If the stool stays in the large intestine for too long, then it blocks the lung energy from sending its energy downward, and this can circle back to cause shortness of breath.

Large Intestine Time is also the time of not letting things go. If you can't move forward emotionally, if you are in a rut or stuck obsessing over something in the past, it can actually cause constipation. It's all connected. (I'll help you more specifically with letting go emotionally in Chapter 9.)

When you get too backed up, eventually your bowels need an emergency evacuation plan, and the energy may get forced violently down into the colon, resulting in diarrhea. (Think about that the next time you crave a cigarette.) Getting re-balanced by working with your internal rhythms and cleansing to get rid of old stuck intestinal matter, as well as old stuck emotions, can help to free you up to make the most of Large Intestine Time.

....

STOMACH TIME: 7 A.M. TO 9 A.M.

You haven't eaten since last night, so it's time to break that fast. Now that your lemon water has prepped your stomach for food, and you've cleared the way with some dedicated bathroom time, your stomach is at its peak energy and ready to take in clean, healthful food. Try some freshly squeezed juice, a wheatgrass shot, a bowl of fruit, or a green smoothie made with a handful of leafy greens, such as kale or romaine lettuce and a cup of berries, along with almond milk or coconut water. The greater the proportion of living, enzyme-rich, raw food to cooked foods, the better.

Chew your food thoroughly and eat it slowly—even your smoothies and fresh juices! Let them spend some time in your mouth and chew them as well as you can. Your stomach may be primed, but you don't want to hurt yourself. Gulping down your food without fully chewing and savoring it will hinder effective digestion. Slow eating and good chewing will keep the stomach energy moving downward, which is the direction it should be going, not upward, back into your esophagus, causing belching and hiccups.

This is how your Stomach Time might go:

7:00 A.M.: Get dressed and start thinking about what you want to have for breakfast.

7:30 A.M.: Put on a kettle for herbal tea (try one of the stomach-supportive herbs, such as cinnamon, ginger, or peppermint). Prepare breakfast. If you need to get the family out the door first so you can have a calm breakfast, do that.

8:00 A.M.: Eat breakfast at the peak of Stomach Time. Eat slowly and calmly, thinking about pleasant things and planning out your day. Relax afterward instead of jumping into your day. Give your body time to get that food safely into your stomach.

....

WHAT CAN GO WRONG DURING STOMACH TIME

If you find yourself belching, feeling nauseous, or having acid indigestion or heartburn during Stomach Time, then your stomach energy is going in the wrong direction—up instead of down. You might have overdone dinner last night, or snacked right before sleeping, so your body had to spend the night digesting instead of healing. There may still be food lingering in there. Try to make it a habit not to eat at least two to three hours before going to sleep at night. By 8:00 to 9:00 P.M., the body is ready to release melatonin to aid your sleep. In the meantime, if you're having stomach distress, keep breakfast on the light side. A freshly squeezed juice might be all you need today. There's no law that you have to load up on breakfast every single morning.

Stomach Time is also the time for worry and pensiveness. If you're worried or your thoughts are too inwardly focused during this time, it can upset digestion. This is a time to think positively about the day ahead. Keep your thoughts light and easy. There will be plenty of time for working out the details later.

SPLEEN TIME: 9 A.M. TO 11 A.M.

You're probably headed to work at about this time of day, and that's good because Spleen Time is a time of high energy. The spleen helps distribute the nutrients from your breakfast throughout your body, so you're getting the full benefit of that healthy food you ate right now. You are also at a creative peak from 9:00 A.M. to 11:00 A.M., so use this time to consider new ideas, take on projects, and brainstorm. You'll also be good at focusing and memorizing things during Spleen Time. Your peak creativity and energy should be right around 10:00 A.M.

This is also a time to stay hydrated so your body functions effectively. Drink lots of water throughout the morning. If you're tired, see if you can forgo the coffee and get to a juice bar on your morning coffee break. Juice is a much better option than coffee for keeping you energized. If you can't leave work, try to bring fresh juice with you. Maybe double the juice amount you need at breakfast and bring half with you. Fresh juice is filled with living enzymes to aid in digestion, as well as healing and general body functioning.

This is also a good time to take digestive enzymes. I'll talk about this in much more detail in Chapter 6 (and recommend some good brands in the Resources at the back of this book). For now, just know that you can purchase digestive enzymes that will help your body to process your food. Normally I like people to take two enzymes with each meal, but if you also take two between meals, this can help move along any undigested food left from breakfast. This will also start cleaning up any unwanted debris in your blood, like excess protein, bacteria, and viruses.

This is how your Spleen Time might go:

9:00 A.M.: Start drinking water. This is an important hydration time.

10:00 A.M.: Focus on projects that require creativity, focus, or memorization. These skills are peaking right now!

10:30 A.M.: Think you won't make it to lunch without a snack? This is an excellent time to hit up the juice bar instead of the coffee cart. Pop a few digestive enzymes along with your juice for maximum detox action.

WHAT CAN GO WRONG DURING SPLEEN TIME

If your spleen is weak, you will have trouble assimilating the nutrients from your breakfast. This can reveal itself if you feel sluggish, tired, or low on energy during this time of day. If your head feels cloudy or you can't concentrate, this is another sign of spleen deficiency. It's a sign that you need to eat a more nutrient-dense breakfast full of living foods, and take digestive enzymes with breakfast to help you use that nutrition more efficiently.

Imbalance in the spleen can also show up as dampness over the body, where a person may have clammy hands and feet and feel swollen over the entire body. This kind of swelling looks more like water weight than fat. If you have bloating after meals, are craving sweets, and feel tired, these are all signs of a spleen imbalance.

For a burst of positive energy, try a cup of Liquid Heaven (my delicious coffee substitute) or Chi City by Truth Calkins or green tea (see the Resources for more information). Also, if it sounds good to you, one square of dark chocolate can add even more pep—but only one square! The combination of coffee substitutes and a little bit of dark chocolate supplies your body with another dose of nutrients, for even more energy and a feel-good morning.

··

HEART TIME: 11 A.M. TO 1 P.M.

Heart time is the peak energy time, as the energy that was being generated during Spleen Time manifests in its full glory at Heart Time. This is when you want to have your largest meal of the day. You need fuel, and you're using the energy to burn it right now. This is also a great time to do any form of easy exercise. A yoga class or a leisurely walk followed by a good hearty lunch is the best way to spend Heart Time. If you're feeling heated during Heart Time, then don't exercise. The heart doesn't like heat. Instead, try meditation to calm and cool your heart.

This is also the most yang time of day, so this is a time of light, heat, activity, and masculine energy. The heart governs the blood and controls the blood vessels, and you might see this in your complexion with flushing, blushing, or a red face. These are further signs of overheating, and signs for you to slow down and relax. Heart Time is also the time of day linked with joy, so let yourself feel joyful during this time, even if you feel like you have things to be sad about. A daily dose of joy is healing for your heart.

Here's an example of what you might do during this time:

11:00 A.M.: Go out for a walk, or take a lunch-hour yoga class.

12:00 P.M.: Have a healthy lunch. Make it your largest meal of the day. Soup, salad, entrée—have all you want of healthy whole food. Eat slowly and chew thoroughly. After lunch, relax and let your food digest instead of rushing off the second you finish your last bite. Let your meal be a calming experience.

12:30 P.M.: Meditate for a few minutes after your meal, to calm your heart and mind.

....

WHAT CAN GO WRONG DURING HEART TIME

Because the heart governs the blood and is also connected with the mind, you might experience flushing and redness as well as sweating during Heart Time. You could also have shortness of breath, palpitations, and circulation-related issues, like cold hands and feet. Some people claim that more people have heart attacks during this time, when the heart energy is strongest, and also at the opposite time of night, from 11:00 P.M. to 1:00 A.M., when the heart energy is at its weakest, so nurture and strengthen your heart with good food and exercise. If your heart feels overwrought during this time, focus on calming.

The heart also houses aspects of the mind, and during the heat of the day, peaking at noon, people tend to show more signs of mental disturbance, often accompanied by sweating. If you're feeling stressed or cold, gentle exercise can help to calm you, but if you're feeling overheated or over-anxious, then this is a good time to meditate to calm the mind and keep it in balance. The heart is naturally heated, being the midday organ, so overheating is more common than being cold at this time.

....

SMALL INTESTINE TIME: 1 P.M. TO 3 P.M.

If lunch is your largest meal of the day (which it should be), all that food will take some time to move through your digestive system, and Small Intestine Time is the time for digestion. This is where most of the nutrients from your food are absorbed to nourish you. If you eat lunch at noon, by about 1:00 P.M. that food will be in your small intestine, and that's where the magic happens. But all this digestion and nutrient assimilation takes energy. That's why, during 1:00 P.M. to 3:00 P.M., the energy is highest in the small intestine, right where you need it.

The small intestine is also responsible for separating the clean and unclean fluids of the body. Unclean fluids go to the bladder where they are excreted as urine. Clean fluids are absorbed into the bloodstream, or move on to the large intestine for further filtering and absorption. Because your body is so busy managing your lunch during this time, you should never eat anything between 1:00 P.M. and 3:00 P.M. Let your body concentrate on absorbing nutrients, not digesting even more food. If you ate a large enough lunch, you won't be hungry during this time. People tend to feel thirsty around this time and might reach for a soft drink when water would be better to hydrate and replenish.

Here's an example of what you might do during Small Intestine Time:

1:00 P.M.: This is a good time to get to work. Sitting at your desk rather than running around will free up energy for digestion, while you busy your brain with the work you need to do. If you don't work during this time, this is a good time to sit down and take care of paperwork, appointment scheduling, and other sedentary tasks.

2:00 P.M.: This is a good time to pop a few enzymes, to keep your digestion humming along and help the body digest any leftover food in the system.

....

WHAT CAN GO WRONG DURING SMALL INTESTINE TIME

If the energy in the small intestine is weak, you may have trouble absorbing nutrients. This can back up the system, moving energy in the wrong direction, and can result in swelling in the face, pain in the lower abdomen, bloating and flatulence, and even pain in the extremities, such as the shoulders and arms. It's also possible for trouble-causing parasites to thrive in the small intestine. According to Chinese medicine, dreaming about being in a crowd is a sign of intestinal parasites. If you have pain or other issues during this time, additional digestive enzymes can be helpful, as well as looking at what you had for lunch. The stronger your health, the better your body will be able to overcome intestinal issues. Focus on more raw living foods for lunch, instead of heavy cooked food. If intestinal issues still seem unresolved, check with your doctor.

....

BLADDER TIME: 3 P.M. TO 5 P.M.

Now that the small intestine has separated the toxins from the nutrients, your bladder can evacuate the unused and toxic elements, so expect to use the bathroom, maybe even a few times, during

Bladder Time, between 3:00 P.M. and 5:00 P.M. During this time of day, people often feel tired and reach for another cup of coffee, or a sugary, caffeinated beverage such as soda or an energy drink. Don't do it! The bladder is expending a lot of energy to release impurities right now, and the last thing you want to do is introduce more. Instead, this is a great time to have a fresh green juice, or a seaweed snack, or coconut water filled with electrolytes that will energize you and keep you hydrated. The bladder is nourished by salty foods, so miso soup broth, veggie broth, or seaweed soup would also be good at this time. Or, have a hot cup of therapeutic herbal tea. Teas that support bladder function include:

Buchu, which strengthens a weak bladder and helps to flush out bacteria.
Goldenrod, which has antifungal and diuretic properties, and is a urinary tonic.
Horsetail, which is high in silica and strengthens bones, hair, and nails more efficiently
    than calcium. It also helps calm an overactive bladder.

Drink lots of fluids throughout the afternoon, to facilitate the bladder's work right now, but keep those fluids pure, clean, and free of caffeine and sugar.

Here's an example of what you might do during Bladder Time:

3:00 P.M.: Prepare a fresh juice, tea with bladder-flushing properties, or salty broth, and savor it slowly.

3:30 P.M.: Urinate.

4:00 P.M.: Drink a large glass of water.

4:30 P.M.: Urinate some more!

....

WHAT CAN GO WRONG DURING BLADDER TIME

Imbalance of the bladder could lead to incontinence, frequent urination, urinary tract infections, and yeast infections for both men and women. Nurture your bladder during Bladder Time with fluids, and see a doctor if you have urinary tract pain or suspect a yeast infection. That afternoon dip in energy can be more exaggerated if you're not well hydrated, so drink up! When there's an imbalance in the bladder, it can also manifest as a feeling of jealousy, holding on to a grudge, or feeling suspicious of others. Pay attention to these feelings if they are uncharacteristic for you.

....

KIDNEY TIME: 5 P.M. TO 7 P.M.

You might think Kidney Time should come before Bladder Time, since the kidneys empty into the bladder. I used to get this wrong all the time on my tests because, to me, it made sense to have Kidney Time and then Bladder Time. However, this system isn't based on the clock or on the linear part of digestion, but on the way energy or *qi* moves through the body.

In Chinese medicine, the kidneys are the origin of *qi* in the body. You first received it from the energy of your parents, but that prenatal *qi* only lasts for so long, without the infusion of *qi* from the food you eat. During Kidney Time, you need to feed your *qi* by having dinner, but not a heavy dinner, as many people have. You're almost done expending energy for the day, so feed your kidneys nutrient-dense but light food for dinner. I prefer a nutritious liquid meal, such as a smoothie or a shake. In the summer, fresh watermelon juice is a good choice. A fresh juice that specifically tonifies the kidneys is made from carrot, cucumber, beet, parsley, and ginger juice, or cucumber, celery, ginger, and lemon juice. Or have a delicious seaweed soup. As a culture we're in the habit of having large dinners, but your dinner should be lighter than your lunch.

If you need more than a liquid meal, have slightly steamed or sautéed vegetables, or soup made with acorn squash or sweet potato, carrots, onions, garlic, and seasoned with rosemary, thyme, and sage, with kelp or dulse sprinkled on top. Simmer until the root vegetables are tender (30 to 45 minutes, depending on how small you chop the pieces), then puree in a high-speed blender until smooth. These are all excellent kidney foods that will nourish and strengthen the kidneys rather than deplete them. Another good option: bone broth, which you can make easily by simmering marrow bones or a chicken or turkey carcass in water for 12 to 24 hours (a slow cooker is good for this). In the last hour, add aromatic vegetables such as onions, celery, and carrots, and some sea salt to taste, then sip it all day. The kidneys help to produce bone marrow, so eating bone broth can support this important function. Black foods and seeds also nourish the kidneys. Try black sesame seeds, black rice, and pumpkin seeds.

Here's what you might do during Kidney Time:

5:00 P.M.: Plan and prepare a light dinner of juice, a smoothie, soup, or steamed or sautéed vegetables.

6:00 P.M.: Enjoy your light dinner. Eat or sip slowly for best nutrient absorption and a feeling of fullness.

WHAT CAN GO WRONG DURING KIDNEY TIME

This is the time when most people finish working, but they may not completely let go of work mentally, even if they leave the office. Maybe you didn't finish a project or you're worrying about something in the future, even if it's something you have no control over. This is common because Kidney Time is also when fear can take over. You may need to blow off steam. Many people go to happy hour and drink to wallow in or forget their problems. Others get a little crazed around this time. Things may seem distorted. People tend to be overly focused on the future rather than being present during Kidney Time, and may even get struck with moments of fearing death during this time.

The kidneys influence reproduction, fertility, growth, and aging. Fear drains kidney energy, so if you're afraid all the time, it can impact fertility as well as aging. Reflecting on the future too intensely, and even having too much sex, can drain kidney energy. (You want to know how much is too much, don't you? It depends on your health and how well you are eating, but anywhere from three or four times per week to once a day is fine for most healthy people. Multiple times per day can be quite depleting if your body isn't in good shape, but super healthy people on a nutrient-dense raw diet can often handle it with no problem. By the way, supplementing with herbs like maca, reishi, and he shou wu make sex even better! You're welcome.) To help restore kidney energy, make a focused effort to be in the present moment and summon your courage during Kidney Time.

PERICARDIUM TIME: 7 P.M. TO 9 P.M.

The pericardium is the protector of the heart. It is the membrane surrounding and protecting the heart with a cushion of fluid, and this is a time to wind down and soothe the heart. Address issues that influence your heart at this time. Intimacy, heartfelt conversations, expressing emotions, talking about your feelings with someone, or meditating to understand your feelings better are all appropriate during Pericardium Time.

This is not a time to do vigorous exercise, watch violent or anxiety-producing movies, or get into stressful situations or conversations. The heart wants to be happy and calm, so let this time of heart protection energy be a time of positivity and joy. Do things that make you happy. Read an inspirational book, or write in your journal about what makes you happy or grateful. Spend good time with positive family or friends. Do not eat anything during this time, but warm almond milk with ashwagandha, an herbal remedy for anxiety, will help to make you feel calm and get to sleep soon. If you add a dash of nutmeg, it will kick in about three hours later to help you stay asleep. Or, try a calming herbal tea, such as valerian, kava kava, or chamomile. I also recommend a little evening aromatherapy. Try smelling the essential oils of bergamot, lavender, chamomile oil, lemon balm, sweet marjoram, or passion flower.

Here's an example of how you might spend your Pericardium Time:

7:00 P.M.: Think about winding down. Do some gentle yoga poses. Write in your journal.

7:30 P.M.: Spend some quiet and/or fun, positive time with people you love.

8:00 P.M.: Meditate, pray, or read or watch something positive or inspirational. Focus on the good and let yourself feel joy.

WHAT CAN GO WRONG DURING PERICARDIUM TIME

If you aren't in sync with your natural rhythms, attempts at conversations about emotions or intimate overtures could go in the wrong direction during this time, creating tension in relationships. This is the time to focus on intimacy, but it doesn't have to mean sex or the deepest conversation you've ever had about your emotions. Touch, be gentle, be supportive, and see where it goes. If your intimate overtures are rejected because your partner isn't in the mood, or your children don't feel like hanging out and talking with you about your feelings, or nobody wants to talk at all, this is no time to get depressed or feel anxious. This is a time to honor your loved ones and yourself with gentle support. If you aren't getting it, try giving it instead. What do other people need? This is incredibly healing for your pericardium.

TRIPLE WARMER TIME (SAN JIAO TIME): 9 P.M. TO 11 P.M.

The Triple Warmer is a unique Chinese medicine concept. It doesn't correlate with a specific organ in Western medicine, but in Chinese medicine it is a system of energy management in the body. It is the communication system between all the organs and the thermostat for the body. A Western perspective might see it as the director of the Circadian clock. It's closely related to the endocrine system (hormones) in Western medicine, but it isn't exactly the same. It's about synchronization and harmony. It's about connection. This is a time to connect after intimacy (sexual or emotional) or just being together. It is cuddle time and calm time. It is about wordless natural biochemical communication.

That means that between 9:00 P.M. and 11:00 P.M., the body is preparing to do its overnight work of processing and assimilating everything you've taken in during that day. This is hard work, and your body needs to devote all its energy to this job, so this is the best time to wind down and go to bed. Yes, that means lights out by 11:00 P.M., and preferably before! Your body begins to produce melatonin now, so you can sleep. Pericardium Time is over, and in Chinese medicine, your heart will hold your mind while you sleep. If you fed your pericardium well, you'll have a calm and relaxing sleep.

This is how Triple Warmer Time might go:

9:00 P.M.: Take a warm bath or shower. This is when melatonin is starting to kick in.

9:30 P.M.: Connect with someone, physically or even on the phone. Say good night. End on a good note.

10:00 P.M.: Get in bed. Read, meditate, or pray. Focus on letting your mind go dormant so you can sleep. For the most rejuvenating and restful sleep, turn off all TVs, computers, and other electronics and screens by 10:00 P.M.

11:00 P.M.: Close your eyes. Breathe deeply. (Remember IF Prep Step #1 on page 26: five minutes of relaxation, five breaths in, and five breaths out.) Let your mind go and let your body relax. You have important work to do, but you don't need to worry about it at all. It all happens automatically, in your sleep. Ideally you will be sound asleep before the clock hits 11:00 P.M., so your body is ready for Gallbladder Time. The work of cleanup and repair starts now.

....

WHAT CAN GO WRONG DURING TRIPLE WARMER TIME

When you can't turn off your mind and you lie awake thinking, obsessing, or feeling anxious, and when you can't even keep your eyes shut because they keep fluttering open again, you aren't in sync with Triple Warmer Time. This is a good time to meditate because your body needs to calm down. Take deep, slow breaths and focus your mind on a single word you can repeat over and over in your mind, or visualize a single object and focus on it. Once you get in the habit of going to bed at this time, it should become easier, especially if you spend Triple Warmer Time winding down rather than stimulating yourself with light, noise, and electronics.

....

GALLBLADDER TIME: 11 P.M. TO 1 A.M.

By this time, you should be sound asleep. Your gallbladder is now gearing up for some important work. In Chinese medicine, the gallbladder drives decision making, initiative, and problem solving, and it also helps to spur change. If you have a dream that helps you solve a problem in your life, it comes from your gallbladder during Gallbladder Time. In fact, this can be the best way to make a big decision. (It's why they tell you to "sleep on it.") If you aren't sleeping during this time—maybe you're out dancing or drinking—then you've lost an opportunity for your body to guide you. Western medicine views the gallbladder according to its more direct and obvious purpose: storing bile from the liver and helping with fat digestion. The gallbladder also helps to detox the body while you sleep. Put the two systems together—Chinese and Western—and you can rest easy knowing it will all come out right in the morning—those tough decisions *and* the accumulated waste from your overnight cleanup. The best thing about Gallbladder Time is that you don't have to do anything at all except be unconscious.

What might be happening during Gallbladder Time:

11:00 P.M. to 1:00 A.M.: You will begin to progress through the five stages of sleep. Your body will cycle from light sleep to deep sleep to REM or dream sleep throughout the night as your gallbladder helps to detoxify the waste from the day.

WHAT CAN GO WRONG DURING GALLBLADDER TIME

If you're chronically awake during Gallbladder Time, your gallbladder won't get a chance to replenish its energy for the purposes of detoxifying the body and the mind. Too much loss of sleep during Gallbladder Time can lead to chronic indecision and timidity, as well as incomplete detoxification.

Sleep is absolutely crucial for internal fitness. It's the final piece in the puzzle of your day. It's also important for long-term health and longevity. Research shows that if you get less than six hours or more than nine hours of sleep per night, you're likely to have a shorter life span. Aim for seven and a half to eight hours and you're golden.

LIVER TIME: 1 A.M. TO 3 A.M.

It's now what most people would consider the dead of night, and you are dead asleep, cycling between deep sleep and REM sleep. This is Liver Time, and your liver, one of your most important detoxifying organs, is hard at work filtering out everything toxic the body has taken in during the day and dumping it into the colon for morning elimination. The toxic waste will sit there, safely encased in the colon, until you're ready to get rid of it. You need enough time to fully clean your body, so keep sleeping! The liver is also accumulating energy at this time.

Here's what might happen during this time of the night:

1:00 A.M. to 3:00 A.M.: You will continue to cycle through light sleep, deep sleep, and REM sleep. Meanwhile, your liver is busy filtering and processing.

....

WHAT CAN GO WRONG DURING LIVER TIME

If you're awake during Liver Time, you miss a crucial period of repair. The cleanup crew can't clean a school or a department store or an office building when everybody is still there learning or shopping or working, and your body can't fully clean your body if you're up and running around. I cannot overemphasize the importance of sleep for internal fitness and mental health. Get to sleep!

....

LUNG TIME: 3 A.M. TO 5 A.M.

During this time, as you continue to sleep, your breath changes with each sleep stage. During REM sleep, your breath is quick and shallow, as if you are walking around living your life, getting excited, and having adventures (which you may be doing in your dreams). During deep sleep, your breath slows down and you breathe from a deep part of your lungs. This is cleansing; during Lung Time, the lungs purge their toxins into the liver, which continues to filter these into the colon, and also sends energy to the colon, in preparation for Large Intestine Time, which starts at 5:00 A.M. And now we've gone full circle, back to the beginning.

Here's what might happen during Lung Time:

3:00 A.M.: You'll continue to cycle between dream and deep sleep. Your lungs are cleansing and sending energy to the large intestine now.

5:00 A.M.: Your large intestine will begin to energize, preparing you for the coming day.

....

WHAT CAN GO WRONG DURING LUNG TIME

It's not exactly a dysfunction, but sometimes when you're sleeping, you may wake up crying or breathing heavily or having a strong emotion, like sadness. This is all part of mental processing. It's normal and natural. You're working out your feelings in your dreams.

....

Now you've traveled all the way around your clock. I hope you're inspired to get into better sync with your body and with the natural cycles of light and dark. You don't have to overhaul your entire lifestyle this second, but consider taking what you can from this and keeping in mind what organ is filled with the most energy at what hour of the day. Do what you can to nurture it, and let your body do its job. The less you get in the way, the better you'll feel, and the more you'll be able to dance to the rhythm of your own life.

WHEN YOUR SCHEDULE IS OFF

I understand that you won't always be able to live in sync with these hours or cycles. Life gets in the way. Maybe you have a deadline, or a new baby, or you do shift work and you have to be up at night and sleep during the day. All these things can interfere with your natural rhythms, and unfortunately, because these rhythms work in tune with nature and the sun, you can never totally adjust your body to (for example) have liver time during the day instead of during the night. If my schedule is off because of a deadline, I know that it is extra important for my diet to be as wholesome as possible, and for me to maintain all my good habits. This can help to balance out the stress the body feels when it is not in rhythm with these natural cycles. It isn't as good as getting to bed by 10:00 P.M. and waking up at 6:00 A.M., but it definitely helps. On any day when you *can* get in sync with this schedule, do it—your body will thank you! As for people who work night shifts, it is even more vitally important to live a healthy lifestyle. At least your organs will get the nutrition they need. A disrupted sleep cycle on top of stress and a poor diet is a disaster down the road, so please take care of yourself, and adhere to the Piper Protocol whenever you can.

In the meantime, take a first step with this next Internal Fitness Prep Step:

....

INTERNAL FITNESS PREP STEP #3

IF you want to get your body back into rhythm, start your day with lemon water. I would like you to begin every morning with a big glass of room temperature or warm water (not cold) with half of a fresh organic lemon squeezed into it. This is a powerful way to get your digestive system moving for the day, but it's easy and you'll learn to love the taste. After your lemon water, wait about 30 minutes before eating breakfast. If you can trigger the reflex to use the bathroom before breakfast, you've got your body into a natural rhythm that will benefit you all day long.

....

PART TWO

Deep Cleaning from the Inside Out

CHAPTER 4

Bacteria Love

DON'T YOU JUST *LOVE* bacteria? What? You don't? I do, and let me make the case for why you should, too. Internal fitness is critically linked to the bacterial content of your intestines. You've got trillions of microorganisms in there, working away, and your gut contains ten times more bacteria than all the rest of your body put together. In fact, you are made up of more bacterial cells than "human" cells! These bacterial cells do many things. Some make you inflamed or sick. Others help produce chemicals you need to thrive, and they keep your digestive system running smoothly. In a healthy body, the nice bacteria far outnumber the nasty bacteria, but if you've been practicing some not-so-nice lifestyle habits (such as stressing out and eating lots of sugar), then the bad guys are going to get a better foothold. We don't want that to happen. We need to keep them in check by following the law of your internal landscape.

In this chapter, I provide all the information you need to give your good bacteria every chance of winning the war against the bad guys and laboring for the benefit of your internal fitness. The more you know about bacteria, the more motivated you will be to get on the side of the good guys, so let's get into it. After you read this chapter, you might just fall in love with bacteria after all.

LET'S JUST CALL IT "FLORA"

Imagine a garden burgeoning with flowers. Now imagine an intestine burgeoning with friendly bacteria. Both pictures are equally beautiful to me, because I love flowers, but I also know how powerful and healthful a heavy dose of good bacteria can be. Another name for the bacteria in your gut is *gut flora*, a.k.a. *microflora*, a.k.a. *microbiota*. These bacteria really are a little bit like plants in the way they grow and multiply. Good gut flora do some pretty good deeds inside of you, including:

- Helping digestion, especially of carbohydrates. The good bacteria actually ferment these foods, which aren't completely digested in the stomach, and then absorb the short-chain fatty acids from the foods, providing you with energy.
- Helping keep your digestion moving along, while fighting and overwhelming the bacteria that contribute to both constipation and diarrhea.
- Shoring up your immune system so you can better fight infections. The better part of your immune system comes from your gut.
- Maintaining healthy levels of vitamin B and vitamin K in the body.
- Regulating metabolism, to keep you at a normal weight.
- Increasing the peristalsis of the intestines to increase transit time and make digestion more efficient.
- Controlling cholesterol levels by slowing down the re-absorption of cholesterol.
- Helping with mood—you have a complex nervous system in your gut, and most of your serotonin is produced there. Serotonin is responsible for that feeling you get when you're in a good mood. Good bacteria will promote healthy serotonin release, helping to relieve issues like anxiety, irritability, and depression. Recent studies even suggest that gut flora are linked to personality, emotions, memory, and IQ.
- ⬆ probiotics = ⬇ weight

You have every reason to cheer for and support those good guys! Here are some great ways to do that every day:

- Reduce your consumption of sugar, sweets, and other simple carbohydrates, such as white flour, white pasta, white rice, sweetened drinks, and even sugary fruits like grapes and bananas.
- Eat lots of fermented foods and drinks, such as almond-milk or coconut-milk yogurt (not from cow's milk), kefir, kvass, sauerkraut, and kimchi.

- Eat living foods, such as raw vegetables, fruits, and sprouted gluten-free grains, including quinoa, brown rice, and black rice.
- Use antibiotics only when you really need them, as for a serious infection.
- Avoid antibacterial washes and soaps, which can strengthen bad bacteria and reduce your body's ability to fight them off.
- Start taking probiotics supplements, or increase your dosage. (I'll talk more about how to do this on page 76, in Internal Fitness Prep Step #4.)
- Manage your stress regularly by making time for yourself and practicing stress-relieving activities, such as yoga, deep breathing, and meditation.

But what happens when the bad guys take over? They're the ones with menacing names like *Candida albicans*, *Clostridium difficile*, *Staphylococcus aureus*, and *E. coli*. If the bad bacteria in your body overwhelm the good bacteria, it can cause a cascade of health issues, from simple to complex. A poor gut flora balance has been linked to the following:

Chronic gas, bloating, and flatulence
Intestinal cramping
Chronic constipation
Chronic diarrhea
Gastritis
Ulcerative colitis
Irritable bowel syndrome (IBS)
Inflammatory bowel disease (IBD)
Leaky gut (intestinal permeability)
Chronic digestive diseases, such as Crohn's disease and celiac disease
Blood sugar issues, including insulin resistance, metabolic syndrome, and diabetes
Leptin resistance (the hormone that tells you when you're full)
Increasing the storage of calories as fat
Strong cravings for sugar or refined carbohydrates, such as bread, pastries, pasta, and rice
Obesity
Fungus in the toenails and fingernails, which shows as discoloration
Autoimmune dysfunctions, including thyroid disease and lupus

Recurring vaginal yeast infections

Rectal itching

Interstitial cystitis of the bladder

Urinary tract infections

Skin conditions like psoriasis, eczema, acne, itchy skin rashes, and contact dermatitis

Foggy brain, poor memory and concentration, lack of focus

Chronic fatigue, exhaustion for no apparent reason

Chronic seasonal allergies

Chronic systemic inflammation

Lowered immunity

Severe chemical sensitivity

Mood swings

Anxiety

Irritability

Depression

Decreased libido

Wow, what a list! You definitely don't want those bad boys in charge, yet many common lifestyle decisions are probably skewing your good guy : bad guy bacteria ratio right now. Some of the things that can give the bad guys the edge by creating an inhospitable environment for the good guys and a party for the riffraff include:

High-sugar, high-refined-carbohydrate diets

Low-fiber diets

Consuming artificial ingredients, such as genetically modified foods and industrial products, including seed oils and high-fructose corn syrup

Taking antibiotics

Using birth control pills

Taking pain relievers, especially NSAIDs (like ibuprofen), on a regular basis

Having a low-grade infection

Experiencing chronic stress

Smoking cigarettes (or anything else, for that matter)

Drinking a lot of alcohol (more than one drink per day)

Too much chlorinated water: drinking it, showering in it, swimming in it

Frequent X-rays, MRIs, CAT scans, and other sources of radiation

If you want to know for sure if you're having issues with bad gut bacteria, there are some tests you can take, including blood tests, an organic urine dysbiosis test, a stool test, or a bacterial count during an endoscopy to test for bacterial overgrowth. You can ask your doctor about getting any of these tests done. Or, you could just start living to feed the garden in your gut, and find out how much better you can feel.

ALL ABOUT PROBIOTICS

Different probiotics live in different parts of our body and exist in just about every part of our internal environment, from mouth to colon. Others like to be on the move, circulating and going where they are most needed. The bacteria most prevalent in the small intestine is *Lactobacillus acidophilus* and in the large intestine, *Bifidobacterium bifidum*. The most important transient bacteria are *Lactobacillus bulgaricus* and *Streptococcus thermophilus*.

The most common probiotic supplement we hear about is acidophilus, which is actually *Lactobacillus acidophilus*. Your doctor may recommend it, or you may see it on TV or advertised at the health food store. There are more than two hundred strains of *Lactobacillus acidophilus*, and each has its unique job. Most acidophilus supplements never mention the strains they contain, but many studies have been done on specific strains called DDS-1 and NAS. (DDS-1 was named by the University of Nebraska Department of Dairy Science, hence DDS.)

L. acidophilus DDS-1 is a superstar, as it has strong antibiotic properties that kill the bacteria that cause diseases, especially yeast infections and eleven other specific disease-causing bacteria. DDS-1 is cultured in milk. The NAS strain is very special, however, as it is dairy free. Made from organic garbanzo bean extract, it's sticky and thus sticks to the wall of the intestines. But chances are, you won't know the particular strains. You'll just see names like *L. acidophilus* and *B. bifidum*.

I personally believe that the more species of probiotics you take, the better. I opt for a rotation of probiotic supplements containing different types, as well as a variety of fermented foods like fermented vegetables (pickles, sauerkraut, kimchi) and non-dairy yogurt (I'll talk more about dairy later). These also contain a variety of probiotic species, depending on which ones you choose. Also, supplements may include multiple strains of bacteria that may or may not conflict with each other, so read your labels. For example, if you put *L. acidophilus* and *L. bulgaricus* in the same capsule, by the time the product gets to you and you take it, *L. bulgaricus* may have consumed *L. acidophilus*, reducing the probiotic variety offered to you. *B. bifidum*, on the other hand, does not compete with *L. acidophilus*, so they can exist together in a supplement product. Another match made in heaven is *L. bulgaricus* and *S. thermophilus*. These strains are great because they're both strong and can survive the harsh acidic environment of the stomach and the harsh alkaline properties of bile in the small intestine.

There are also a broad number of species and strains that do specific things in the body, so you can also customize your probiotics supplement to your individual issues: for example, general health, gastrointestinal discomfort, viral diarrhea, traveler's diarrhea, vaginal yeast, irritable bowel syndrome, *C. difficile* diarrhea, urinary tract infection, allergies, autoimmune issues, antibiotic associated diarrhea, cold and flu, and eczema. Here's a probiotics cheat sheet:

....

GUIDE TO COMMON PROBIOTICS

Bacillus subtilis: This bacterium is one of my favorites. It's the active ingredient in Nattokinase enzyme supplement, and it's well known for secreting extracellular enzymes that help to regulate blood viscosity in cases of deep vein thrombosis and embolism, and for cardiovascular health. It eats up the protein fibrin, which makes blood clots.

Bifidobacterium animalis: This one is good for general health and gastrointestinal (GI) health.

Bifidobacterium bifidum: This is a very common strain of probiotics found mainly in the large intestine. It synthesizes vitamin B complex as well as vitamin K (which helps your blood clot and improves your bone health). *B. bifidum* helps to regulate and improve digestion and phagocytosis of bad bacteria in the body by enhancing the immune system. It controls the production of histamine release to reduce allergic reactions and, in turn, inflammatory response. Taking *B. bifidum* in a supplement can help a damaged liver, heal gut permeability (leaky gut), and reduce diarrhea. It also helps the body stop healthy cells from turning into cancer cells. Drinking too much alcohol kills off *B. bifidum*, so remember all the good this important probiotic does for you the next time you want another round.

Bifidobacterium infantis: This one is also good for general health, GI health, and in relieving irritable bowel snydrome (IBS) symptoms like bloating, gas, flatulence, constipation, and diarrhea.

Bifidobacterium lactis: Also good for general health, GI health, and viral diarrhea.

Lactobacillus acidophilus: One of the most popular probiotics, it's used to control diarrhea, especially in the case of lactose intolerance. It aids in the reduction of LDL (bad) cholesterol, fights *Candida albicans* (yeast), and strengthens the immune system. It has also been shown to help with IBS symptoms and viral diarrhea. This one is a superstar.

Lactobacillus bulgaricus: This probiotic helps to promote the growth of other beneficial bacteria in the body but doesn't colonize in the GI tract. Selfless, isn't it. All about the others not about itself. It just makes the environment in the GI tract inhospitable for the bad bacteria. It also aids in digestion, controls intestinal infections, reduces lactose intolerance, and helps lower the "bad" LDL cholesterol. It's also very beneficial for constipation or diarrhea, or alternating constipation and diarrhea.

Lactobacillus casei: One of the more popular probiotics for intestinal infections and strengthening the immune system, it helps to maintain the balance of the flora in the GI tract and increases the immune system by stimulating its natural killer (NK) cells. Take it for general health, GI health, inflammatory bowel disease (IBD), antibiotic-associated diarrhea, allergies, and autoimmunity.

Lactobacillus plantarum: This is a probiotic with the beautiful benefit of helping tremendously with bloating and flatulence. It produces lactic acid, and one of its strains has had clinical studies showing how effective it is for IBS. It also preserves omega-3 fatty acid in your body, allowing it to stay in the gut longer, where it reduces inflammation.

Lactobacillus rhamnosus: This probiotic is very effective in supporting the mucosal lining of the intestinal tract, attaching easily and protecting the lining from infections. Take it for general health, GI health, IBD, IBS, viral diarrhea, antibiotic-associated diarrhea, *C. difficile*, traveler's diarrhea, eczema, and autoimmunity.

Saccharomyces boulardii: This bacteria is good for general health and GI health, and has also been shown to help relieve the symptoms of IBS, IBD, viral diarrhea, antibiotic-associated diarrhea, *C. difficile*, traveler's diarrhea, eczema, and autoimmunity. This is another one of my favorites because it's a bad-guy killer, helping to make the intestinal environment uninhabitable for those shady characters.

Streptococcus thermophilus: This probiotic is great for traveler's diarrhea. It can stop it immediately. It's also good for acute diarrhea from other causes, including lactose intolerance. I think of it as the diarrhea probiotic. Maybe you think that's a yucky name, but when you need it, you're going to be glad you remembered it!

VSL#3: This one can help relieve IBS and IBD symptoms. It's often prescribed by a doctor for serious gastrointestinal situations like ulcerative colitis. It has a large number of strains.

Some other advice I often give clients and follow myself regarding probiotic supplements:

1. Consider brand reputation. When choosing supplements, go with a reputable brand that has been extensively researched, and that lists the genus, species, and strain, as well as the number of probiotics in the product, if you can find a brand that does this. Reputable companies have better quality control, so the product is more likely to contain viable live cultures at the time it reaches the consumer, not just at manufacture. If a product says "proprietary blend," you don't know what you're getting. (I recommend several excellent brands in the Resources, all available online.)

2. Take probiotics daily. Taking one probiotic a week or remembering to take one every once in a while isn't going to help. To be effective and actually impact health, probiotics must be taken every day. If you have a health challenge, such as an infection or a chronic disease, you may want to take them even more often, like two or three times per day. They're best taken on an empty stomach because less acid will be present and the probiotic can adhere more easily to the intestinal wall.

3. Rinse your mouth. Don't let your stomach and intestines have all the fun. Your mouth needs good bacteria, too. There are more bacteria in the mouth than anywhere else. If I was a bacterium, I would prefer the mouth because I would have endless access to food and water and a comfortable environment to keep me growing and happy. Most of the bacteria in your mouth do the very important job of eating up the excess food left behind in your gums and teeth after you eat, so it doesn't rot away in there. Without it, you'd have a lot more cavities and probably some yucky mouth ulcers, too. Your dentist probably already told you that when you eat too much sugar, this feeds the bad bacteria—the ones who like to drill into your teeth and make those cavities. But don't forget the good guys. To give them a boost every morning, open a capsule or two and mix it with a little water, then swish it around in your mouth, getting it between your teeth and into your gums. See IF Prep Step #4 on page 76 for more information about how to do this.

4. Add calcium. You can also take probiotics with calcium. Probiotics help the body absorb calcium by making some of the co-factors necessary for building bones, and calcium also helps probiotics cling to the wall of the intestines better, thus crowding out the bad bacteria. The calcium that works best for probiotic colonization is a calcium phosphate supplement. Taking these together also helps to reduce LDL ("bad") cholesterol.

5. Add protein. If you take your probiotic with protein, the probiotic enhances protein utilization in the body. This increases strength as well as lean muscle mass. Normally, I have you take probiotics on an empty stomach, but taking additional probiotics when you eat protein will give you a boost, especially if you are trying to increase your muscle mass.

PROBIOTIC SUPPLEMENT SURVIVAL STRATEGIES

Probiotics are delicate, and easily denatured by heat. To keep your supplements viable longer, keep them refrigerated, even if the packaging says it's not necessary, for better preservation. Probiotics can typically stay alive for about two weeks at room temperature, but under refrigeration they'll last longer. When you travel, you may not be able to keep your probiotics refrigerated, but if you bring a fresh batch at the beginning of your trip, they should be fine for two weeks. Just keep them out of extreme heat. Always check the expiration date on the package to be sure you can finish them all before they expire. If your package is running out, double up so that you're not left without. You can't overdose on probiotics, and even taking them three times a day won't do any harm and may actually keep your body flush with the good guys. The most that happens is they may make your stool softer. This is a welcome change for the constipated crew.

FEEDING PROBIOTICS WITH PREBIOTICS

The other important piece to consider is how to keep those probiotics you're taking alive and thriving inside of you. If conditions aren't right, they aren't all going to take up residence and have families. In fact, conditions have to be right for those supplements to do anything at all! And what's the first way to keep anything alive? Feed it.

To do this, it is extremely important to consume *prebiotics*. Prebiotics are the food for probiotics, and without them, your expensive probiotic supplements are going to pass on through town with an eye out for a better place to eat. With plenty of food, on the other hand, the probiotics you take will have a better chance of settling in and multiplying.

Most of this happens in your small intestine—90 percent of the prebiotic soluble fiber you eat gets digested there. Remember when I said that probiotics metabolize undigested carbohydrates in the small intestine? This is what I was talking about! It's food and thus energy for them. Some common prebiotics your gut flora may be enjoying right now include the following types. As you will see, many of them exist in foods you are already eating. Others are available in supplement form. Taking in a wide variety of prebiotics is the best way to ensure a healthy colony of probiotics:

Alpha-lactalbumin: This prebiotic makes up more than 20 percent of the protein in human breast milk (but only 2 to 5 percent of the protein in cow's milk). It makes peptides that protect the newborn from harmful bacteria it may be ingesting from the environment or the mother, thus reducing overall infant infections.

Galactooligosaccharides (GOS): Like the probiotics that feed on it, GOS has been shown to benefit people with IBS. It's a commercially manufactured prebiotic, made from the enzymatic conversion of lactose from cow's milk.

Glycomacropeptide (GMP): Found in the protein in milk and its curds (casein), GMP is rich in sialic acid, which increases the growth of beneficial bifidobacteria and improves digestive function. GMP specifically makes it difficult for bad bacteria to adhere to the intestinal wall. In order for good and bad microflora to survive in the GI tract, they must be able to adhere to the wall of the intestines, and if they can't, they're destroyed. Go, GMP!

Inulin: These are starchy carbohydrates with a low glycemic level, so they are good for diabetics. Find them in root vegetables like onions, garlic, and leeks, and other vegetables like asparagus, dandelion greens, chicory root, and Jerusalem artichoke (sunchoke). Bananas also contain inulin. Not only is inulin good for feeding probiotics, especially the *Bifidus* species, which prefer it, but it also helps to reduce blood fat, cholesterol, and triglycerides.

Lactoferrin: This is a milk protein that binds to iron. In order for the microflora (both the good guys and the bad) to grow and multiply, they need iron. But lactoferrin gives the good guys an advantage because only probiotics have the keys to unlock the iron in lactoferrin. The bad guys can't unlock it.

Oligosaccharides: A carbohydrate naturally found in plants like chicory root, Jerusalem artichoke, onions, garlic, and asparagus.

Pectin: This one is found under the skin of apples, pears, oranges, and grapefruits, and it's used as a thickening agent in jams and jellies. It's great at removing toxins and heavy metals from the body as well as helping to eliminate drug residue.

Polydextrose: This is a synthetic indigestible prebiotic made from glucose and sorbitol. It's artificially made and found in things like sugared cereal. It's actually a prebiotic to avoid because it is synthetic, but I want you to know about it so you will recognize it when you see it on a processed food ingredients label.

Xylooligosaccharides (XOS): XOS is a new prebiotic that is made from xylose. XOS uses lignocellulosic materials (LCMs), which are rich in xylan. XOS fermentation causes acidification of the contents of the colon and forms short-chain fatty acids that become the fuel for different tissues and regulate cellular processes. A recent study published in the *Journal of Nutrition* linked XOS with the prevention of precancerous lesions in the colon.

These all sound like pretty fancy names, but here's what most of these really are: fiber, starch, and protein, and you can get them from the food you eat so you really don't have to take any additional supplements. The good prebiotics that will feed you and your probiotics can be found in many delicious things you should be eating, such as:

Most vegetables

Lots of fruits

Many herbs and spices

Dark chocolate

Non-dairy, unsweetened yogurt and kefir (like coconut—homemade is best)

Fiber supplements, like psyllium seeds and chia seeds

FIBER FACTS

It's important to take in at least 35 to 50 grams of dietary fiber every day. Not only does the bulk in fiber speed up the release of waste through the colon, and not only does fiber have no calories, but it also makes you feel full so you'll be less likely to overeat. It also provides a Thanksgiving feast for your friendly gut flora. Fiber essentially passes through your system undigested. It has no vitamins or minerals, but it is found in all plant foods, such as fruits, grains, nuts, seeds, and vegetables. There are two types of fiber: insoluble and soluble. Both are important:

Insoluble fiber is like a sponge when mixed with any type of fluid. It never dissolves—it just expands, which is why it makes you feel full after you eat it. This is what people mean when they talk about "roughage." Insoluble fiber stimulates the intestines to move the stool along its tract. This aids in the relief of constipation because it increases peristalsis, the wave-like movement of the intestines that keeps things moving along. It also makes it unnecessary to strain to push in the bathroom (straining can cause hemorrhoids and diverticulosis). Because insoluble fiber speeds up the transit time of the stool, it's known to be an integral factor in preventing colon cancer. Because it is a bulking agent, it also sweeps through the colon, picking up toxins, bacteria, parasites, and carcinogenic substances and shuttling them on their way.

Soluble fiber is like a powder that absorbs water and then turns into a gel. It's not digested by you but by your microflora (which is why it's considered a prebiotic). This gel also makes you feel full, which helps with appetite control. Soluble fiber does your blood sugar a favor, too. It slows down the rate of sugar entering the bloodstream from the food you eat, to keep your blood sugar levels from getting too high or too low. It also controls cholesterol levels by absorbing bile salts and cholesterol that are in the intestines during digestion. This is a conservative and safe way to reduce cholesterol levels in your body.

Both types of fiber offer you benefits far beyond feeding your friendly flora!

WHAT IF YOU ARE ON ANTIBIOTICS OR ANTIFUNGAL MEDICATION?

There are *pro*biotics, and the opposite of those are *anti*biotics. If you are on antibiotics for an infection, know that they will kill the good bacteria as well as the bad bacteria. The only good bacteria they don't kill is *Saccharomyces boulardii*, but it will be killed as well if you have to go on an antifungal medication.

If you're taking antibiotics or antifungals, double up on your probiotics, taking them two to three hours after you take your medication. Some people believe that this will somehow negate the effects of the antibiotic, but this is untrue. Your antibiotic medication is slaying all the bacteria in order to get the bad guys. All you're doing is sending in replacement troops of good guys. And be sure to increase your fiber consumption to feed your probiotics.

I recommend taking multiple strains of probiotics, switching types every month or two to get as many types as possible and cover all the bases. If money is not an object, then get two different kinds with different strains and take one kind in the morning and another in the evening. If money is an issue, try making your own coconut kefir, a delicious drink with a natural population of friendly bacteria. You can get a culture starter kit from Body Ecology (www.bodyecology.com), or try making your own Rejuvelac with the recipe from the Ann Wigmore Natural Health Institute (www.annwigmore.org), or look for any book about making fermented food at home.

ABOUT FERMENTED FOODS

A discussion about probiotics wouldn't be complete without information on fermented foods. Probiotic supplements are a fairly recent invention, but people have been eating fermented foods for thousands of years, and they have been benefiting the human body and contributing to survival long before we had such modern conveniences as refrigerators and freezers. In fact, they were a major part of life in those days.

Back then, people had to find other means of preserving their foods. One common preservation method was salting. I remember my grandmother doing that before we were able to afford a refrigerator. Another was to cook food, which didn't spoil as quickly as raw food. And yet another way was to ferment food. Each one of these methods prolongs freshness and extends the life of food, which helps humans survive in times of scarcity. Fermentation is one of the most effective methods of food storage.

Fermentation is a process in which lactic acid–producing bacteria break down the nutrients in the food. These bacteria, which are actually probiotics, are natural residents that live on fruits, vegetables, and grains, in milk, and even in the air. You probably already eat some popular fermented foods: yogurt, sauerkraut, pickles, miso, cottage cheese, nattō, relish, kimchi, tempeh, soy sauce, beer, and old-fashioned root beer. These foods contain not only probiotics but also their own built-in prebiotics.

I suggest eating fermented foods as often as you can get them, and in as natural a form as possible, without added sugar, coloring, and binders. Plain organic non-dairy yogurt, unsweetened kefir, natural sauerkraut, other fermented or cultured veggies, and kombucha tea are all easy to find and enjoy. Double up on them if you're taking antibiotics. Fermented foods in your diet every day will help keep your microflora blossoming, which in turn will make your immune system strong, your digestion fit, and your weight stable.

Are you ready to incorporate probiotics into your life, along with the first three Internal Fitness Prep Steps? Here's your assignment:

....

INTERNAL FITNESS PREP STEP #4

IF you want to start populating your gut with an army of friendly bacteria (trust me, you do!), begin a daily regimen of probiotics. Always take them on an empty stomach. In the morning after using the bathroom but before breakfast is the perfect time. Here's what I want you to do:

- Purchase probiotics capsules with 50 billion bacteria. It should say on the bottle how many bacteria they contain. Some brands have enteric coating, so make sure the coating is not synthetic. The supplement should be all natural.

- Take one capsule with a glass of room-temperature water, for your stomach and intestines.

- Open a second capsule and put it into 3 to 4 ounces (⅜ to ½ cup) of room-temperature water. Mix it in. Put it in your mouth, but do not swallow. Hold it in your mouth and swish it around for 30 seconds to 1 minute. This is so the bacteria can get into all the cracks and crannies, and permeate the gums and mouth. Then swallow slowly, a little at a time if you can, so your esophagus gets coated, too.

Do this every morning from now on, as part of your new internal fitness routine.

....

CHAPTER 5

Your Acid/Alkaline Balance

YOU MIGHT HAVE TESTED the pH of a swimming pool or an aquarium, or seen someone else do it, but did you ever think of testing yourself? Swimming pool water has to stay within a certain pH for the safety of swimmers and to control bacterial growth. Fish tank water has to stay within a certain pH for the health and survival of the fish. Soil has to stay within a certain pH for plants to grow in it. And *you* have to stay within a certain very narrow pH range in order to stay alive.

What's so important about pH? For one thing, acidic substances aren't very amenable to most life forms. How many critters hang out in battery acid, or hydrochloric acid? Not many. You certainly wouldn't want acid running through your veins. Highly alkaline substances aren't safe, either. Lye and bleach are highly alkaline, and you don't want to be taking a bath in either of those. So let's learn just a little something about pH.

WHAT'S YOUR PH?

The term *pH* is actually an acronym that stands for potential hydrogen (or *power of hydrogen*, historically). It's called pH because it technically measures a substance's ability to potentially attract hydrogen (chemical symbol H) ions. For our purposes, this translates to a measure of acidity or alkalinity or basicity. The pH scale runs from 1 to 14. Pure water, which is neutral (neither acidic nor basic, *basic* being another word for "alkaline"), has a pH of 7. With every step up on the scale, such as from 7 to 8, the concentration of whatever you are measuring is 10 times more alkaline (and more likely to attract hydrogen). With every step down on the scale, such as from 7 to 6, the concentration is 10 times more acidic (and less likely to attract hydrogen). Lye has a pH of 13, making it extremely basic or alkaline. Bleach has a pH of almost 13, and ammonia has a pH of about 11.5.

On the other end of the pH spectrum, battery acid has a pH of about 0, and your stomach acid has a pH of just over 1; that cola you like to drink has a pH of about 2.75, and vinegar comes in at about 3.

All your tissues, the water in your body, your blood, your sweat, your urine, your saliva—each one has a particular pH. In general, your cells and tissues are bathed in an alkaline environment for best functioning, but all their metabolic functions produce acid. Your body is constantly balancing, adjusting, and monitoring its pH by secreting acid through the skin via sweat, exhaling it through the lungs via breath, processing it out through the kidneys in the form of urine, and eliminating it through the colon as solid waste, all in order to keep your body pH approximately neutral, and in particular, in order to maintain a steady pH in your blood.

Your blood is the focus of all this methodical acid elimination because the blood pH has to stay in a pretty narrow range for you to survive. For most people, that is right around 7.35 to 7.45, or just slightly alkaline. If your blood pH dropped even a little below this or rose even a little above this range, you would be in big trouble. Your body knows this, so in order to maintain the blood's pH and keep the body in homeostasis or a stable state, your other fluids—urine, sweat, saliva, and so on—can become more acidic or more alkaline in order to take on the extra burden and preserve the blood.

Saliva is naturally between 6.5 and 7.5; on the other end, urine pH is about 4.5 to 8, depending on what you need to excrete. In the middle, your stomach acid is super acidic (because it has to digest your food), with a pH from around 1.5 to 4.0. Once your food moves into the small intestine, it gets more alkaline again, from about 6.0 to 8.0. It rises and drops as it moves through the gastrointestinal tract in its constant quest for equilibrium.

WHY YOUR PH IS CRITICAL

There's a timeline in our bodies with the development of any health issue. During the early stages, we often don't see or feel anything. By the time we begin to notice problems, it becomes much harder to correct the problem. When it comes to pH, either extreme can become dangerous, although getting too acidic is a more common problem than getting too alkaline.

When someone's body is too acidic, we call that *acidosis*. This can happen for various reasons: diet, environmental stress, physical stress, emotional stress, mental stress, even spiritual stress. These can all raise acidity levels. When tissues become overly acidic, it makes the body more susceptible to inflammation, which is the core cause of all disease.

When body fluids become too acidic, the body uses its buffers to create balance. No one specific food will cause acidosis; the scale is tipped by a series of foods and events in combination over a period of time. Chronic acidity will eventually deplete the body's buffers if they aren't replaced via the diet and supplementation. When buffering stops, acidity can rise suddenly, having an adverse effect on the entire body, all the way down to the cellular level. Acidity isn't obvious at first. You can eat a high-acid diet and feel just fine for a long time. But as acidity starts to build up, you'll begin to notice the effects in stages.

Stage one is the basic acidic state, when the problem is just beginning. During this stage, you may get a cold or notice flu-like symptoms or a mild headache. This is the stage people tend to shrug off and ignore. Maybe they pop a pill because of a disruptive headache, and then move on with their (acid-promoting) routine.

As your body becomes more acidic, you move into stage two. Maybe now that headache is a bit more pronounced. Instead of a sniffle, you're now coughing up mucus or feel congested in your head and/or chest. Body aches are a bit more noticeable. You're tired and start slowing down on your duties or lose interest in things you like. Your libido might diminish, and for women, PMS symptoms like irritability and acne might become worse. Bowel patterns may shift, or you might develop alternating diarrhea and constipation, flatulence, or bloating. Some people go to the doctor at this point to get a prescription for a pill to mask whichever of these symptoms is most bothersome. This might temporarily relieve the headache or body aches, or temporarily restore the sex drive or reduce the PMS symptoms, but all this does is drive the condition further into the body, where it can cause even more harm. You haven't taken care of the problem. You've just told it to "shush."

This is where chronic systemic inflammation takes hold. You might develop cold sores, impotence, or difficulty walking. You might notice that your memory has become spotty or you have concentration issues that are negatively affecting your life. Suddenly, you need glasses to read. You might develop rashes or hives on your skin, or diagnosable skin conditions like eczema or psoriasis. You might get a more serious viral infection, migraine headaches, or depression. Instead of a chest cold, you're more at risk of bronchitis or pneumonia.

Insomnia is common at this stage. So are urinary tract infections, cystitis, recurrent yeast infections, and endometriosis.

Stage three is full-blown disease. By now, the inflammation has gone on for an extended period of time and the body has used up all its readily available buffers. You are on acid overload, and the result is often a chronic disease—cancer, Parkinson's disease, multiple sclerosis, lupus, Lou Gehrig's disease, bipolar disorder, schizophrenia, rheumatoid arthritis, and many more.

Becoming too alkaline is just as dangerous as becoming too acidic, but it's a lot less common. In fact, often when people believe they're too alkaline, they're actually too acidic. When someone is legitimately too alkaline, this is called *alkalosis*, and these people tend to go into a catatonic state, then fall into a coma and eventually die. Before it gets that severe, however, the person may complain of nausea, involuntary muscle spasms, confusion, light-headedness, hand tremors, numbness, and tingling in the face, arms, and legs.

But as I said, this is very rare. It's usually due to low carbon dioxide in the bloodstream from hyperventilation, altitude sickness, a high fever, poisoning, or liver or lung disease. Disease can (rarely) cause alkalosis, since diseases love acidity. In unusual cases where someone actually eats too much alkalizing food, it can result in an overabundance of potassium salts. This can cause rapid weight loss and an emaciated look, with dark circles under the eyes. This is when you know you've pushed your body too far in the alkaline direction. Slow it down, incorporating more sodium (such as sea salt) into your diet to get your potassium : sodium ratio back into balance. However, I'm of the opinion that even if your diet is almost totally alkaline foods, the stress and chemical impact of living in the modern world are likely to shift your body back to acidic, so in most cases, a mostly alkaline diet will be beneficial.

Have you ever noticed a slight hint of ammonia on your breath after exerting yourself too much? That is your body trying to throw off acid via the lungs. I remember when my sister-in-law was dying of cancer, her room always smelled like ammonia. At the time I didn't understand why. That ammonia smell is a highly alkaline substance, but it's a red flag for acid.

You may have heard about alkaline diets. A lot of popular books and plans emphasize alkalizing foods, and for good reason. A primarily alkaline diet and proper hydration with adequately alkaline water are incredibly important in helping the body deal with excess acidity and keep the blood pH safe and stable. A key part of the Piper Protocol is the consumption of 80 percent alkalizing food, but even before we get there, you can start nudging your body in a more alkaline direction by shifting some things around on your dinner plate.

YOUR PERSONAL PH ANALYSIS

Are you acid or alkaline? You can find out, easily and inexpensively. I recommend that my clients test their saliva and urine every morning, using a test kit you can buy from your pharmacy or health food store. They're inexpensive—you can usually get a box of 80 to 100 test strips for $5 to $15.

I like people to test first thing in the morning because at night, your body has been busy self-cleaning and is flushing out acid from everywhere on your body that releases any kind of fluid. During the night, the parasympathetic nervous system is working its hardest to rebuild, funneling waste products down to the excretory organs for release first thing in the morning. The moment you put anything in your mouth, even water, the pH of your saliva will become more alkaline, so you always test before eating or drinking anything to give you a more accurate result. This is the best way to monitor the effect of your diet and lifestyle.

Typically, morning urine should have a pH of no lower than 6.8 to 7.2 and morning saliva should have a pH of right around 7.2. (Usually urine is slightly more acidic than saliva first thing in the morning.) Anything below 6.8 is considered too acidic. A little higher than 7.2 is fine—it means you have lots of good mineral stores to manage future incoming acid. The best way to determine true pH is to take your pH measurement every day in order to get an average and see how it progresses over time.

Increasing acidity over time is a sign that you need to be eating a more alkaline diet. You should also watch for sudden, unexpected spikes of alkalinity. If the pH test on your saliva and urine shows up as suddenly too alkaline, it's actually a sign of excess acidity. When the body is trying hard to adjust to the constant influx of acid, whether from food or environment, it must release large amounts of buffering minerals, such as potassium, calcium, and magnesium. When these minerals become depleted, our kidneys have a backup system. They begin to produce a hormone/enzyme called glutaminase, which allows ammonia to be excreted from the amino acid glutamine. This by-product is extremely alkaline, so it can raise your pH dramatically, in a last-ditch emergency effort to help the body neutralize acid before it affects the blood.

I also want you to test your urine more than once during the day. Remember when we discussed Liver Time as being between 1:00 and 3:00 A.M.? As the body rounds up all the toxins from the day before, it prepares to dump them all out of the body with the morning's first bathroom visit. The morning urine will be more acidic than at any other time of day, since your kidneys are responsible for most of your acid elimination. If you test a few times throughout the day, you will see how your pH fluctuates. The second urine of the day should be less acidic than the first, ideally 7.2 or higher. Your saliva pH should be between 7.2 and 8.4 right after meals and between 6.8 and 7.2 a few hours later.

Your average throughout the day should be slightly alkaline, at about 7.2. If it is still low/acidic during the day, after the first morning urine, then you may be in what Dr. Robert Young (co-author of the wonderful book *The pH Miracle*) calls "a state of latent tissue acidosis." This is common in people who eat a high-protein diet made mostly of animal proteins and/or a lot of acidic foods and beverages like coffee, soda, and junk food. You need alkalizing food, and you need it ASAP! If your pH is higher than 7.2, then you have more than enough alkaline buffers to handle the acid in your body. You may have a better balance between your sympathetic and parasympathetic systems. Good for you! Keep up the high veggie intake!

So what's the verdict? Acidic? Alkaline? Neutral? Whatever it is, you can maintain or improve your pH through lifestyle, and no lifestyle change is more dramatic and more influential than diet. Diet can have a direct and almost immediate effect on pH. A lot of meat, dairy, grain, and sugar will add more acid and deplete your acid-buffering minerals. A high percentage of fresh raw vegetables and a little fresh fruit will replenish your minerals so that your body has everything it needs to keep acid in check.

One thing to recognize about food is that it's not the pH of the food itself that matters as much as what the food does in your body. Take lemons, for instance. They seem acidic, right? Yet they have an alkalizing effect. The first thing to focus on when working to alkalize your body is to reduce the acidifying foods (rather than acidic foods) and add more alkalizing foods (rather than alkaline foods). Let's look at which foods do what for you.

· ·

WHAT'S YOUR PH PERSONALITY?

Over the years, I've noticed that people who tend to be more alkaline have grounded, calm demeanors and move slowly and deliberately. They tend to have more dominant parasympathic nervous systems. They are rarely rushed, and they are attentive listeners. They tend to be creative, and good team players, but slow movers. They also tend to have champion digestive systems and can eat anything. They're usually in a repair-and-maintenance state. They sleep well and wake rested. They exist on an even keel and aren't easily rattled. They also tend not to get sick too often. When someone is overly alkaline (which is rare), they can seem to exist in a dazed state all the time and are slow to react. Their speech sounds sluggish and monotone.

Acidic people, or more sympathetic-dominant types, tend to be loud, leaders, controlling, get angry quickly, talk fast, and are less patient. They tend to be more gaseous, bloated, and constipated, and are generally more reactive. They tend to have a weak digestive system. They are often tired, especially in the morning, and may feel like they need coffee, a cigarette, or some other stimulant to get going and deal with life. This is because their body is in a catabolic state—a state of constant breaking down with no time to repair. They often catch every illness going around and are frequently on antibiotics. They often have poor bowel habits and restless sleep and wake up tired. Joint and muscle aches are prominent, and the hair breaks easily and is slow to grow. They're often but not always heavy meat eaters, drinkers, or smokers, or are frequently stressed out.

Being in a long-term acidic state can cause people to become underweight and over-medicated and to develop a strange odor. They may lose teeth and eventually develop chronic diseases such as multiple sclerosis, lupus, Parkinson's disease, Alzheimer's disease, cancer, arthritis, osteoporosis, and candidiasis. They're burning the candle at both ends, so they burn down faster. If you are a naturally acidic type, alkalizing foods will be extremely therapeutic for you!

ACIDIFIERS: THE BAD GUYS

These are some of the primary acidifying offenders. Try not to consume these foods and drinks, or at least use smaller portions:

Coffee. I know, you love your cup of joe, but joe is no friend to your pH. Shade-grown organic cold-brewed coffee is better than the stuff at the gas station (or your favorite coffee house), but it's still more acidic than water. New to the market is alkaline coffee with a pH of 7.2 to 7.6 (Longevity and Bulletproof are two popular brands; see Resources). If you just can't give up your morning coffee, consider switching to an alkaline type.

Soda. Don't get me started. There are about a thousand and one reasons to quit drinking it, but acidifying your internal environment is darn near top of the list. Diet soda is just as acidifying as regular soda, and both are full of chemicals your body will have to labor to remove from your system. Step away from the soda can!

Alcohol. A glass of wine after a long day can be nice, but regular alcohol consumption can definitely increase your acidity in a big way. Don't give disease that foothold!

Meat. Sorry, steak dinner, but you're not doing anybody any favors. Meat is highly acidic and too much can wreak havoc on your body's delicate balance. Cured meats like bacon and salami are the worst, but even fish is acidic. If you're overly acidic, it's a no-no. If not, moderation is key. Increase your alkaline food with it to create balance. (This is what we'll be doing in the initial weeks of the Piper Protocol.)

Sugar. Sweeteners such as cane sugar and corn syrup drive acid levels up, up, up. Sadly, chocolate is also an acidifier. Dark chocolate is okay, but again, moderation is key. Don't have more than 1 ounce per day. Try low-glycemic sweeteners like stevia, luo han guo fruit, or coconut sugar. The more you stay away from the sugar, the better. Less sugar = less inflammation.

Salt. Too much sodium increases acidity and causes the cells to swell. Try to limit your salt intake to less than 1,200 mg per day, and stick to good salts such as Celtic salt, Himalayan salt, and natural sea salt, or dulse and kelp, which are naturally salty sea vegetables. These contain valuable minerals and are not highly processed and toxic, like regular table salt.

Dairy products. Pretty much anything made from or coming out of an animal is acidic, including cheese, butter, milk, and ice cream. Ironically, even though yogurt and sour cream taste more acidic, they have more of an alkalizing effect on the body, but I still don't recommend any dairy products because they tend to be mucus-forming and difficult to digest for most people. Instead, I recommend homemade non-dairy yogurt or kefirs, like the kinds made from coconut and almond milk.

Grains. Wheat, corn, pasta, oatmeal, even quinoa and whole wheat bread are acidic in the body. Quinoa and amaranth are better choices than wheat because they are gluten-free. (See page 185 for more about why gluten is not conducive to internal fitness.)

Nuts. Most nuts and nut butters are acidic, so while they contain protein and good fat, don't overdo it. Nuts contain enzyme inhibitors that protect them but destroy our digestive enzymes. The only way to remove these is by soaking the nuts (see page 101). By the way, peanuts and peanut butter are highly acidic, often mixed with sugar and fillers, and full of pesticides—they are not nuts but legumes. Avoid them!

Legumes. Lentils, pinto beans, black beans—these all have an acidifying effect on the body. They also have enzyme inhibitors, so if you eat them, soak them first, according to the instructions on page 101.

"Whoa!" you might be thinking. "What's left to eat?" It's not that you can't ever let an acidic food pass your lips. In fact, you need a certain level of acidity in your body, but to balance most of the food you usually eat, you should also eat an equal or higher amount of alkalizing foods (on the Piper Protocol, you'll work up to 80 percent alkalizing foods).

But there are other bad guys, too, that have nothing to do with food. Environmental chemicals can tip the body into an acidic state. These are harder to avoid than acidic foods—you don't always have a choice about exposure—but be aware that these things can create additional problems. They settle into the fat and muscle tissue, aggravate the body, and cause inflammation, and this leads to a rise in acidity:

Antibiotics	Pain medications, such as NSAIDS
Cleaning supplies	Paints (both for interior housepainting
Deodorants	and for art)
Detergents	Perfumes
Dry-cleaning chemicals	Pesticides and herbicides
Hair dyes	Toothpastes
Mouthwashes	Treated wood
New carpets	

Chemicals in these products penetrate our cells and can actually change the structure of our DNA. Smell the chemical, rub it on your skin, or inhale it, and it can acidify you (not to mention introduce more toxins your body has to work to process and remove). Often, we do it to ourselves—we want to smell nice, get clean, have a clean house, have nice dry-cleaned and pressed clothes, look younger, and have nice breath, but when we use traditional products to do many of these things, we poison ourselves!

Of course, I'm not telling you that you have to stop brushing your teeth, wearing deodorant, getting rid of your gray hairs, and cleaning your home (although there are people who have opted not to use any chemicals to do these things). I live in the real world, and I know how most of us want to live (and look, and smell!). However, you can definitely modify the toxicity by looking for more internally friendly products that will not wreak havoc on the body. Whenever you can, choose natural materials for your home, organic products for your beauty supplies, and organic or natural cleaning supplies.

Many of the old-time recipes and remedies our grandparents and great-grandparents used can work perfectly well and will be much less harmful than products with industrial chemicals. We get caught up in the next marketing hype that we see on TV or on the Internet, and we think that some new product will be the next best thing to make life easier for us. Just consider that easier and newer isn't always better. Sometimes, it is much, much worse.

Just the other day, I saw a television commercial in which a baby was crawling on a brand-new carpet. In my head, I was saying, "Nooooo! That baby's immune system and neurological system are still developing, and she's crawling around on that chemical-laced carpet!" It's amazing what the human body can survive, but it's also no wonder we so quickly become acidic.

THE ALKALIZERS: THE GOOD GUYS

In order to bring the body back into balance, foods rich in certain minerals, including calcium, magnesium, potassium, and bicarbonate salts, will replenish the body's supply of natural acid buffers. These minerals can be found in fresh fruits and vegetables. Examples of food high in potassium are asparagus, potatoes, tomatoes, zucchini, bananas, raisins, and spinach. Another way to reduce acidity is to stay hydrated with pure water and eat food with a high water content, such as watermelon, cucumber, and celery. Fresh green juice not only alkalizes the body but also provides it with plenty of minerals, vitamins, and nutrients. This is part of the reason people who have chronic diseases and go on green-juice cleanses often have such positive results.

These delicious natural foods all increase alkalinity in your body, so try to eat more of them. This is the stuff you want to pile on your plate:

- Almost all fresh vegetables, especially leafy greens and sea vegetables. The only exceptions are corn, olives, and winter squash, which are all more acidifying.
- Fermented vegetables, such as sauerkraut, kimchi, and pickled vegetables (look for naturally fermented foods that say "lacto-fermented," not the mainstream processed,

pasteurized pickles you find in the aisle with the ketchup and mustard). You can ferment these foods yourself.

- Almost all fruit (except for cranberries, plums, currants, and blueberries, which are more on the acidifying side—still fine to eat but balance them with alkalizing fruits). Even though they taste acidic, citrus fruits are especially alkalizing—yes, lemons, limes, and grapefruits all increase alkalinity, not acidity.
- Fermented soy products such as tofu, tempeh, and miso (be careful of the soy if you have been diagnosed with problems with estrogen dominance).
- Almonds and chestnuts (best if soaked in clean water for 24 hours first, to start the enzymatic reactions that will help you digest them—see page 101 for directions).
- Millet (a gluten-free grain).

There are ways outside of diet to help alkalize the body and shore up the body's acid-buffering reserves. Try to incorporate as many of these into your life as you can:

- Exercise and an active lifestyle. Regular exercise moves acid out of the body by moving the lymph, increasing respiration to expel acid through the lungs, and sweating. Even moderate exercise such as walking and yoga accomplishes acid removal. Vigorous exercise is acidifying because of lactic acid build-up in muscles.
- Stress reduction. Stress hormones encourage acidity, but relaxation is alkalizing. Meditation is an excellent alkalizer.
- Positive thoughts. Optimism actually has an alkalizing effect on the body, and negativity has an acidifying effect.
- Water. Drinking coffee, soft drinks, and sweetened beverages acidifies, but water is alkalizing—especially alkaline water.

....

DON'T DRINK AND EAT

Never drink water while eating a meal. Drinking water—especially alkaline water (which is preferable to drink in most situations)—with your food dilutes your stomach acid, which you need to properly break down your meal, especially if you are eating animal protein. You already know how important digestion is, so don't mess with it by mixing a bunch of water into the equation.

....

THE MAGIC OF WATER

Growing up in the Caribbean surrounded by some of the most crystal-clear water in the world, I have vivid memories of the fresh smell of earth during the intermittent bouts of rain on an otherwise sunny day. My grandmother and I would go to the well together to fetch water. When I was older, I drank from the cistern at my parents' home, and the water was always fresh and clean.

But I never really appreciated or understood water until much later, even though I drank it, bathed in it, cooked with it, played in it, and swam in it. Our bodies are about 70 percent water, and parts of us contain even more, so we must all consume about 70 to 100 ounces per day to survive (including water in our food, like juicy fruit and soup, and other beverages like tea). Water not only helps to rebuild tissue but also regulates temperature, keeps the blood fluid, flushes out waste through urination, and protects our vital organs, especially the brain and spinal cord. It lubricates our joints and keeps the whole system running smoothly, like the oil in a car engine. We wouldn't get very far without it.

Maybe you think you know water. Two hydrogen atoms and one oxygen atom, right? You probably learned that in school. But water isn't quite so simple. Did you know that some water is dry and some water is wet? Sometimes, my clients complain that they drink two or three liters of water a day, still feel thirsty, *and* spend the whole day in the bathroom. "That's because you're drinking dry water," I tell them.

Dry water? What could that be?

You see, water isn't all the same. Depending on its chemistry, and on the condition of your body, some water will be absorbed by the body, hydrating it. Other water will pass right through without helping you very much. I call this second type "dry water" because you drink it, but you still feel thirsty and you can even become dehydrated. Many things can impede your absorption of water, but two of the most dramatic reasons are the pH of the water and your own biochemistry. If you're lacking sufficient levels of certain minerals, especially magnesium, you may not be able to absorb water as well.

When it comes to water, there are two common problems:

- You aren't drinking enough.
- Your water is too dry (see page 92).

(see page 92)

....

THE EMOTIONS OF WATER

Did you know water can hold emotions? In his best-selling book *The Hidden Messages in Water,* and in his other books, Masaru Emoto writes about this. He took pictures of water crystals and saw the changes in the water structure based on the emotions of the person holding the water. The water structure even changed when the words *love* or *hate* were written on the glass the water contained. When he wrote "Thank you" and "You fool" on two batches and froze them, the results were astonishing. The "Thank you" bottle formed beautiful hexagonal-shaped crystals. The "You fool" water showed no pattern at all—just shattered fragments. The study was repeated many times in order to replicate the results.

My conclusion from this is that not only are our emotions important while drinking water but also that they can influence both the nutrition and the very structure of everything we eat and drink. I believe it is essential to give thanks for the food and drink we have, and to keep good thoughts in our minds while we eat and drink, in order to get the most benefit. Chinese medicine counsels that we should never eat while upset because the distress will affect digestion and disturb the spleen's function, causing bloating, gas, and indigestion. I also think this applies to cooking—cook the food with love and positive thoughts, and it will be more nourishing. I have noticed that in my personal life, when I cook a meal I've made a hundred times and I am happy, then everyone raves about how amazing it tastes. If I'm not in the best mood while cooking, it never tastes quite right. Food for thought!

....

WHY YOU PROBABLY AREN'T DRINKING ENOUGH WATER

Thirst is not a reliable indicator of your body's hydration needs. The hunger signal is much stronger than the thirst signal, and sometimes we confuse the two, thinking we're hungry when our bodies are actually crying out for water. Because the voice for hunger is loud and strong with great *qi* and the voice for thirst is a fragile whisper, you may not be attuned to it. Listen: You need water, so drink up! Orange juice, coffee, tea, and wine with dinner don't count. Yes, they contain water, so you won't die of dehydration as long as you're drinking fluids, but these drinks won't give your body the pure, plain, crucial hydration it requires for true internal fitness. As soon as you mix in other substances—fruit sugar, coffee beans, tea leaves, and so on—what you're drinking is no longer water because its properties have changed.

Because your brain is made mostly of water, dehydration can also result in impaired brain function. At first you might just feel tired. Then your thinking might get foggy, you might lose your ability to concentrate, and you might even notice memory loss. The brain is also directly linked to your pain receptors. Have you ever felt pain somewhere but you can't remember injuring that area? It could be what we call local dehydration—that area is dying of thirst, and that pain is a cry for water. When you're dehydrated, your body actually starts rationing its water stores, moving water to the most vital organs to preserve life. The rest of your body will begin to dry out and suffer. Think of wrinkles!

In response, your brain will signal the body to release a neurotransmitter called *histamine*, which causes inflammation. The longer you're dehydrated, the longer histamine stays around and the more inflamed your body becomes, until the inflammation is systemic. This can also cause central nervous system (CNS) pain. Initial local thirst can manifest as pain in a particular area, such as lower back pain. If you take a pain killer to numb that pain, or you choose to ignore it, then the pain can spread until you hurt all over. Your body is crying out: "Water, water, *water*!"

What's the first thing that happens when you're admitted to the hospital? They hook you up to an IV and give you fluids—salt and water (saline solution). Doctors know the importance of hydration for basic function as well as healing.

Here are some signs that your water is not hydrating you and is likely too dry, and/or that you aren't absorbing enough water. Dehydration is certainly not the only cause of the problems on this list, but it's often a contributing factor. You're probably dehydrated if you have the following:

Any chronic disease
Bladder infections
Constipation
Dry, brittle hair and nails
Dry skin, eyes, ears, nose, throat
Gallstones
High cholesterol

Kidney stones

Local pain with no obvious explanation

Malnutrition

Premature aging

Shortened menstrual cycle and discoloration of blood (brownish, burgundy, or clots are all
   signs that you aren't getting enough fluid, causing stagnation)

Toxemia

Urinary tract infections

Weight gain

Wrinkles

Yeast infections

To combat chronic dehydration, drink about 8 cups of water a day if you're a woman and about 9 cups a day if you're a man. If you're an athlete or a larger person, you will need more. Always sip water while you exercise and drink an additional full glass on top of your daily recommendation after hard, sweaty exercise to replenish what you've lost. And make sure you replenish your electrolytes and minerals—unsweetened coconut water is a good staple. (It's naturally sweet.)

....

"BUT I DON'T LIKE WATER!"

I hear this all the time. People say they don't like the taste of water and they want to sweeten or flavor it. Water is the natural drink for humans, so why don't more of us crave it on a regular basis so we can get all we need? There's a very serious culprit that has caused many people to become completely out of touch with their natural thirst. His name is Mr. Sugar.

Most of us first encounter Mr. Sugar as children, and we soon become addicted to sugar-sweetened drinks. It starts innocently enough, with Kool-Aid and lemonade, then progresses to processed juices that contain only a little real juice, and then to sweetened soda. Some people think they're being good by drinking so-called electrolyte drinks like Gatorade, Powerade, and Vitaminwater, but these are also filled with sugar. Sugar causes inflammation in the body, and to combat inflammation, you actually need even *more* water. As we become chronically dehydrated and eat drier food (things like bread, pasta, pizza, meat, and processed food) and then drink less and less water, we seriously impair our internal fitness.

But what about diet soda? Isn't that okay, since it doesn't contain sugar? Aspartame contains three main ingredients that can cause health issues: The amino acid phenylalanine presents issues in people who do not have the enzyme to break it down, causing phenylketonuria (PKU). This leads to impaired mental functions. However, even people without this genetic disorder can suffer neuronal damage by consuming too much phenylalanine—it is a neurotoxin, particularly dangerous to pregnant women, and may be a trigger for attention deficit hyperactivity disorder in some people.

Another ingredient in this delicious pack of sweetness is methanol, a wood alcohol, which in large doses is poisonous. The Environmental Protection Agency (EPA) says we should not consume more than 8 mg a day. Well, a liter of diet soda contains 55 mg. Two other ingredients are excitotoxins: aspartic acid and the famous glutamate that is found in MSG. These can cause neurons in the brain to die. After years of diet soda, we might think our slowing of our mental capacity is due to old age. Think again (if you can!). Some claim the liver can take care of these toxins, but I'd rather spare my liver the trouble, thank you very much. I choose not to take the risk, and I hope you won't, either. Your body needs pure, clean water to run efficiently. Stop drinking sweetened drinks and artificially sweetened drinks, and start drinking water. Do it as a gift to yourself. I promise you that in a few weeks—for some, it takes only a few days—you'll stop craving sweet drinks and will actually begin to crave water again, the way you were meant to. You can also put a few drops of lemon juice or food-grade essential oils in your water to give it a taste you may enjoy. Some favorites are pink grapefruit, cinnamon, peppermint, and ginger.

HOW TO MAKE YOUR WATER WETTER

You want two things from your water. You want it to be clean, and you want it to be wet. You can test your own tap water, as well as your favorite brand of bottled water, using the same pH strips you use to test your urine and saliva. For people who eat a highly acidic diet, I believe it is best to drink water with a pH of 9.5 for about a month, then taper down to a pH of 8, then 7.6 or so. Keep testing your urine or saliva to guide you.

There are several ways to alkalize your water to make it easier for your body to absorb. There are water alkalizing machines and equipment, which are nice but expensive, or you can add pH drops or freshly squeezed lemon to your water. Also consider your source, which impacts not only water's pH but also its cleanliness:

Tap water. Tap water is preferable to beverages with sugar, artificial sweetener, caffeine, or alcohol, but you can do much better. Despite the best efforts of your local water treatment plant, your tap water likely contains hundreds of pollutants, toxins, and carcinogens, so unless you have no other option, tap water should not be your source for drinking water. If you do use tap water, filter it first. An easy way to do this is with a tabletop filter or pitcher with a filter in it. Most of these units use granulated charcoal to remove contaminants like chlorine. They make the water taste much better. Unfortunately, they don't remove heavy metals and endocrine disruptors, but it's certainly better than not using anything at all, and is much more affordable than other types of water filtration systems. Or consider a water purification system in your home.

Reverse-osmosis filtered water. Many people invest in a reverse-osmosis water purification system for their homes. This system filters out many contaminants, but it also filters out minerals. You can compensate for this, however, by adding minerals to your water. I like Dr. Patrick Flanagan's Crystal Energy, or ConcenTrace Trace Minerals (see the Resources for information on where to find these products). You can also add ¼ to 1 teaspoon powdered dulse or kelp to your water for added minerals, if you don't mind the taste. A squeeze of lemon can help to modify it. We are so easily depleted of minerals that it is useful to replenish them as often as you can.

Bottled water. Bottled water seems like a good option, but there are problems with it. You have no idea where that water came from. Is it from a clean source? A polluted source? Many bottled water brands are just tap water, or water filtered through reverse osmosis. You have no idea what might be in there. You also have no idea how long that water has been sitting in those bottles on the supermarket shelves and what has leached into it from the plastic. This happens at an even greater rate when the plastic is heated, such as if you leave your water bottle in a hot car—and you have no idea how the bottles were stored at every stage before you bought them. There's no guarantee that bottled water is pure, and many bottled water brands also tend to be on the acidic side. Plus, plastic bottles are a real and serious threat to the environment. Water bottled in glass may have the same quality issues, but at least it won't leach plastic chemicals into your beverage. Look for reputable water companies and check if the water bottles are BPA-free.

There are a few bottled water brands that I like. The better ones in plastic are:

Evian, with a neutral pH of 7
Fiji Water, with a neutral pH of 7

Eternal, with an alkaline pH of between 7.8 and 8.2

Essentia, with a lovely pH of 9.5

In glass, I like Mountain Valley Spring Water, with a pH of 7.6. If you're out and about and thirsty, you can almost always find Fiji Water and Mountain Valley Spring Water.

Your best choice is to purchase a glass jar to carry your water from home. Buy some pH drops, drop a lemon slice in your water, or use one dropperful of liquid chlorophyll (I like ChlorOxygen brand).

Distilled water. This is water that has had the minerals removed via vapors collected from the boiling process. It's not meant for drinking often or over the long term. It's mineral deficient and can pull toxic heavy metals out of the body during a short-term detox, but there are better choices for long-term uses.

Hard water. This water contains dissolved minerals, but if it comes from the tap, it has all the other problems common to tap water.

Spring water. The ideal way to drink water would be to scoop your own water every day straight from a naturally alkaline spring coming from an underground source that rushes over rocks, picking up minerals along the way. Unfortunately, this isn't possible for most people in the modern world, so do the best you can to source your water.

....

HOW TO USE DRY WATER

Dry or acidic water has its place. It's good for beauty and cosmetic purposes. Shampoo your hair, shave, wash your face, and soak in acidic water. It also makes a good makeup remover and skin toner. It can help cool the inflammation from a sunburn and disinfect skin abrasions, and it even cleans fruits and vegetables and sanitizes cookware more efficiently than alkaline water. Your acidic tap water is great for washing your counters and floors because it is a disinfectant. Forget dangerous chemicals—acidic water is all you need for cleaning. Alkalize your drinking water and cooking water, but the stuff straight out of the tap is fine for everything else.

....

YOUR ALKALINE LIFE

Internal fitness is so impacted by pH that I hope you'll think about this whenever you make a dietary choice, wonder about skipping your daily walk, or spend too much time stressing over something unimportant. Life is too short to be acidic—and being acidic can make life shorter. Let's toast with a green juice and start living more alkaline today, with Internal Fitness Prep Step #5:

INTERNAL FITNESS PREP STEP #5

IF you want to increase your alkalinity, do two things:

- Get some test strips and start testing your saliva and urine every morning, and throughout the day, to monitor your pH.

- Every day, starting today, start drinking more alkaline water. If you are a woman, aim for 8 cups of the purest possible water you have access to. If you are a man, aim for 9 cups. You can work up to this amount, but try to get there by the time you start the Piper Protocol, so your body is fully hydrated and able to take full advantage of the dietary changes you'll introduce starting in Chapter 12. If you can test your water, do so and take steps to keep it on the alkaline side. The easiest way to do this is to squeeze ½ fresh organic lemon into every 8- to 12-ounce glass. If you use a big water bottle, such as 24 to 32 ounces, add the juice of a whole lemon. Drink up, and start feeling better by tomorrow!

CHAPTER 6

Living Foods and the Magic of Enzymes

ENZYMES ARE MY FAVORITE topic, yet I find that most people, even if they've heard of enzymes, have no idea what they are or what they actually do. Let me tell you, enzymes do *a lot*. In fact, they pretty much run your entire system. They aren't in control. They aren't calling the shots, like the nervous system and some of the major organs. Nevertheless, enzymes are the catalysts for life itself. They run things. They're like the workers in the factory that is your body, doing the work to keep your metabolism humming along. Enzymes make digestion, repair, and healing happen. You wouldn't last very long without them.

Most people think about enzymes in terms of digestion or food. They know on some level that enzymes help digest food. You may have heard that cooking destroys the enzymes in food, which makes food harder to digest. Enzymes do help with digestion and cooking does kill the enzymes in food; and it's also true that enzymes are instrumental in much of the power behind raw food. However, the power of enzymes extends far beyond these jobs.

There are two groups of enzymes: enzymes produced inside our bodies (endogenous enzymes) and enzymes that come from outside, through our food (exogenous enzymes). Enzymes are like tools in a tool kit. Each tool has its specific function that allows it to do its job well. For instance, a Phillips-head screwdriver is for screws with a Phillips head, and a slotted screwdriver is for screws with a single slot in the head. A wrench (at least the non-adjustable kind) is used to loosen or tighten a specific size bolt. I remember my dad would be working on his truck and he'd say, "Give me a one-sixteenth wrench." If I gave him the wrong size, he would show me that he asked for that specific size, because it's the only one that would fit the bolt he was trying to loosen. Funny how a Saturday afternoon hanging out with your dad under his truck can teach you something about enzymes years later.

A one-sixteenth wrench fits around a one-sixteenth bolt in much the same way that the enzyme amylase "fits" or is able to break down and extract energy from carbohydrates. The enzyme protease is one of the enzymes that "fits" protein. All the enzymes that break down protein are called *proteolytic enzymes*. The enzyme lipase is one of the enzymes that "fits" fats. All the enzymes that break down fat are called *lipolytic enzymes*. The enzyme cellulase is one of the enzymes that "fits" fiber, and all the enzymes that break down carbohydrates are called *amylolytic enzymes,* and so forth.

Food consists primarily of three macronutrients: protein, carbohydrates, and fat. Think about a fabulous entrée of grilled New York strip steak with sautéed mixed vegetables and a romaine lettuce salad. Different enzymes will break down each part: proteolytic enzymes will break down the protein in the steak; lipolytic enzymes will break down the fat in the steak, salad dressing, and cooking oil; and amylolytic enzymes will break down the carbohydrates in the vegetables.

Everyone is born with a certain store of enzymes—millions of them that you use throughout life and that should last you to old age. You are also born with a body that has the potential to continually manufacture enzymes to help break food down, repair, and rejuvenate you. However, like an inheritance you were born with, you can grow it or you can squander it. You can make your enzymes work for you and turn what you have into an even more powerful factory of chemical workers through healthy lifestyle habits and regular deposits of even more enzymes via raw living food and supplements, or you can exhaust your stores until you don't have enough to sustain you. Being hard on yourself, living with chronic stress, and eating a poor diet (especially one made primarily of cooked food, which is like a deposit of $0 into your enzyme account) are all enzyme-depleting habits. You can still survive without depositing more enzymes, but you won't thrive.

Think about the older folks you know. Some of them are still alive but ill or incapacitated, often taking many medications. Others are vibrant, sharp-minded, and full of life. When will you run out of life-sustaining enzymes? In a decade or two? Or never? I was recently chatting with a man on the train I take to go to my house in upstate New York. I thought he was at least forty-five, but then he mentioned he was thirty-two. *Oh no!* I thought. *He's running through all his enzymes! He's not putting anything back in!*

Metabolically, enzymes repair and digest unwanted debris in the blood and body, like bacteria, cellular debris, and viruses. If this debris isn't cleaned up, we can get sick, or at the very least, begin to look and feel older, less energetic, less radiant, and less alive than we might with a full tank of enzymes.

ENZYMES AND FOOD

So how do you make deposits into your enzyme bank? You eat the right food, and you take the right supplements. Food is the best place to get enzymes because the enzymes in a food are customized to digest that particular food, plus do much more good in your body. But in the absence of sufficiently enzyme-rich food (the situation for most of us who don't live off the land), supplements can fill in the gaps.

The best, most enzyme-rich foods are fresh, whole, raw food just plucked from its source. Imagine a beautiful orange tree in Florida. The oranges are attached to their source of life, the tree that's getting its nutrients from the earth. When you pick that orange, you detach it from its source of nutrients, so there's no longer an influx of enzymes, but enzyme activity still exists inside the orange.

As soon as you peel that orange, the enzymes are now exposed to the elements, and they start breaking down. This is why the freshest, most recently picked produce has the highest enzyme content. Recently, I was on a trip for a few weeks and I left an apple in my fruit bowl. I came back to an apple that looked just fine until I picked it up. On the other side of the apple, where it was touching the bowl, it had started to rot. This is enzymes at work. This is what happens to live, raw food: It disintegrates. Processed food can sit in a bowl for months (sometimes even years!). You want to eat plenty of food that rots—not after it rots, of course, but fresh food that *would rot* if you didn't eat it within a few days.

Highly processed food is "dead" and devoid of enzymes, but even seemingly innocent cooking of fresh foods can destroy most of the enzymes in food. Cooking isn't all bad. It makes many nutrients more available. But when it comes to enzymes, cooking is a death sentence. Other enzyme-relevant conditions: how fresh the food is and how long it's been stored, how it's been handled before you eat it, the conditions under which it was grown or raised (such as soil quality and feed), and your body's ability to utilize the enzymes.

First, let's talk food.

....

THE DENMARK EXPERIMENT

During World War I, when food was scarce in Denmark, the government had to come up with a plan to feed the people, so they limited the production of livestock and placed a quota on meat. The government enforced the production of more fruits, vegetables, and whole grains to feed the people because these were cheaper to produce and buy. Grain was no longer processed, and meat was substantially reduced. The accidental result of this wartime measure was that the death rate in Denmark dropped 40 percent!

....

The closer to nature your food is, the more abundantly rich in enzymes your food will be. A piece of fruit or a crisp ripe vegetable plucked from the plant is brimming with the enzymes your body needs to digest that food and to help with all the other processes enzymes accomplish in their journey through your digestive system. Raw fresh fruits and vegetables from local sources are also good choices, and raw organic supermarket produce is good, too. Living food that has been fermented, sprouted, or soaked is just as wonderful as it is raw and full of enzymatic activity.

Once you cook food, the situation changes. Cooking food destroys the enzymes, putting a burden on the liver and pancreas to use more endogenous (internal) enzymes for digestion, since they aren't coming from the outside. This is like telling the front-line soldiers in a war to go clean up the kitchen—it's not the optimum use of your best troops! Several studies support this. One showed an increase in white blood cell count (a marker of inflammation or infection) after eating cooked food. Another showed that proteolytic enzyme deficiency (the enzymes that digest protein) was linked to an increase in cell division, which is a sign of cancer-like activity. I'm not trying to scare you, but I want you to understand how crucial it is for you to get enzymes from real, fresh, whole food. They take care of all kinds of things in your body that could result in poor health down the line, before you even know they're happening.

Some people have a hard time digesting raw food, especially if they aren't used to eating very much of it, but blending and juicing are good ways to make raw food more digestible. Raw blended smoothies, soups, and juices reduce the inflammation in the body that can be produced by too much acidity and cooked food.

Every plant food that can be eaten raw and/or juiced is full of valuable enzymes. For example, pineapples contain an enzyme called bromelain that has powerful anti-inflammatory effects. Papayas contain papain, which is a great enzyme for digesting food, especially meat. It is most concentrated in the unripened green papaya, which is much less sweet. When I was small growing up in St. Thomas, we had many fruits and vegetables growing in our yard. If my parents were cooking meat, they would have us pick an unripened green papaya from the tree. We would peel it and cut it up and place the pieces in the pot with the meat. When the meat was done, it would fall off the bone—the enzymes helped to soften it during cooking, so it was more digestible, even if the enzymes were then destroyed by the cooking. I also like to use green papaya when making bone broth because the enzymes help pull the nutrients out of the bone.

WHAT ABOUT ORGANICS?

Whenever possible, choose organic produce. The fewer toxins you put into your body, the easier it will be to clean things out. Organic foods are generally raised in more natural conditions, which can also increase their nutrient content and availability. Better yet, find local organics that are freshly picked and haven't traveled far to get to you. The enzymes in these fruits and vegetables will be even more vibrant and available. However, if you find organics to be too expensive to buy all the time, keep an eye on the annually updated Environmental Working Group lists: the Dirty Dozen and the Clean Fifteen. The first lists the 12 fruits and vegetables most contaminated by pesticides in any given year—the things you definitely want to buy organic—and the second lists the 15 cleanest fruits and vegetables, least contaminated with pesticides. It's generally okay not to choose the organic version of these. Find the lists at www.ewg.org/foodnews, and check it yearly.

Fermented foods are also enzyme-rich. Foods like sauerkraut, Worcestershire sauce, soy sauce, and kimchi are ancient—people probably developed these methods by accident and used them for preservation, but the enzymatic benefits are huge. I remember when I was growing up, everybody put Worcestershire sauce on their steak. Maybe they thought it was for the flavor, but it gives the steak an enzymatic boost, too. I suspect that the reason so many people now have undigested meat in their colons is that they aren't eating meat with enough enzymes to help digest it.

ENZYME INHIBITORS AND HOW TO NEUTRALIZE THEM

Raw seeds, nuts, legumes, and grains are valuable sources of protein, fat, and carbohydrates, and potentially rich sources of enzymes, but there's a problem with eating them raw. Nuts, seeds, and legumes contain protease inhibitors or enzyme inhibitors, such as phytates, polyphenols, and goitrogens, that inhibit enzyme activity. These have a purpose—they help the seeds remain dormant until they are ready to sprout. When growing conditions are perfect (such as when the seeds land in soil and are soaked by a spring rain), water dissolves these protease inhibitors and the seeds can sprout. Sprouting produces a host of enzymes and turns the seeds, essentially, into plants.

This is why it's very important to soak nuts, seeds, and legumes before eating them. Otherwise, the protease inhibitors can make them more difficult to digest, and will also inhibit your body's ability to access the potential enzymes and valuable nutrients. Soaking and sprouting allow the carbohydrates to turn into simple sugars, which are easiest to digest, and break down the protein into its simpler amino acid form. Soaking also removes mucus-forming and toxic enzyme inhibitors so you digest the food better, and it activates both digestive and metabolic enzymes. Sprouting (soaking until the seeds sprout) also makes the grains more alkalizing. Here's how to do it:

- Put your nuts, seeds, dried legumes, and grains in a glass jar or ceramic crock and cover them with pure water. Do not used distilled water. Spring water is best.

- Let them soak overnight at room temperature to break down the enzyme inhibitors and allow the life force of the seeds and nuts to be released. Essentially, you're doing what nature would do—creating ideal growing conditions in order to turn those nuts, seeds, legumes, or grains into plants. This turns on the spark inside the seeds, and then you get the benefits from that spark when you eat them.

- After 2 to 24 hours (see list on page 102), drain and rinse your nuts, seeds, legumes, or grains. Spread them out on paper towels on the counter or on a baking sheet. Pat them dry, and then store them in the refrigerator for up to 1 day, or use immediately (such as with grains or legumes that you will be cooking or dehydrating).

- For foods you want to eat raw, such as nuts and seeds, soak and then dry them in a dehydrator or in your oven on the lowest possible setting to give them a more pleasing, crunchy texture (soaked nuts can be a little chewy). Spread them out on a baking sheet and dehydrate or bake until they are chewy or crunchy, depending on your preference. This can take as little as 2 hours in a warm oven or up to 12 hours in a dehydrator.

If you want to get really precise, follow this guide, which tells you the minimum amount of time to soak different foods to ensure that the enzyme inhibitors dissolve and the enzyme-increasing sprouting action begins:

Adzuki beans: 8 to 12 hours (overnight)

Almonds: 8 to 12 hours (overnight)

Amaranth: 8 hours

Black beans: 8 to 12 hours (overnight)

Brazil nuts: 3 hours

Buckwheat: 6 hours

Cashews: 2 hours

Chia seeds: 3 hours

Flax seeds: 30 minutes

Lentils: 7 hours

Macadamia nuts: 2 hours

Pecans: 6 to 8 hours

Quinoa: 5 hours

Sesame seeds: 8 hours

Sunflower seeds: 8 hours

Walnuts: 4 hours

Wild rice: 9 hours

From a more mystical perspective, enzymes are also the life force or *qi*. As enzymes are depleted, life energy wanes. You can spot the people who are full of life energy, radiating *qi*, and you can probably also spot the people who are drained of life energy. Enzymes are at the heart of this difference. Most people would say I have strong *qi*, but if I eat a gluten-filled meal, I become like a zombie. It's as if gluten sucks the *qi* right out of me, but what is really going on is that all my readily available enzymes have to try to digest all that gluten, using up more than a meal's worth of enzymes. I become depleted. If you notice how you feel after eating particular foods, you can sometimes determine whether that food is increasing or reducing your *qi*. Take that as a signal from your body about what foods you should and shouldn't be eating.

The bottom line is that raw food is enzyme-rich food, and cooked food isn't, so I'd like you to begin incorporating more fresh, high-quality raw food into your diet. Some people eat 100 percent raw, or nearly so. Full disclosure: I do not eat 100 percent raw, but I try to hit that Piper Protocol 80 percent most of the time (you'll read about this in Chapters 13 and 14). If you begin a meal with enzyme-rich raw food, then the cooked food you eat will be processed more thoroughly and efficiently. Have a fresh vegetable juice about 20 minutes before your meal, then include a raw salad with your meal. Replenish your reserves!

ENZYME SUPPLEMENTS

If you could get enough enzymes from the foods you eat, that would be fantastic, but the truth is that in real life, that's not always going to happen. People don't always make the best dietary choices, but even when they eat in a way they think is healthy, the foods available to us aren't usually freshly picked, and most people don't eat very much raw food.

For this reason, I recommend enzyme supplements. The journey through the digestive tract is rough terrain for the enzymes, with all kinds of obstacles. You can't overdose on enzymes, so the more enzymes you take in, the better you'll be able to digest your food, support your reserves, and help your body along in doing all its work. The best time to take digestive enzymes is right before a meal. Take metabolic proteolytic enzymes between meals, on an empty stomach, so they can start scavenging and cleaning up unwanted or stuck proteins and other cells that have a protein shell, such as bacteria, viruses, and even cancer cells. Cancer cells are covered in a tough protein, so proteolytic enzymes can attack the cell walls of bacteria, viruses, and cancer cells, break them down, and then allow the body's killer cells to destroy them. This is a natural process that keeps disease in check, but it can't work if you don't have sufficient enzymes on hand to accomplish the task. They are like the cleanup crew.

Let's get to know your key enzymes.

Amylase is the first enzyme in saliva to begin digesting carbohydrates; eating a diet that's too high in carbohydrates can exhaust amylase supplies. It also breaks down dead white blood cells from things like pus and abscesses. Amylase is anti-inflammatory and is a good remedy for skin and lung conditions. Amylase supplements can help to resolve respiratory conditions like allergic reactions, asthma, emphysema, and shortness of breath. Also, try them to support the treatment of skin conditions like atopic dermatitis, eczema, hives, psoriasis, and even herpes. Don't ignore other medical treatments, but take amylase supplements to support the healing of these conditions.

Cellulase is generated by the gut flora's fermenting action in your large intestine. It has the very important job of breaking down the cellulose walls in plant foods so your body can get to all the nutrients.

Lactase is the enzyme that digests lactose, the protein in milk. When people are lactose intolerant, it means they don't have enough lactase to digest milk. In these people, dairy products cause uncomfortable symptoms like abdominal cramps, diarrhea, and asthma. Taking lactase can resolve this issue (although I don't recommend consuming dairy products in general).

Lipase is an enzyme that digests fat and fat-soluble vitamins. If there's a deficiency of lipase enzyme, then the body will store cholesterol and excess fat, causing high cholesterol in the blood and a rise in triglycerides.

ENZYMES AND YOUR INTERNAL FITNESS

You require good enzymatic activity to be internally fit. External beauty is great, but it can come with internal weakness, like beautiful furniture made from particle board. It might look great and you might be able to put it together with a few screws and a diagram, but it won't stand up to the wear and tear of everyday use and time. Solid wood from an oak tree can be carved into a beautiful piece of furniture, and it will last a long time because it's not pieced together from junk. It has substance, and although it might cost more, the long-term investment will pay off in years of use and beauty.

This is why you want to choose real, whole, living food: to build a body that can stand up to time and daily wear and tear. When the majority of your food is raw and enzyme-rich, you are partaking of *qi* in its highest form, coming from Mother Earth, taken up by the roots and permeating the cells of the plants you consume. You're eating quality, and you're building quality, so that your living can be of the highest quality as well.

As you gradually incorporate more raw and living foods into your diet (the Piper Protocol will help), you'll notice some wonderful benefits: an immediate energy boost; more mental clarity; a noticeable difference in your skin quality; natural weight loss; more complete and easier bowel movements; a happier attitude and a more positive outlook. You'll have more pep in your step; more stamina in everything you do, from exercise and work to the bedroom; reduced junk food cravings and a more sophisticated palate; and a refined sense of beauty and quality in regard to every aspect of your life. That's a whole lot of benefits you're going to get from the happy addition to your diet of more big bowls of salad, delicious green juices, and succulent smoothies. That sounds pretty win-win to me.

Let's start infusing your body with enzymes right now, with the next Internal Fitness Prep Step.

....

INTERNAL FITNESS PREP STEP #6:

IF you want to infuse your body with enzymes, I have a new enzyme-rich healthy habit for you. Every day, whip up a smoothie made from fresh raw food. Smoothies are easier to digest than chomping on raw fruits and vegetables, and they're an easy and delicious way to add more super-powered enzymes to your system. Maybe you'll always have one for breakfast, or a mid-morning snack, or even for dinner. I don't care when you have one, but don't ever miss an opportunity for a smoothie.

One caveat: Smoothies should contain veggies and fruits only, and you may add some plant milk. Nix the extra ingredients, such as dairy and sweeteners. Eventually, you will be working toward making your smoothie with more veggies and just a tiny bit of fruit, if any at all. The purpose of this is to keep your blood sugar even and stable and not to encourage the sugar-loving gut bacteria.

It's time to start getting your taste buds accustomed to pure plant-based smoothies, so you'll be ready for the even more powerful smoothies you'll be having on the Piper Protocol. For now, begin with 1 cup of fresh or frozen berries (strawberries, blueberries, or sliced peaches or green apples, but these tend to be pesticide-heavy, so go for organic), a small handful of any leafy greens (such as romaine lettuce, baby spinach, or kale), 1 cup water or coconut water, the juice of 1 lemon, and ¾ cup ice. You can add a dash of ground cinnamon if you like the taste. If this is really not sweet enough for you, you could also add a few drops of pure stevia. If you want a thicker smoothie, add avocado or protein powder. Blend until smooth and savor until satisfied.

Once you get into the smoothie habit and start enjoying the enzyme-fueled high-energy benefits, you'll never go back. Remember to have one every day because, you know what they say: A smoothie a day keeps the doctor away! (That *is* the saying, isn't it?)

....

CHAPTER 7

Food Combining

NOW THAT WE'VE TALKED about gut bacteria, acid and alkaline foods, and enzymes, you have some idea of the kinds of foods that feed your body and the kinds that cause problems. What we haven't yet discussed, however, is something incredibly important and central to the entire concept of the Piper Protocol. No matter how good a food is, it can become detrimental to your body if you *combine it* with other foods that don't harmonize digestively. On the flip side, even not-quite-perfect foods can become less damaging if you *combine them* with other foods that help your body to digest them more easily.

This is called *food combining*, or the science of trophology, and it is based on the principle that different food groups require different levels of digestive juices to break them down. Some juices are acidic and some are alkaline. Different kinds of foods also take varying amounts of time to digest. When you mix up a bunch of foods that require different kinds of digestive juices and have different digestive transit times, your whole GI tract can get confused, cramped, and inefficient. Poor food combinations can cause gas, bloating, stomach pain, constipation, and/or diarrhea. In other words, your digestive issues might have nothing to do with the foods you choose to eat, and everything to do with how you combine them. Break down an innocent sandwich, and there might be nothing wrong with any of the parts, but put them all together, and they can spell disaster.

Food combining can be very confusing because there's a lot of conflicting information out there, but I'll try to simplify it for you the best I can. Let's talk about the basics.

WHY FOOD COMBINING AFFECTS YOUR DIGESTION

When you eat a complex meal full of different kinds of foods, there are ways to do it so that it works, and ways to do it so that it doesn't work. Ideally, foods that digest quickly go in first, and after some time, foods that digest slightly less quickly go in next. Foods that take the longest to digest should be last. This keeps everything in line in the right order, and also involves some time. No scarfing down a five-minute meal, please. This is one of the reasons people used to spend a long time at the dinner table, enjoying different courses, with time (and palate cleansers) in between. Quick-digesting foods such as bread and crackers might come first, then vegetables, and then after some time, lighter meats like fish, and finally, the meal would end with heavier meats, and perhaps a cheese course at the very end.

These days, we tend to cram it all in and then run, and what can happen (what *often does* happen) is that food that should digest quickly (such as grains and fruit) wait in line behind food that takes a long time to digest (such as meat and cheese). While it's waiting, it ferments and rots, creating gas and toxic by-products of fermentation. Even if you don't feel the stomach upset (you probably don't get stomach issues after every single meal, although many people actually do and are just so used to it that they ignore it or don't notice at all), your digestion isn't working as well as it could or should.

When you combine foods that digest similarly, however, then digestion works much better. Not only will you avoid digestive pains and problems, but the nutrients in the food will be better absorbed because they're digesting in the proper environment and at the proper rate. They have time to go through the process, and your body has time to recognize them and utilize the nutrition they provide.

Unfortunately, gas, bloating, abdominal discomfort, and hiccups are all considered "normal." Just eat some antacids and you'll be fine, right? Wrong! Sure, the pharmaceutical companies are making billions off of antacids, but you don't need to be spending that money on drugs. You could be spending it on food, in the right combination. Otherwise, poor digestion can lead to excess weight gain, increased acidity, inflammation, and the buildup of cholesterol in your arteries.

Still, people fight against proper food combining, often because their most beloved meals—the things they've been eating since childhood—combine foods improperly, and they don't want to give up those foods. A simple roast beef sandwich is the perfect example. The bread is a grain, which requires an alkaline medium to digest it. The roast beef requires acid. The lettuce requires alkali, and the tomato requires acid. Also, the lettuce and tomato digest quickly, the bread digests less quickly, and the roast beef digests the slowest. Food traffic jam! The poor stomach is playing eeny meeny miney mo. It doesn't know what to do first because everybody showed up at the same time!

Let's look at some other so-called perfect meals that are anything but. Let's say you go out for dinner. You have a delicious, juicy little filet mignon with a side of rice and mixed vegetables. You enjoy it with a glass of red wine, and then you indulge in a dessert of crème brûlée and a cup of coffee. Sounds pretty good, right? Wrong! This meal might taste good, and you might have eaten it many times, and you might even cook meals like this for yourself, at least on special occasions. Maybe your doctor or your nutritionist even gave you a similar meal plan: lean protein, starch, vegetables, maybe instead with fruit for dessert.

But despite what your favorite cookbook or even your nutritionist tells you, this meal is a digestive disaster. I, too, danced the dance of "Oh, this won't hurt me and it tastes so good," even when I knew better, and I paid the price. You might say, "Come on, all of America can't be wrong," but I would have to argue that one. Your body's performance is directly influenced by what you put in your mouth, and when, and in what order, and the simple fact is that your body can't digest steak, rice, vegetables, wine, crème brûlée, and coffee all at the same time. It's going to have problems just with the steak and rice, let alone all those other things.

But what if you like your steak and rice? Your roast beef on rye? Your bacon and egg biscuit? Your chicken Alfredo? Your yogurt with blueberries and walnuts? Everybody eats those foods, and everybody can't be wrong, so why should you change what you do? Okay, let's think about this another way.

Let's say you just bought a brand-new car. Let's say it's a brand-new shiny, beautiful Infiniti. You love your beautiful new car. It turns heads. Everyone admires it. The first time you go to the gas station, you notice that the sticker by the fuel tank says you should only put high-octane, premium gasoline in the gas tank. But let's be honest—you spent a lot on that car, and now you're looking to save a few pennies. Does it really make that much of a difference? Gas is gas, right? So you decide to put regular gas in the tank, and it's almost a dollar cheaper per gallon. You saved about ten dollars on one tank of gas. Score!

Over time, you might notice that your car is slowing down a bit, the performance not quite what it was at first, but you don't think it's anything to worry about. You're in the habit of using the regular gas now, and it seems like a splurge to go for the fancy stuff, and really, your car works, so why bother? Then one day the gas station is out of gas and all they have is diesel. Hmm, that's probably okay, you think. Better than driving five extra miles to the next station. So being the resourceful person you are, you decide to put diesel into your lovely, brand-new Infiniti. (Okay, I know they don't have the same nozzles and you couldn't and wouldn't really do this, but bear with me—it's a metaphor!) Diesel is going to wreck your car, and you probably knew that in the back of your mind, but it was just "easier." "Quicker." "More convenient." Then the trouble really starts. Why is your car making those weird noises? Why isn't it working? And then boom, the car dies.

So you have it towed to the mechanic, and you tell him what happened and he just stares at you. "You put *diesel fuel* in your Infiniti?" You're afraid to tell him that not only did you do that, but you've never filled that car with premium fuel, even once in its short life. Because now you need a new engine, and now you're talking a *major* expense that you can't afford. Not even with all those dollars you saved on gas. At least you learned your lesson. You won't make that mistake again.

So here's my question to you: If you can learn that lesson with a car (and let's hope that story never actually happens to you!), then why can't you learn it with your own, beautiful body? Maybe you object that you would *never* put the wrong fuel into your beautiful new car, but then why are you doing it to yourself? If you're like me, your pets eat like kings. Once someone commented in the grocery store that I ate such great food, and then the store owner chimed in that the food wasn't for me, it was for my dog. It's true—my dog, Niko, and my cat, Tucan, eat excellent diets. Do you fuel your car and feed your pets better than you fuel and feed yourself?

If you think about it for maybe two seconds, you'll see how nonsensical this is. What good is a great car and healthy pets if you aren't around to enjoy them?

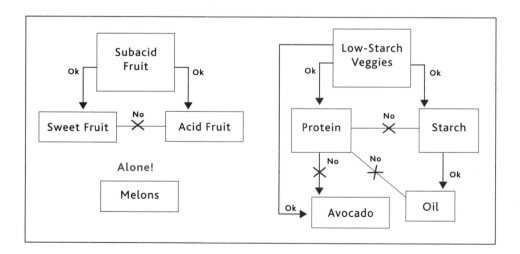

So let's get you back on track. The diagram on page 109 describes some basic and indispensable food-combining rules to utilize during the Piper Protocol—and any other time, whenever possible. This is *not* the highest, strictest level of food combining, which can get very complex. I know that a lot of these principles aren't practical for most people, especially families, unless they have the time and money to invest in a specific and regimented diet. Instead, these are some loose food-combining basics I would like you to adhere to *most* of the time. Do the best you can and you'll see the difference in how your body digests and responds to food.

THE PIPER PRINCIPLES OF FOOD COMBINING

Always eat fruit alone, or with other fruit. Fruit is delicious, sweet, and full of nutrients, such as vitamins and antioxidants. However, it's also full of natural sugars, especially fructose. Fruit should make up only about 15 percent of your diet (and even less if you have certain sugar-sensitive conditions like cancer). Fruit didn't used to be so sweet—years of hybridization have increased its sugar content. Fruits can be subdivided into three groups:

Acid fruits: Citrus, strawberries, cranberries, kiwi, lemon, kumquat, pomegranate, tangerines, oranges, and pineapples
Subacid fruits: Cherries, mangoes, plums, peaches, some grapes, apples, blackberries, and blueberries
Sweet fruits: Bananas, some grapes, dates, figs, papayas, and all dried fruits

When it comes to food combining, the cardinal rule about fruit is to *always eat it alone*. Preferably, eat a single fruit for a snack with nothing else, not even other fruit. If you do decide to mix fruit, mix acid fruits with subacid fruits, and subacid fruits with sweet fruits, but do not mix acid fruits and sweet fruits. They are digested differently. This rule is *especially* important as it applies to melons. Melons can be mixed with other melons but *never* with other fruits or any other foods. Melons are highly therapeutic foods for the body and are made mostly of water, so they take only 15 to 30 minutes to go through the digestive system. Anything else combined with them will interfere with this swift digestion, causing the melon to slow down and ferment in your digestive tract. Rule of thumb: *Eat melon alone, or leave it alone.* Eat sweet fruit when you know you'll be burning off the energy, such as before you exercise. Always eat fruit ripe—many commercial fruits are picked before they're ripe so they don't spoil. Unripened fruit lacks the full nutrient profile of ripe fruit, and can be more difficult to digest. Note that you can use acid or subacid fruits (like lemons, limes, and green apples) in a smoothie with leafy greens and even avocado (which is technically a fruit, although I classify it as a fat).

Don't mix protein and starchy carbohydrates: When protein and starchy carbohydrates such as rice, pasta, and bread are combined, they create toxic by-products just by existing in the digestive tract together. Sulfur is one example. Sulfur is one of those gases that gives *you* gas—really stinky, rotten-egg gas. These toxic by-products can slow down and impair digestion, distend your intestines with gas bubbles, impair proper elimination, and cause a backup in your body.

The best time to eat protein is in the middle of the day, between 11:30 A.M. and 1:30 P.M. Eating the largest meal and the most protein-rich meal is common in many other cultures in Europe, Latin America, and the Carribean, and is also a tenet of the Ayurvedic system of medicine from India. Lunch is a big deal, and should be. Have most of your calories while you are active and need them. It's also easier to digest protein during the day and harder to digest it at night, when you have less hydrochloric acid in your stomach. Animal protein takes about four hours to digest, so when you have your steak dinner at 8:00 or 9:00 P.M. because you worked late, you're still actively digesting when you collapse into bed at 10:00 or 11:00. This makes it harder to enjoy a deep and rejuvenating sleep.

As for those starchy carbs, save those for dinner and skip the meat. A little bowl of rice or gluten-free pasta with vegetables makes an excellent light dinner that will take only about 2½ hours to digest. By the time you're ready to go to sleep, your body will be, too.

Don't mix too much fat with meat or starchy carbs. Fat is okay in small amounts to add flavor to a salad with some meat on it, or to add a little flavor to a grain dish like brown rice with veggies, but if you plan to eat a lot of fat, keep it with greens only—a big green salad with lots of mixed veggies and olive oil dressing, or a green smoothie with avocado or nut butter are good examples.

Don't mix meat with beans, eggs, or dairy products. In fact, don't eat *anything* with meat except non-starchy vegetables like salad greens or steamed veggies. Anything else is a recipe for gastrointestinal distress. Beans are too close to meat in protein but also too full of starchy carbs to mix with meat. Eggs are completely indigestible for some people, and I don't recommend that you eat them very often. Dietary cholesterol in the body contributes to inflammation. If you do eat them now and then, don't mix them with meat. They're too high in protein, and you should not mix different proteins together. If you want eggs, combine them with vegetables only, as in a veggie omelet or on a salad.

As for dairy products such as milk, cheese, and ice cream, they really have no place in the adult diet, in my opinion. Milk is for baby cows, not humans at any stage of life. I prefer that you don't ever eat dairy products, but I know some people will choose to do so anyway. If you do eat dairy products, stick to organic, preferably raw dairy, and preferably from goats and sheep rather than cows. Never eat dairy products with any kind of meat! This is toxic to the body. There's a reason it's prohibited in kosher meals. Dairy goes with eggs and vegetables only, as in a veggie omelet with cheese (please hold the bacon) or a salad with feta or Parmesan cheese. It would be my preference, however, for ideal digestive health, to eliminate dairy foods entirely.

You can eat non-starchy veggies with just about anything. With the exception of sweet fruit, veggies are your key for enjoying any protein or grain. Mix meat or fish into a big salad. Mix steamed veggies into quinoa or rice or amaranth or millet. Flavor with just a little lemon juice and zest and enjoy! The more veggies in your diet, the more enzymes and nutrients, and the better your internal fitness will be.

....

WHY YOU SHOULD DITCH DAIRY

You probably grew up drinking milk, and maybe you can't imagine life without cheese, but I strongly urge you to ditch dairy products right away. In my opinion, dairy products are the worst foods for humans! Milk comes from a cow, and so it's great for a calf, but we're not calves. We have been brainwashed by the dairy industry, as they tell us that milk "does a body good." Really? How? We all need calcium, but not as much as the dairy companies say we need, and there are much better sources of calcium than dairy products, such as dark leafy greens, sea vegetables, broccoli, Brussels sprouts, almonds, butternut squash, sweet potatoes, black beans, white beans, lentils, kidney beans, oranges, figs, raisins, blackstrap molasses, and plant-based milks like rice milk and almond milk.

Let's go into some of the reasons why dairy should be avoided at all cost, despite the fact that the USDA tells us we should drink three glasses of milk a day:

- **Dairy increases insulin in the body,** which can lead to blood sugar issues, metabolic syndrome, and eventually diabetes.
- **Calcium does not strengthen bones,** and can actually cause them to become brittle. Vitamin D and silica are better at strengthening bones and preventing fractures than calcium.
- **Calcium has been linked to increased cancer risk,** especially prostate cancer in men. It increases insulin growth factor 1 (IGF-1), which is a known cancer promoter.
- **It's estimated that 75 percent of people worldwide are lactose intolerant.** For them, dairy can cause IBS, spastic colon, and other digestive upsets.
- **Dairy has been linked to acne,** allergies, sinus and ear infections, and anemia.
- **Dairy is filled with saturated fat,** which can cause clogged and hardened arteries and other heart disorders.
- **Raw milk might seem to be better because it's unpasteurized,** doesn't contain antibiotic residue, and is not homogenized, but it's still mucus-forming. The few benefits don't outweigh the negative effects.
- **You can get more calcium from seaweed,** dark green leafy vegetables, gluten-free whole grains, seeds, and nuts than you can from dairy products.

It can be a little bit difficult at first to understand how to put together a meal after knowing which foods to combine and which to avoid combining, but that's usually because people are creatures of habit and it's hard to imagine new ways to combine food. Permit me to assist you. You will see, once we start the Piper Protocol, that this way of eating follows food-combining principles, but you can start now with this basic guide to the kinds of meals that are most beneficial to your internal fitness:

BREAKFAST

Forget eggs and toast or bacon with waffles—but that doesn't mean you have to forget any of those items on their own. Breakfast could look like any of these:

Veggie omelet or scrambled eggs with spinach, mushrooms, and onions
Quinoa cereal with almond milk

A big bowl of berries

A whole-grain muffin or two pieces of whole-grain toast (preferably from a gluten-free grain; I'll talk more about gluten in Chapter 11) and a cup of herbal tea

Green smoothie with kale, lemon, green apple, and avocado

LUNCH AND DINNER

Meat sandwiches and wheat-based pasta with meat sauce are off the menu, but you can design many other delicious combinations.

Big salad with protein, like chicken, steak, or salmon

Any grain, such as brown rice, quinoa, or amaranth, with chopped, steamed, or sautéed veggies or on a salad

Zucchini and yellow squash "pasta" with turkey meatballs

Zucchini and yellow squash "pasta" with raw pesto sauce

A big bowl of veggie soup with rice or gluten-free pasta in it

Chicken or turkey breast or even a steak with a salad and as many steamed vegetables as you like

When you understand what to eat together and what not to eat together, you will create an ease and flow in your digestion that you may never have experienced before. Foods that you thought didn't agree with you might get digested just fine if you combine them properly. Keep this in mind, on the Piper Protocol and afterward: If you don't want digestive issues to be a way of life for you, then make proper food combining a way of life instead. Gas and bloating may soon be a distant memory.

Ready to start practicing with one very easy new habit? Try this IF Prep Step:

INTERNAL FITNESS PREP STEP #7

IF you want to make a big difference in how well you digest your meals, start with one very simple new cardinal rule: *Never drink and eat at the same time*. I mean it! This might be hard to get used to at first, but drink lots of water and green juices between meals, and when it's time to eat, just focus on your food. Take small bites, use the salad fork, chew thoroughly, and don't drink anything until one hour later! You will give your body the best chance to digest your food properly if you don't dilute your digestive juices and enzymes.

CHAPTER 8

Physical Cleansing

THE TERM *PHYSICAL CLEANSING* often brings to mind external improvement—the idea of losing weight, reducing cellulite, and adding a glow to the skin. These are seductive promises. We all want to look beautiful, fit, and radiant. However, the part that entices me the most is internal fitness, and that's the true goal of physical cleansing.

You can look amazingly "hot" according to society and be rusting and rotting inside. I see it all the time. I had a beautiful and quite famous woman come to see me, who shall remain nameless. She had long, flowing hair and fair skin with a little bit of acne and some red blotching that she covered with makeup. In our intake interview, I learned that her main complaints were acne and severe constipation. She had been having just one to two bowel movements per week for her entire life. This was normal to her, but she was addressing it now because being newly in the spotlight, it was becoming harder and harder to hide her skin issues with makeup, and she felt constantly bloated and in pain. She barely ate when she was out with other people because of the severe pain she would get in her stomach. No one knew her personal drama.

What was so interesting to me was that she had a body that was, by any standard, "hot." She had a flat stomach, was in great shape, and looked stunning. However, she felt miserable. I had to see her four times in a row to get things moving again because her colon was extremely sluggish. I referred her to a GI doctor to rule out any other issues I wasn't seeing, because she was so impacted. Fortunately, she didn't yet have anything extremely serious—just colitis and some leaky gut issues. After six colonics, I put her on Week Four of the Piper Protocol (her diet was already pretty clean, so she was ready for it). She drank fresh juices and blended soups, and I gave her some specific supplements to heal her gut and reduce her inflammation, including high doses of omega-3 fatty acids, probiotics, fiber, and lots of enzymes. She now has one to two bowel movements per day and no reoccurrence of her bloating and pain, except for mild bloating when she doesn't follow the food-combining rules. Every four to six weeks, she does anywhere from three days to a week of Week Four of the Piper Protocol. She finds that this keeps her body running optimally. To me, this was a classic case that reflects many of my patients—fitness and beauty on the outside, suffering on the inside.

We focus so intently on appearance that we can destroy our internal fitness in a quest for quick external results. The cover of a book may sell copies, but it won't sustain anybody's interest for very long if the pages are empty. If you look great but you're growing more acidic (rusting) by the moment and heading toward chronic disease, that beauty won't last. Start with internal fitness, with all your organs working optimally, so you can live a long, fulfilling life. Then you can worry about the outside. The magic is that, when you're internally fit, the outside looks better than ever before! Internal finess radiates from within. It's the secret key to external beauty and a radiant life.

I've already gone through many steps with you about how to achieve internal fitness via lifestyle habits, but in this chapter I want to get serious about some physical cleansing techniques you can do for yourself to give your internal fitness a jump-start. Cleanliness is the first step to internal fitness, so I provide some tools for you to work with: techniques like lymph massage, sauna, skin brushing, castor oil packs, and turpentine packs, oil pulling, and customized enemas. Don't be afraid! I'll show you how to use them safely and comfortably, including a special section on how essential oils and herbs can keep you in the right emotional space for maximum effectiveness.

I don't expect you to do all of these, but I want you to know about them because I use them in my clinic or recommend them to my clients, and I've seen how every one of these practices has a big impact. Look them over, read about them, and choose the ones you want to try. I recommend trying a new one about once a week. Move on from those that you don't love, and keep the ones that make a difference in how you feel, how well your digestive system is working, how much energy you have, and how much you enjoy them. Every one of these therapies will improve your internal fitness if you adopt it as part of your regular routine.

LYMPHATIC DRAINAGE MASSAGE THERAPY

The lymphatic system is made up of lymphatic vessels, nodes, organs, lymphocytes, and fluid (called lymph) that flows through the body, picking up waste and directing it through the lymph nodes and into the kidneys, then up through the cisterna chili, into the left thoracic duct, and into the bloodstream for removal. It's a system-wide waste-removal system. The lymphatic organs and glands are the thymus, spleen, tonsils, adenoids, appendix, mucosa-associated lymphatic tissues (MALT), and the Peyer's patches in the small intestines.

Many things can cause lymph to thicken, slow down, and block the lymphatic pathways: eating too much processed foods, too much sugar in the diet, not enough exercise, dehydration, too much salt, chemical exposure, shallow breathing, wearing tight-fitting clothes, constipation, liver congestion due to alcohol consumption, and even wearing a bra for more than twelve hours and then sleeping in it. Emotional stress can contribute to the problem, too.

Lymphatic drainage therapy (LDT) is a gentle massage technique that encourages this process in profound ways. The therapy works on the body's lymphatic system by activating and moving the fluid manually. The massage therapist uses specific hand placement, depth, direction, and rhythm to manipulate the lymphatic flow in the body. The network of lymphatic vessels is just under the skin, so they're easily manipulated manually by people who are trained to do this. Lymphatic massage detoxifies the body, reduces swelling, and facilitates healing systemically or in a specific area, reducing the stagnation of lymph anywhere in the body.

What LDT can help with:

Reduction of edema (swelling) and lymphedema, common after mastectomy or other
  lymph-node removal surgery
Reduction of puffiness (bags) under the eyes, cheeks, and overall face
Reduction and alleviation of cellulite
Reduction in the symptoms of chronic fatigue
Alleviation of congestion in the breast
Alleviation of constipation and diarrhea
Facilitation of healing during fasting
Alleviation of insomnia by increasing deep relaxation
Alleviation of stress
Reversing the effects of aging on the face and body

There are many "spa" lymphatic therapists, but when you're looking for quality work, especially if you have a health problem like cancer, you need someone who has been trained properly. This person will know what to do if you have had lymph nodes removed; he or she will shunt the lymph from the injured area to another area. The therapist must know the proper pathways of the lymphatic system because, if the massage is performed incorrectly, it can make serious swelling even worse. Because the lymph massage is a gentle massage, people who are used to deeper massage may not immediately understand the benefit, but it's one of the most powerful therapeutic massages you can get.

CASTOR OIL PACKS

A castor oil pack is essentially a folded piece of fabric soaked in castor oil that you place over any injured or ill body part, then cover with heat, like a hot water bottle or heating pad. The castor oil soaks into the skin and has a medicinal effect on the area and/or the underlying tissues, including organs like the liver.

Castor oil comes from the castor plant (*Ricinus communis*), also known as the "hand of Christ" or "Palma Christi," because it's so intensely healing. The oil is pressed from the castor seed, and it has been used therapeutically in several ways for decades—usually in the form of a pack (as described above) or ingested as a purgative (your grandmother or great grandmother might have made her children take their spoonful every night). Castor oil packs in particular became popular through the work of Edgar Cayce (the father of holistic medicine).

Many holistic healers use castor oil, usually for these conditions, among many others:

Calluses and bunions	Moles and warts
Cerebral palsy	Parkinson's disease
Cholecystitis	Pelvic cellulitis
Cirrhosis of the liver	Poor circulation
Constipation	Psoriasis
Eczema	Ringworm
Gynecological issues	Scleroderma
Inflammatory conditions	Tumors and cysts
Liver and gallbladder issues	Toxemia
Mastitis	

How can the oil from one little bean make a difference in conditions as wide-ranging as moles and cirrhosis? Castor oil is a triglyceride fatty acid that contains about 90 percent ricinoleic acid, as well as undecylenic acids. These immune-specific fatty acids are the key to castor oil's great healing power. Castor oil fights infections and increases blood circulation in the area where the pack is applied. It is anti-inflammatory, anti-microbial, and an immune-stimulant, drawing impurities into the lymphatic system so they can then be removed from the body. The small intestines then break down the castor oil into ricinoleic acid, which activates the intestinal lining and makes it a purgative.

I remember when I was a child, every Friday night my grandmother gave me a "pot spoon" of castor oil to move my bowels for the weekend. It was a thick, viscous oil that was hard to get down, but I must say it worked—what came out of me I thought was the end of the world!

You can use castor oil to treat a problem such as constipation, or you can use it even when you feel great. It is an excellent preventive. I like castor oil packs in particular because you can place them over the area where you are having a problem, and the skin absorbs the oil so it can get right to work. When purchasing castor oil, though, pay attention that you purchase organic oil, not chemically processed. Baar is a safe brand (see Resources).

There are a few situations in which you should not use a castor oil pack:

- Do not use a castor oil pack if you have undiagnosed abdominal pain that feels hot to the touch, as the heat from the heating pad or hot water bottle (not the castor oil) could exacerbate the condition. You can, however, use the castor oil pack without the accompanying heat.
- Do not use the heated castor oil pad on the abdominal region during pregnancy.
- For the ladies, do not use a castor oil pack at all during menstruation.

Otherwise, I hope you'll try this healing therapy!

HOW TO MAKE AND USE A CASTOR OIL PACK

You can buy premade castor oil packs for about $10, or you can make your own if you plan to use them regularly. To do so, first gather your supplies:

Cotton or wool flannel in a square large enough to fold two to four times into an
approximately 4- to 6-inch square. A 1-foot square should be about right.

A bottle of good-quality cold-pressed castor oil

A roll of plastic wrap or a garbage bag

Two large towels and one washcloth dedicated to your castor oil pack therapy; they will get
stained, so find ones that you don't mind delegating for the job

A glass container for storing your castor oil pack in a cool, dry place

An electric heating pad or hot water bottle

Now you're ready to prepare and use your castor oil pack. Here's what to do:

1. Collect everything you will need and choose an area to work that will be easy to clean up. Soak the flannel with castor oil, not so much that it drips everywhere but enough to moisten it. Do this over a sink or a basin or put the flannel in a container to minimize mess.

2. Select a good place to relax. If you find it hard to stay still without doing anything, have something to read or watch within reach.

3. Lay out one of the towels. Sit or lie on it. Place the castor oil pack over the area you want to treat. For example, if you're working on the colon, place the soaked flannel over the abdomen. If you are working on the liver, place it over the liver area, which is over your right rib cage.

4. Cover the castor oil pack with the plastic wrap, or just use a plastic bag. Place the heating pad or hot water bottle over it, and cover it with the remaining towel to help retain the heat.

5. Sit or lie there and relax for 45 minutes to 1 hour, allowing the castor oil to penetrate the skin.

6. Repeat daily or every other day, especially when treating a serious health issue. Do this for one or two months (or according to the advice from your health-care practitioner). Then, reduce the usage to every other day for a week or two. Then, reduce to once or twice a week, rest a week, and repeat every other week for health maintenance.

7. After using a castor oil pack for about three days, follow up with olive oil therapy: Combine equal parts olive oil and lemon juice, and drink this mixture every night for one week on an empty stomach. This will encourage the liver to dump its toxins. For the quantities, start with 1 teaspoon of each and work up to 2 tablespoons of each.

DETOX BATH

This bath is excellent for stimulating the lymphatic system, alkalizing the body, and general detoxification, because it pulls toxins out of the body. To a very hot bath, add 4 to 6 cups magnesium salts (Epsom salts), 1 bag of Bob's Mill aluminum free baking soda, and 32 ounces hydrogen peroxide 3%. Soak for at least 20 minutes.

DRY SKIN BRUSHING

Dry skin brushing is an effective way to stimulate lymphatic drainage. It also removes the dull, dead layers of skin and encourages the generation of new skin cells, which completely regenerate monthly. It's easy to do and only requires a dry, natural bristle brush. The best time for dry skin brushing is first thing in the morning or right before your evening bath. Here's how to do it:

1. Begin at your collarbone and brush down around your neck. This will help activate the large lymph nodes in your neck.

2. Move down to the chest, but do not brush breast tissue. Brush around the chest, outward toward the armpit, where you have more lymph nodes.

3. Move to the arm. Brush from elbow up toward the armpit, then brush the lower arm from the hand to the elbow. Then, brush all the way from fingertips to armpit. Repeat on the other arm.

4. Brush the rib cage, above the navel outward and upward toward the armpit.

5. Brush from the navel down, into the lower abdomen, where you have lymph nodes that lead to the colon. Brush the abdominal area in a clockwise motion.

6. Move to the legs and do them the same way you did the arms, brushing knee to groin, then foot to knee, then all the way from toes to hips. Repeat on other side.

7. Do your back, as well as you can reach. Direct the brushing toward the armpit. (It's nice to get someone to do this for you, if possible.)

That's all there is to it! It should take you only a few minutes, but your skin will glow, your lymphatic system will move more freely, and you will feel energized.

REBOUNDING

All cardiovascular exercise is good for your circulation and lymphatic flow, but one of the best is rebounding. Rebounding is simple to do, as long as you have a mini trampoline. Get a sturdy one with a bar to hang on to if you have any balance issues, and jump to your heart's content. How awesome is that? Every day, jump up and down on the trampoline for a few minutes. This shakes your lymph loose and gets everything flowing.

Gradually work up to 20-minute sessions. Not only will this help your lymphatic flow, but it's good exercise for your muscles and lungs. And it's fun, so you'll finish with a smile! Note: For women, if you feel floppy on the trampoline, wear a good sports bra and also contract your pelvic floor muscles (as you would if you were doing Kegel exercises). This can strengthen your pelvic floor and prevent organ prolapse.

HEALING CLAY AND ZEOLITE

Healing with clay is certainly nothing new—clay baths and poultices have been used for many centuries because clay pulls impurities from the body. Clay can be beneficial for healing when used both externally—as a poultice, mud pack, bath, and facial cleanser/toner/mask—and internally, although this is less common and usually for use in the case of poisoning, as clay can absorb poison.

Two healing clays that are widely available are bentonite clay and montmorillonite clay. These commonly found smectite clays have specific chemical and physical properties, including the ability to expand dramatically when wet. They are alive and raw, totally unprocessed, and filled with an enormous amount of minerals and enzymes. They absorb 30 times their weight in toxins—incredible! They also have an electrical charge when water is added, which enhances their ability to absorb toxins.

When taken internally, bentonite clay is particularly good for upset stomach, digestive disorders, food poisoning, detoxification, tooth cleaning (oral health), and skin issues. It easily releases its minerals to the body; the silica strengthens hair, nails, and bones, and the iron enriches the blood. Bentonite clay also supplies the body with the alkalizing minerals it requires for acidity buffering: calcium, potassium, magnesium, and sodium. It's a great way to help your body maintain a more alkaline environment. There is also evidence that bentonite clay can kill *E. coli*, MRSA, and salmonella. (Maybe an instinct about this is the reason why some people feel compelled to eat soil!)

Zeolite is a mineral that traps toxins within its honeycomb structure. It's very similar to clay, but is made from volcanic ash and sea salt. I find zeolite a nice and easy alternative to clay for detoxifying. You'll see in Chapter 16 that I use zeolite in the Piper Protocol during the advanced stage.

HOW TO USE CLAY EXTERNALLY

Raw clays like bentonite and montmorillonite clay are versatile detoxifiers. Here are some of my favorite ways to use them:

For oral health: Mix ⅛ teaspoon clay with a fluoride-free, sulfate-free toothpaste, or just use it alone to brush your teeth. This will clean your teeth, kill bacteria in the mouth, whiten and re-mineralize the teeth, and freshen breath. To use it as a mouthwash, mix ½ teaspoon clay with ½ cup lukewarm water in a jar. Cover and shake to mix well. Hold it in your mouth for a few minutes if you can, to help re-mineralize your teeth along and under the gum line, where a toothbrush might not reach. Spit it out, then rinse out your mouth. This is great to do after oil pulling (see page 127).

As a facial mask: Mix a small amount of clay—about 1 tablespoon—with four to five times as much filtered water to get a paste-like consistency. Mix and apply to blemishes, acne, or over your entire face to cleanse and tighten the skin. Leave the mask on for 20 minutes, or until it is completely dry and you feel it tightening the skin. Rinse it off and then moisturize your skin with a touch of pure baobab oil, coconut oil, or argan oil. (Nothing with chemicals, please!)

As a poultice: To use for bites, bruises, burns, chicken pox sores, cuts, eczema, psoriasis, shingles, and stings, make a paste with clay and water and put it on the affected area. Cover it with a crushed brown paper bag to help draw out impurities even more (crushed brown paper can conform to different body parts and its absorbency helps draw the toxins away from the skin). Cover with an Ace bandage or wrap in cloth. Repeat several times a day, especially for burns.

....

MEDICATION WARNING

Clay can actually absorb medications and ingredients in supplements, so please take clay treatments two to three hours after taking any supplements and medications. This will allow them to do their job, and then the clay can do its job without interfering.

....

As chafing powder: Babies tend to experience chafing in their chubby areas, and so do adults, especially athletes, when thighs rub together or in the underarm area. Instead of using toxic talcum powder (*especially* on babies!), dry clay powder is a great alternative because it's completely nontoxic. Rub it into the chafing areas or apply with a powder puff or cotton to soothe and speed healing.

As a detoxifying bath: A bath takes the power of a poultice and applies it to your whole body. Clay baths are good for pulling heavy metals and other toxins out of the body. Bentonite clay is the best for bath use. Fill a tub with water as hot as you can take it, pour 1 to 2 cups of bentonite clay into the bath (depending on the size of your tub, your size, and the size of your condition needing treatment), step in, and relax for 20 minutes. (Use a fine-mesh strainer in your drain to prevent clay from clogging your tub.) You may notice as you soak that the clay changes color. This is a sign the clay is doing its job. Rinse off with a quick shower, and notice how much softer your skin feels now.

As an internal detoxifier: For mild cases of digestive upset after eating something that might have been old or spoiled (but of course if you suspect a serious case of food poisoning, please go to the emergency room!), mix ½ teaspoon bentonite clay with ½ to ¾ cup warm water. Mix well and drink. The clay will expand and absorb the toxins that you ingested. For heavy metal removal, candida, or a parasite detox, mix 1 teaspoon bentonite clay with 1 cup water, or for a stronger dose, mix 1 tablespoon bentonite clay with 1½ cups water. Add 1 tablespoon psyllium husk and drink. This acts like a broom through your digestive system, sweeping up toxins and moving them out of the body.

For morning sickness: Some women experience morning sickness during their first trimester, and a common remedy is to eat crackers. The reason this can work is that the crackers absorb excess bile, which can cause nausea. But wheat flour isn't good for your colon—it has a clogging effect; the high sodium content in crackers doesn't do you any favors, either. A better choice is bentonite clay for easing the morning sickness right on the spot. Stir ½ teaspoon into 1 cup water and drink. It absorbs bile and other toxins, and flushes them out of the bowels without clogging the system, triggering food sensitivities, or bloating you with salt.

For your pets: Pets have the habit of eating things that don't necessarily agree with them. Often, you don't even know it happened, until your pet throws up something on your carpet. Sometimes you aren't sure why your pet is sick, but you can tell there is digestive upset—the pet won't eat, seems woozy, or is throwing up or having diarrhea. If you suspect a serious problem, you should definitely contact your veterinarian, but you can also try a clay remedy to ease the pet's discomfort while waiting to go to the vet. Mix ⅛ teaspoon for dogs under 40 pounds and ¼ teaspoon for dogs over 40 pounds, stirring it into the water bowl. If your pet is finicky and won't drink it, you can use a dropper or syringe to put some of the clay water directly in your pet's mouth. Remember, you cannot poison your pet or yourself with clay, so don't worry about that. There have been studies to test this—tremendous amounts of bentonite clay have been administered to people with no side effects (other than a good cleansing).

OIL PULLING

This practice is easy to do and extremely detoxifying, and I highly recommend that you give it a try because it's so easy and so powerful. It involves putting oil in the mouth and swishing it around for 20 minutes, then spitting it out and rinsing out your mouth with water. An ancient practice that seems to have come from India, and is part of Ayurvedic medicine, oil pulling is enjoying renewed popularity. There are more than 500 species of bacteria in the mouth, and some are bad and some are good. These bacteria are responsible for the sticky film on our teeth called plaque. Plaque releases toxic material that causes the gum line to slowly separate from the teeth, leaving a perfect space for more bacteria to grow and wreak havoc. These pockets can become infected over time, but oil pulling is a great way to foil that bacteria growth.

Here's how to do it:

1. Measure out 1 tablespoon of safflower, sesame, or melted coconut oil. For added benefit, add 2 or 3 drops of oil of oregano, tea tree oil, peppermint oil, or basil oil.

2. In the morning, first thing after rising and pH testing your saliva, put the oil in your mouth and swish it around without swallowing. Try to keep it in your mouth for 20 minutes. If this is too difficult at first, go as long as you can, and try to add another minute each morning until you work up to 20 minutes.

3. Spit out the oil, rinse out your mouth with water, then brush your teeth. Follow with a probiotic rinse (see page 76).

Personally, I recently had a bad toothache—one of those that feels as if it goes all the way to the root. I prepared a mixture of 1 tablespoon safflower oil and 2 drops of oil of oregano, and I swished it around between my teeth and up around my gum line. I left it in my mouth for 20 minutes, spat it out, and rinsed my mouth thoroughly, then brushed my teeth. Not only did my whole mouth feel clean and refreshed, but my toothache was gone. I repeated it twice and the toothache has not returned.

Teeth are interesting—in fact, your teeth are connected to all the organs of the body through energy meridians; in much the same way, all the body's organs are connected to spots on the foot, as reflexology has shown us. If you're having a dental issue, oil pulling can help relieve the discomfort, but also pay attention to where that issue is and look to the corresponding organ for dysfunction. Here's a chart showing your teeth meridians:

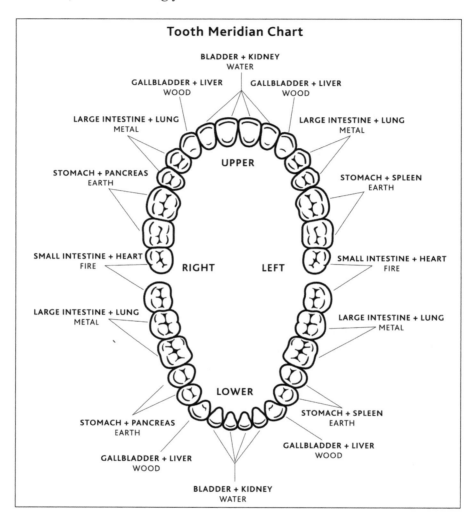

And on that same subject, I highly recommend finding a holistic dentist who does not use mercury fillings, which introduce mercury into your system, especially when the fillings are going in or coming out. Mercury can cause a cascade of harmful effects. To find a holistic dentist, search your state's website or that of the Holistic Dental Association (www.holisticdental.org).

And pay attention to your teeth! Oil pulling is an excellent place to begin.

MASSAGE THERAPY

Massage might sound like a luxury, something you do to treat yourself once in a while, but it's actually highly therapeutic for the body, increasing circulation to injured areas and generally improving both musculoskeletal and organ function throughout the body. The feel-good part is just a happy side effect. I recommend a weekly professional massage, but this isn't in most people's budgets, so between appointments you can massage yourself in ways that will be helpful. I particularly like self-massage to increase circulation, reduce pain, and deal with kidney and bladder issues. Just hold and rub your own body wherever it feels discomfort, or exchange massages with a loved one. A trained massage therapist will do the most therapeutic job, however, so determine how often you can fit a professional massage into your budget. Remember, it's not a luxury—it's preventive health care!

INFRARED SAUNA

Infrared saunas are smaller and heat differently from traditional saunas. The heat tends to be lower but more penetrating, so you can typically stay in an infrared sauna longer. This is a well-known treatment for removing toxins, weight loss, relaxation, pain relief, and to improve circulation, as well as to lower blood pressure, heal wounds, rejuvenate cells, and combat the signs of aging. I also like it for skin purification. The skin contains many types of bacteria and toxins, and an infrared sauna gently opens the pores and allows the toxins to leave the body via the sweat. This pulls toxins from as deep as the cellular level.

Not everyone will have access to an infrared sauna, but sometimes they're available at health clubs or health centers; if you're really lucky, you have one at home (see Resources). Sit in the sauna for 10 to 15 minutes at a time. You may be able to increase this amount as you get used to the process, but increase by just a few minutes at a time. If you have a high tolerance, you could work your way up to 30 minutes or even more, but always leave the sauna if you start to feel dizzy or nauseous.

It's very important that you're adequately hydrated before, during, and after your sauna. Be particularly vigilant about replenishing water and minerals after your sauna, especially with a liquid mineral supplement added to water. Coconut water is good for this, as it contains electrolytes. To enhance the treatment, take a teaspoon of powdered kelp or dulse in ¾ cup water. You can use an infrared sauna for detoxification purposes on a daily basis, even twice a day if you're having serious health issues. The best times to do a sauna treatment are first thing in the morning and before retiring, when you're most relaxed, as this helps you to sweat faster, thus releasing more toxins.

A few cautions:

- If you feel dizzy or faint, leave the sauna immediately, rest, and drink some water.
- If you've never tried a sauna before or aren't used to heat, approach this therapy slowly, acclimate your body to the heat, and get used to sweating.
- Do not consume any alcohol or caffeinated drinks for 3 hours before a sauna. Most practitioners say 2 hours, but I say 3 only because some people are slow metabolizers and may take a bit longer to clear these substances from the body.
- There are some reactions that may occur while doing sauna treatments, such as mild to moderate body odors, rashes over the body, headaches, and changes in bowel patterns. Memories of past emotional traumas may come up, and you may experience temporary depression or anxiety. This is all part of the detoxification process. Your body is releasing these negative things—physical as well as emotional toxins—so let them go.

ENEMAS (PLEASE READ THIS EVEN IF YOU THINK YOU'LL NEVER TRY ONE!)

Depending on where you live, who you hang around with, and to some extent your personality, you may think enemas (and by extension, colonics) are no big deal. I often travel to southern California, an environment where colon cleansing is widely accepted as just one more wonderful, holistic health practice. But for many people (including people in New York City, where I live), the whole notion of cleansing the colon is suspicious. Shouldn't things *come out* down there, rather than *go in?*

Actually, that's exactly the point.

Ideally, the human body works perfectly, with food moving smoothly through the digestive tract, the toxins and by-products of digestion neatly eliminated, and the bowels moving easily and painlessly. In reality, however, sometimes the body needs a little help. You can get that help from a professional (see Chapter 10), or you can get that help on your own at home, using an enema.

Enemas are nothing new—in fact, they've been around for centuries. It's a simple concept: liquid is inserted into the rectum under low pressure to clean out and empty the lower part of the colon, sigmoid colon, and rectum by inducing movement. Different enema techniques and amounts of fluid can get the water or other liquid to flow up further, as far as the hepatic flexure (the bend between the ascending colon and the transverse colon, under your liver). The more you do enemas, the stronger your muscles become and the longer you're able to hold the liquid in, reaping even more benefits. It's somewhat of an art, in my opinion.

Enemas are useful for helping with many types of digestive system dysfunction, as well as other health issues that may not seem (but are) related to digestion. These are just a few of the conditions that enemas may help to alleviate:

Acne	Fatigue
Allergies	Hemorrhoids
Anxiety	Infertility
Body odor	Irritable bowel syndrome (IBS)
Candidiasis	Leaky gut syndrome
Chronic pain	Liver toxicity
Constipation	Parasites
Depression	Psoriasis

WHAT DO YOU NEED?

You don't need too much to do an enema (see Resources):

1 quart of purified (filtered or boiled and cooled) warm water.

An enema bag or enema bucket with tubing and clamp. You can purchase these online or at any pharmacy.

Catheter to add on to tubing (this will be inserted into anus). You can get an enema catheter online for a few cents. It's more flexible and comfortable than the plastic insert that comes with the enema kit, and it's easier to wash, so I prefer to use it.

Towel

Chuck pad (a disposable pad for any spills).

Yoga mat or exercise mat.

Pair of gloves to clean up (optional).

A little olive or castor oil for lubrication.

Essential oils, especially lavender, peppermint, clove, thyme, and/or bergamot (optional but useful).

A small stool for squatting on the toilet, as you might find at your local Target, Walmart, or Bed Bath & Beyond, or a Squatty Potty or Welles Step (see page 155 and the Resources).

HOW TO PERFORM AN ENEMA

Although it may seem complicated the first time you try it, you'll soon see that enemas are easy to do, and can even be pleasant, after you get over any initial mental blocks you may have about them. The first time you try an enema, it probably won't take very long because you aren't used to holding the water and you will likely need to use the toilet soon. As you get better at it, you can try retention enemas (implants), in which you hold water containing therapeutic substances such as coffee or wheatgrass for up to 15 minutes before using the toilet (see page 136). (Sometimes they don't come out again—your body "steals" them for its personal use!) The whole process for me takes about one hour.

Your first time, block out an hour to use the bathroom, just because you will be figuring everything out. As you get better at it, the basic enema will take less time, but therapeutic enemas will take longer because of the retention time. Playing some relaxing music in the bathroom can make the experience nicer and also help to pass the time while you are holding.

Here are the basics:

1. Put your warm, filtered water into the bucket or enema bag.

2. Connect the tubing to the bag or bucket, with clamp in place close to the other end of the tube. The clamp controls the flow rate, so keep it closed.

3. Cut the end of the tube that came with the enema kit below the hole. It's lubricated with petroleum jelly, and you don't want to put that into your body. Attach your enema catheter to the end of the tube.

4. Hang or place the enema bag or bucket 3 to 4 feet high (height of a doorknob)—no higher, because you don't want the water to enter the body too quickly. You could also use a towel rack or put the enema bucket on the sink counter.

5. Put the end of the tube over the sink or bathtub. Run some of the water through the tube to remove the air in the passageway by opening the clamp. It will flow downward with gravity. Once some of the fluid comes out of the hole, close the clamp.

6. Make yourself a comfy spot with the yoga mat. Place a towel over the mat and put the chuck pad on top of the towel to avoid any spills. Lie on your left side with the chuck pad under your buttocks area. Your colon makes a 90-degree turn after the rectum, so lying on your left side facilitates the water flow.

7. Lubricate the catheter tip with olive oil or castor oil up about 3 inches. This is how far it will go into the anus. Next, lubricate the anus. Slowly and gently insert the tip of the catheter into the anus. I know this seems daunting and maybe even a bit scary at first, but it's only because you aren't used to doing it. All you're doing is entering the rectum with a pencil-size tube—you won't do any harm. Go slowly until you find a smooth entrance. If you feel as if you're forcing it, stop! Relax and go with the flow of your body shape. It's really worse in your head than it is in reality. Persevere! It will be so worth it in the (ahem) end.

8. Once the catheter is in, release the clamp for just 3 to 5 seconds, allowing the water to flow in. Close it, and hold it in, to get used to the feel of it. Are you comfortable? Do you feel cramping? If you feel any cramping, don't add any more water. Massage your abdomen in a clockwise direction. Breathe normally and relax. The cramping should subside. I'd like you not to use the toilet yet, but if it's your first time and you really need to, go ahead. Whenever you feel you can't hold it anymore during this process, use the toilet. If you can keep holding it, however, proceed with the next step.

9. When you feel ready, open the clamp for 3 to 5 more seconds, then close it again. If you feel more cramping, massage your abdomen again to relieve it. Here is where you

can inhale some essential oils to help you relax and move things along. Continue this pattern two more times and continue to massage the abdomen, trying to feel intuitively where you need to be touched. Hold those areas and breathe into them. Don't use the toilet yet unless you really need to.

10. When you're ready, turn onto your back, add more water—let it in for maybe 5 to 7 seconds or more. Hold and massage. Repeat two to three more times.

11. If you're up to it, turn onto your right side. This allows the water to travel down to the ascending colon. Do you feel full? A bit crampy? Can you hold the water longer so it can moisten the stool to make its exit much easier? If not, get up and go to the bathroom. If you can retain the fluid, roll onto your back again and put more water in, then turn on your right side again. Try to retain the liquid as long as you can—for some it will only be a minute or so. Others might be able to hold it for up to 10 or 15 minutes, or even more.

12. When you're ready to evacuate, then get up. You'll know because your body will experience a strong peristalsis (the feeling that you have to go *now*). This is your body telling you that it's ready. Make sure the clamp is closed, slowly turn onto your back, pull the catheter out, and get to the toilet.

13. When you're on the toilet, put your feet up into a squatting position (place them on the small stool), and let your body release naturally. What comes out will vary, depending upon what's in there, but expect water and stool, either liquefied or in pieces. It should all come out easily. Sometimes you will also see phlegm or mucus and even bits of undigested food.

14. If all is well, and especially if you're getting experienced, you can now repeat the whole process to get more out. If you do this, open one or two probiotic capsules into the water, to replenish the good bacteria that were rinsed away. Or, if you're done for now, relax and congratulate yourself for a job well done. Now, go have a big glass of water and a probiotic capsule or two.

If this is the first time you've ever tried an enema, don't be frustrated if you can't hold the water in for very long. The muscles you use for this will become increasingly conditioned, and you'll get more and more used to the feel of the whole process. No matter how much fluid you used, be proud of yourself. You did it, and your body will thank you.

If you're having a serious health problem, you can do up to three enemas per day, tapering down to one or two as you start to feel better. Severe constipation can benefit from this regimen, which releases impacted feces and toxins that may not come out right away. Taper down to one a day, and eventually one per week for maintenance, after the constipation is resolved. Coffee enemas and wheatgrass enemas can also be particularly therapeutic. (I will talk about how to do these on pages 136 and 137.)

Three coffee enemas per day can help cancer patients with pain and help to speed detox in patients with multiple sclerosis. Wheatgrass enemas are incredibly nourishing for people who cannot take in enough nutrition. They are great for MS patients, as well as others who are having trouble eating enough, for any reason. The fastest way to get nutrients directly into the body is anally because the enterohepatic circulatory system, via the hemorrhoidal vein in the sigmoid colon, absorbs nutrition so efficiently. As an example, a friend of mine had a grandmother who stopped eating and drinking. Her doctor told us she had about three weeks to live. We started giving her three wheatgrass enemas per day to nourish her. Within about ten days, she started eating again, and she lived for another year.

During an intensive cleanse, two enemas a day to jump-start your progress is excellent. Work your way down to one a day. You can do one enema per day all the time if you choose, but most people who do regular enemas aim for once a week on the weekend, when they have time to relax, or even one per month. Remember, both health and death begin in the colon, so please try to keep it clean, at your own comfort level.

ENEMA TROUBLESHOOTING

If your first enema didn't go well, or if you want a little more encouragement and information before you try it, here are some more tips:

- Always start out with a warm water enema first before trying any additions to the water.

- Do not use chlorinated water (as in tap water) for an enema. Chlorinated water will deplete the body's supply of good gut flora. Instead, use spring water or filtered water.
- Sometimes, depending on how backed up you are, you may need to use 2 quarts of warm water instead of just 1 quart.
- Don't be in a rush. It's not a competition. Slow and steady wins the race.
- Make sure you have the bathroom to yourself, so you feel comfortable and not rushed. Take time for you and your health.
- Have a regular bowel movement, then if you're still up for it you can go straight into the retention enema (see below). After that, evacuate and clean up. With the retention enema added, you'll probably spend about 90 minutes total. Do not do the retention enema until you have had a bowel movement.

THE RETENTION ENEMA (IMPLANT): BUILDING A BETTER ENEMA

As mentioned, the first time you do an enema, it's a good idea to use warm water only. You're getting used to how the enema works, how it feels, and how well you tolerate it. Once you know what you're doing, however, you can take it to the next level, infusing the water you use with herbs and other substances that will increase the power, effectiveness, and therapeutic nature of the enema. Most people are somewhat depleted of minerals, and so adding at least some chlorophyll or wheatgrass can significantly replenish mineral stores. But the possibilities don't end there. Here are some other enemas you can try. For each one, add the substance to warm water as explained, then proceed with your retention enema or implant in the usual way, per the directions on page 132. You can also use an enema implant syringe. This allows you to put the additive in separately. These are easy to use—if you purchase one, follow the package directions.

The following are all retention enemas, so once you fill up with the liquid, try to hold it for 15 to 20 minutes so that your body can fully absorb the beneficial components of the enema.

Chlorophyll/Wheatgrass Enema: This is what I use most in my enemas because it is so mineralizing, and it also helps to balance pH and expel gas. Add 2 ounces of liquid chlorophyll or wheatgrass to the enema bag (or in the implant syringe). Look for chlorophyll brands without glycerin or parabens (DeSouza's and World Organics are good brands; see Resources) or pure powdered wheatgrass. Fresh wheatgrass juice is the best, if you can find it.

Apple Cider Vinegar Enema: This is extremely alkalizing, very soothing, and so great for stomach issues and intestinal spasms. It can also help to reduce your blood pressure and stabilize your blood sugar. Just add 1 tablespoon apple cider vinegar to the syringe or enema bag and repeat as before.

Aloe Vera Enema: This is a soothing and healing enema. Because of its astringent properties, it can help stop any bleeding of hemorrhoids. Just add ¼ to ½ cup aloe vera juice to the enema bag or syringe. I like George's brand aloe vera juice (see Resources).

Coffee Enema: Coffee enemas are particularly therapeutic and are one of my favorite enema therapies. Most people drink coffee for the energy they get from caffeine, which stimulates the sympathetic nervous system. But most people tend to drink too much, stressing the nervous system and causing jitters, stress, and irritability. Eventually, the caffeine and the many other toxins present in coffee (especially non-organic coffee) can build up in the liver and cause damage. The great thing about coffee enemas is that you get the benefits of coffee without the harmful effects, because the coffee never goes through your digestive system. Coffee enemas are also particularly effective for pain relief.

The colon absorbs all the nutrients and antioxidants in the coffee. It can also help the colon shed a thick mucus lining. The palmitic acid in coffee enhances the enzyme glutathione S-transferase, which is important in the body's mechanism for killing cancer cells. Also, when coffee is administered rectally, it dilates the bile ducts and stimulates bile flow. The theophylline and theobromine present in coffee dilate the blood vessels and reduce inflammation in the gut. Coffee implants also stimulate peristalsis to help the body release toxic bile from the duodenum to the colon, and the coffee is absorbed by the hemorrhoidal veins (or enterohepatic circulation). These are located in the sigmoid region of the colon that delivers the caffeine straight to the liver, causing it to contract and thus release bile. You can see why I love this powerful therapy!

To do the coffee enema, use a special kind of coffee called S. A. Wilson (see Resources), or use organic coffee. The blond roast is the strongest, but the organic medium roast works great, too. Coffee specific for enemas like S. A. Wilson's has more caffeine and other beneficial properties for the purpose of the enemas, but is not meant for drinking!

To make an enema coffee concentrate, bring 2 quarts of purified water and 1 cup enema coffee grounds to a boil. Boil for 3 minutes, reduce the heat, and simmer for 15 minutes, covered. Let the coffee cool and then strain it into a container. Add 1 cup of this coffee concentrate to 3 cups warm purified water, which is enough for 4 enemas. Store in a glass container in the refrigerator for up to 2 days.

For a single coffee enema, bring 1 quart of water to a boil. Add 2 tablespoons ground enema coffee and boil for 3 to 5 minutes. Turn off the heat and let steep until it cools to 100 degrees F, or room temperature. Strain into a container.

....

COFFEE ENEMA LORE

How the heck did anybody ever think of using coffee in an enema? The story goes that during World War I, doctors and nurses always kept coffee around to keep them awake for the grueling tasks of tending to the wounded soldiers. They would also regularly perform warm water enemas to help the soldiers move their bowels, as they suffered chronic constipation from anesthesia use. One day, an overworked and tired nurse accidentally poured an old, cool cup of coffee into an enema bag instead of water. The soldier who was the recipient of this accidentally "adulterated" enema had been in a lot of pain, but he noticed that after the enema, his pain diminished significantly. He mentioned this to the nurse, who then realized her mistake. She had accidentally discovered a natural pain reliever, and the coffee enema was born.

This was a fortuitous discovery because pain medication was in short supply during the war and was reserved only for postsurgical patients. The discovery of the coffee enema helped the medical teams to stretch the pain medication even further. Soldiers benefited not only from relief of constipation but also from relief of pain.

Up until about fifty years ago, the *Merck Manual* mentioned coffee enemas along with colonics. Then they began removing these holistic therapies from the *Merck Manual.* My theory is that they interfered with pharmaceutical profits. If enemas are effective, why take drugs? (Why, indeed?)

....

Castor Oil Enema: Castor oil is a great oral therapy, but it also makes a therapeutic addition to an enema. Add 2 to 4 tablespoons castor oil and ½ teaspoon ox-bile powder (sold in health food stores or on amazon.com) to your coffee enema solution and stir or blend until the powder dissolves. Administer immediately.

Epsom Salt Enema: Epsom salt, or magnesium sulfate, is commonly used to relax muscles in a bath or is used orally as a laxative or during a cleanse. This particular enema helps to relax the smooth muscles of the colon, thus allowing the waste content to exit more easily. Combine 1 tablespoon Epsom salt (magnesium sulfate) with 1 quart warm water for your enema. This is not a retention enema; eliminate as for a regular enema.

Garlic Enema: I personally love this enema because of its results. You probably already have fresh garlic in your kitchen, but if you don't, just grab it at the supermarket. Garlic enemas cleanse the colon of mucus congestion that may or may not be hardened over time in the colon, and its antiseptic properties make it an ideal therapy for tackling various types of bacteria, parasites, and worms.

I've prepared this enema two ways. The common way is to place 3 or 4 freshly peeled and crushed garlic cloves into 1 quart water. Bring to a boil and boil for 3 minutes, then turn off the heat and let it cool. Strain it and use for your regular enema.

The other way I do it (the Piper way) is to make a garlic concentrate. Place 6 or 7 peeled garlic cloves in a high-powered blender. Add 1 quart hot water. Blend until the liquid is completely smooth and the garlic liquefied. Strain through a fine-mesh sieve or use a nut milk bag (that you reserve specifically for this) into another container. Press the garlic to get out every drop of juice. Add 3 or 4 ounces of garlic concentrate to 1 quart warm water for your enema. This can be used as a retention enema as well.

Lactobacillus **Implant:** Even if you take probiotics and eat fermented foods, this is yet another way (and a direct route) of getting good bacteria into your colon. Too much bad bacteria in the colon can cause yeast infections, IBS, and malodorous flatulence. Probiotics administered via the rectum have a better chance of surviving and thriving in your colon because they don't have to endure the rigors of the entire digestive tract. I even find it beneficial to end all enemas with an acidophilus implant so as to replenish any of the good bacteria that might have been washed away during an enema.

To make an acidophilus implant, combine 2 teaspoons powdered acidophilus blend (look for one that includes other probiotics like *L. casei* and *L. bulgaricus*) with 2 ounces filtered lukewarm water (very warm or hot water will kill the probiotics). Mix well and implant immediately.

Catnip Enema: Catnip doesn't just soothe cats—it can soothe humans, too. In enema form, catnip can energize you, improve circulation, and relieve gas. Steep a catnip teabag in 3 cups water and let it cool. Use this for your enema. This can also be used as a retention enema/implant.

Pau d'Arco/Cat's Claw Enema: Pau d'Arco tea has intensive healing properties and makes a great addition to an enema. It's good for inflammation, stops the growth of candida, and helps purify the blood via the liver. It's also anti-bacterial, antifungal, and anti-microbial. I find it useful to combat parasites and effective against *E. coli*. It also helps to dissolve mucus and phlegm, and has an anti-tumor effect and a neutralizing effect on leukemia cells and other abnormal cell growth. I like to add cat's claw to Pau d'Arco leaves because it also has an anti-bacterial and antiviral action and can help to prevent healthy cells from becoming cancerous.

To make this tea, put 3 tablespoons Pau d'Arco and 3 tablespoons cat's claw herbs into 1 quart water in a glass or stainless steel pot. Bring to a boil, reduce the heat, and simmer for 15 minutes. Cool, strain, and use for your enema.

These are just a few of my favorite physical cleansing techniques, but now you have things to choose from, so take what resonates with you and give it a try. You might just discover a therapy that supports your health in a way you never imagined it could! All these therapies are safe if done as I have instructed, so enjoy and don't worry. And if you aren't quite ready to try any of them yet? Just keep reading. I'll help ease you into a few of these once we begin the Piper Protocol in Chapter 11.

For now, let's just jump in with one easy one:

....

INTERNAL FITNESS PREP STEP #8:

IF you want to try physical cleansing, start with oil pulling. Oil pulling may sound unusual to you, but it's easy and painless to do, and it has a great detoxifying effect, not just for your mouth but also for all your organs, since as you learned, your organs are connected to your teeth. Follow the instructions on page 127 and try oil pulling every morning, just before you rinse with your probiotics.

....

CHAPTER 9

Emotional Cleansing

PHYSICAL CLEANSING IS ESSENTIAL for internal fitness, but it might surprise you to know that emotional cleansing is essential, too—and inextricably linked to physical cleansing. I see this all the time in my practice. Emotional blockages translate to physical ones, and vice versa, so it makes no sense to clear one without clearing the other.

From the time we are very young, we internalize messages from our environment about what to do with our emotions; if we all let our emotions go as freely as infants do, well, frankly, not much would get done in the world. Can you imagine teachers and CEOs and police officers and doctors having temper tantrums and crying whenever they were hungry? We all need to learn to master our emotions, but for many people, mastery becomes repression. We learn to bottle up our emotions. We learn that "men don't cry," or that excessive emotion in a woman is a sign of weakness. We bury what needs to come out.

In my line of work as a colon hydrotherapist, I see where this emotion gets buried—and often, it's in the colon. In many belief systems around the world (if not in conventional Western medicine), emotions have a real place in the body. We all know this instinctively. You probably recognize the feeling of butterflies in your stomach, or what it feels like to be scared or anxious and feel your heart racing. Maybe you get headaches or diarrhea when you're under stress, or stiff painful joints when you're feeling depressed. Repressed hurt, pain, anger, refusal to forgive, grudges, hate, pettiness, bitterness—all of these emotions, when held inside and unexpressed for too long, can fester and even encourage the development of more serious chronic diseases, such as heart disease, cancer, and autoimmune disease. It's not that any disease is your fault. It isn't even your fault that you didn't know how to release those emotions. It's the fault of the negativity and the way it acts on your physical body.

What's more, your digestive tract actually contains neurons, just like your brain. This concept is fascinating to me. Most of your serotonin, which regulates mood, is produced not in your brain (10 percent) but in your small intestine (90 percent). You can "feel things" in your gut, in a very real way. (For a lot more great information about this, I suggest you read the fantastic book *The Second Brain* by Michael D. Gershon, M.D.; see Resources). In my practice, what I see in particular is how emotion impacts the large intestine. When we don't let go of things like anger, grief, or emotional pain, they stick here, and the result can be holding on to waste that should be evacuated.

But this goes both ways. In traditional Chinese medicine, there's something called liver *qi* stagnation. This is a common problem that happens when the liver is overburdened with toxins (which can come from foods like dairy products, wheat, and sugar, or from other toxins like caffeine, alcohol, medication, and environmental pollution). Liver *qi* stagnation can cause anxiety, anger, and depression. In other words, physical harm can cause emotional harm, just as emotional harm can cause physical harm.

Sometimes during a colonic, I may be massaging a certain area of the body, say along the spine around the bra line, or at the bottom end of the scapula. There are acupuncture points there that influence the liver and the gallbladder. Maybe I feel a knot in the muscle in that area. The client may say it's painful as I try to work it out. Sometimes the client gets upset at me or calls me names. Sometimes the client gets silent or begins to cry. I ask the client if it hurts and sometimes he or she says it's uncomfortable, or tells me that it's bringing up some hidden emotion or memories. What I notice at this time is a darkening of the colonic water, more mucus, and an increase in the flow.

If the client talks about what's bothering him or her at this time instead of holding it in, then a greater colonic release occurs and the client feels it physically and emotionally. A burden has been lifted. It's a pretty amazing phenomenon, and I might not believe it if I didn't see it for myself, time and again.

Our thoughts make our lives, plain and simple. If you think negatively, you'll manifest negativity. If you're always getting into bad situations, pay attention to your attitude about life.

Sometimes my clients say, "But of course I'm angry/sad/depressed/anxious, because X, Y, and Z have happened to me." But I counter that argument: Perhaps X happened to you, and then your thoughts turned negative, and that is part of the reason Y and Z happened to you next. If you think trouble always follows you, consider whether you keep a metaphorical GPS activated inside you that shows trouble exactly where to find you.

So how do you redirect that emotional GPS? How do you stop the negativity and begin to channel more positive thoughts? You need an emotional detox. Physical cleansing can help to get this started, but then you need to take it the rest of the way. You very well might not be responsible for the source of your negative emotions, but you must be responsible for processing and healing them if you want to remain healthy and at peace within yourself. Here are some strategies:

FORGIVE

Forgiveness is a form of letting go. In Chinese medicine, the time for letting go is autumn, when we clean out negative thoughts and old hurts, but you can forgive any time. Forgiving is not forgetting, and it's not condoning someone else's bad behavior. It's simply setting yourself free from the pain of hate, anger, hurt, and grudge. It's not an easy thing to do, and if you need the guidance of a professional counselor or therapist, seek it. If you think you can forgive on your own, spend some time each day in quiet contemplation, working on letting go of the negative feelings about someone else (or even yourself) that you've been clinging to. You'll feel an immense weight lifted when you are actually able to let these thoughts go.

Forty-three-year-old Michael was sexually molested as a child by a family member. He suffered from longstanding social withdrawal and was haunted by his experience. He never had any serious relationships growing up because he was too afraid to let anyone get close. He had major trust issues. To protect himself from the pain, he piled on the pounds until the scale hit 300. He had terrible acne, alternating constipation and diarrhea, and skin rashes, which all contributed to his low self-esteem. But to Michael, that was better than trusting someone else who might then hurt him.

Michael was referred to me by a friend and he reluctantly came to my office. I could tell from the moment he walked in that we had emotional work to do. Even with all his pain, Michael had a good sense of humor, but it was always aimed at himself. That is, if he made fun of himself, then nobody else would. During our first session, we laughed and I tried to create a bond with him, but he didn't release much from his colon during his first or second colonic.

During the third colonic, however, he had a pep in his step when he came in to see me. He suddenly wasn't shy or self-deprecating. He gave me a huge hug and said he was ready to work. He told me he had already lost 3 pounds, just from pooping daily! We laughed and began the session.

As we got deeper into the session, I asked him about his childhood and when he started to gain weight. Then I asked if he thought any emotional challenges had led to his weight gain. Suddenly, wow—an avalanche. As he told me his story, his body released continuously. Interestingly, it was mostly mucus, which in Chinese medicine means the body suffers from too much dampness. This is a quality we often see in "mother" types who are round and juicy looking—the kind of people you just want to hug. They take on a layer of fat as protection, to isolate and shield them from physical and emotional toxins.

After twenty minutes of nonstop release, Michael slowed down. He said he felt exhausted and asked if we could stop. I said yes, but let's try just one more time. I filled him again and the blackest sludge I ever saw came out with a crawl through the tube. During this release, he began to sob quietly. I held space with him, not talking but letting him know I was there with him with a gentle touch. When it all had passed, he not only looked exhausted but also looked younger, as if he'd lost ten years off his face. After freshening up and meeting me outside in the waiting area, he said, "Guess what? I weighed myself in the bathroom. I just lost eight pounds in forty-five minutes."

By the next visit a week later, he'd lost an additional 5 pounds, and said he no longer harbored any ill feelings toward himself or his attacker. He realized it was hurting him, not helping him, to hold on to the pain and fear for so long. He's now in a committed relationship, and I treat his partner, too.

There is the power of forgiveness. Sometimes physical cleansing can lead to emotional cleansing, but emotional cleansing can also lead to physical purging and the loss, quite literally, of the weight and baggage you've been carrying. We all have people we can forgive, whether they've severely harmed us or just hurt our feelings. Not all forgiveness will be as dramatic as Michael's, but it can always be profound, at any level. Forgiveness, I have found, is alkaline, and anger, fear, and hate are acidic. Work on forgiveness, either on your own or with a therapist, and you will experience miracles.

AROMATHERAPY FOR FORGIVENESS

In my practice, I like to use aromatherapy to help people with particular emotional issues during colonics. You don't have to have a colonic to benefit, however. The essential oil product I use for this purpose is Forgiveness, an oil by Young Living Essential Oils that contains frankincense, sandalwood, lavender, coriander, bergamot, lemon, Roman chamomile, geranium, ylang-ylang, rose otto, jasmine, melissa, palmarosa, and angelica in a sesame oil base (see Resources). You could also pick just three or four of these oils and make your own mix. Smell them while taking in deep breaths and thinking about your emotional issue. With each inhale you bring in good energy and with each exhale you let go of what you no longer need or want in your life.

SPEAK YOUR TRUTH

Sometimes, the best way to release a buried emotion is to speak it out loud. This can be as simple as telling someone that your feelings are hurt, or that you're angry, or admitting that you're depressed or anxious. Or, it can be more complex and difficult.

Laura was in her mid-thirties and she struck me at first as a positive, happy person, but she suffered from alternating constipation and diarrhea. Typically I do an intake questionnaire, and I learned in talking with her that she didn't have a good relationship with her mother, but she said she couldn't remember the reason why. During her third colonic session, this client became very angry with me for no apparent reason and wanted to end the session. Her anger surprised me, but I asked her to just stay with me as I talked her through the discomfort. She was intermittently releasing hard pebbles of stool and mucus, and then quite suddenly she began to release a thick, dark brown sludge. She began to cry at this moment, and then told me that as a little girl, she had been molested for years by an uncle who was her caregiver while her mother worked. She said that when she told her mother about it, her mother didn't believe her and instructed her to stop telling lies. Her mother continued to take her to this man's house every day.

Remembering this experience was a dramatic moment for her, and it gave her the energy and conviction to take action. She went home during the holidays that year and confronted her mother and the uncle. She was rejected and told to leave, but just as she was leaving, a younger cousin stopped her, yelling out that the uncle had done the same thing to her. This forced the family to listen, and my client was validated. The event allowed her to let go, finally, of all the hurt, betrayal, and pain that had consumed her for all these years. After that, her gastrointestinal symptoms disappeared.

Whatever you're holding in, tell someone, whether it's a friend, a therapist, or the person who has (perhaps unknowingly) hurt you or made you angry. This is an important practice. Truth holds great power, and allowing yourself to have a voice can be just the emotional detox you need. Metaphorically, the thyroid deals with "speaking your truth." If you are not being honest with yourself or saying how you really feel, this could be a subtle sign of thyroid issues. In Chinese medicine we call it *plum pit qi,* a knot in your throat.

....

AROMATHERAPY FOR TELLING THE TRUTH

To help with telling (and recognizing) the truth, I like to use a blend of essential oils containing cypress, frankincense, lavender, and black spruce, in jojoba or grapeseed carrier oil. Put a few drops on your hand and inhale deeply. Imagine with each inhalation that you breathe in truth and exhale lies. Imagine a vibrant blue color surrounding your throat, which is the center of your fifth chakra and the place for speaking truth. This can help you to heal and recognize what is true for you in that moment, and it can help you speak it out loud when you're ready.

....

LET GO WITH DEEP BREATHING

People hang on to things with such intensity that it can become a great burden that they don't recognize because they're so used to carrying it. My forty-one-year-old client Brenda was in a marriage in which she gave everything and received very little back. She had no emotional or financial support from her husband, and no mental or physical connection with him. She felt a deep responsibility as a wife, so she did not leave him for many years. However, the lack of love caused her to gain an enormous amount of weight. Through work with a therapist, she finally recognized that she was not benefiting anyone by holding on to the marriage. A week after her divorce, she weighed herself. She had lost 15 pounds! The marriage had actually been a physical weight on her. Over the next few months, she lost another 10 pounds, as she gradually let go of that painful experience and stepped into her new life.

Letting go is extremely difficult for some people, while others do it easily. We hold on to what's familiar, even when it doesn't serve us. The practice I find the most beneficial for letting go is deep breathing.

Deep breathing calms the mind, slows the breath, brings more oxygen to the brain, and moves the lymph by exercising the diaphragm. It also calms and centers the emotions for more clarity. There is a direct link between respiration and emotion. Calm, serene emotions cause the breath to become slower and deeper, whereas aggravating, anxious, or excited emotions cause the breath to become more rapid and shallow. Purposeful deep breathing can actually reverse a panic attack, whereas purposeful rapid, shallow breathing can cause aggravation and anxiety. There's a reason people tell others who are upset to "just breathe." Deep breathing really does impact your emotional state in a positive way. Here's how to do it:

1. Sit in a quiet place, in a comfortable position, with your back straight to give your lungs and diaphragm plenty of room. You can use a straight-backed chair if you find it difficult to sit straight without support.

2. Close your eyes and breathe normally for a few breaths, then slowly begin to lengthen and slow your inhales and exhales.

3. Once you're ready, inhale fully to a slow count of 5, and exhale fully to a slow count of 6. Repeat ten times. This is a calming exercise. (Five is the number for change and six is the number for love in numerology.)

4. If you want an energizing exercise, do the opposite: Exhale fully to a slow count of 5, then inhale fully to a slow count of 6. Repeat ten times.

This is the basic deep breathing exercise, but you can customize it according to what you're trying to let go of, like this:

To let go of grief: In Chinese medicine, the organ that stores grief is the lungs. People who are having trouble letting go of grief often experience breathing difficulties, decreased oxygen availability in the body, and a sunken chest, as well as constipation, because of the association between the lungs and the large intestine. To help yourself let it go, on the exhalation, make the sound of *Sssssss,* the sound that's the antidote for grief. Visualize the color *white,* the color that's the antidote for grief. As you do this, think about the emotion that counteracts grief: *courage.* With every inhalation, imagine you're filling yourself up with courage.

To let go of worry: We tend to store worry in the stomach. Signs of holding on to worry are butterflies in the stomach or a knot in your stomach, the way you feel when you know you're in trouble. To help yourself let go of worry, on the exhalation, make the sound *Whooooo,* the sound that's the antidote to worry. Visualize the color *yellow,* the color that's the antidote for worry. As you do this, think about the emotion that counteracts worry: *trust.* With every inhalation, imagine you're filling yourself up with a sense of openness and trust.

To let go of anger: Anger is a liver emotion, and that's where people tend to store it. If you're holding on to anger, you may experience insomnia or disturbing dreams. Liver *qi* stagnation can also lead to PMS, irregular menstruation, and bouts of anger and rage. Other signs of holding on to anger are the inability to fully detox, too much bile production, impaired digestion, and poor circulation. Anger takes so much metabolic energy that it can drain you of the energy to do anything else. This can also lead to blood sugar spikes, as the body releases too much glucose in order to meet the body's increased energy needs. To help yourself let go of anger, on the exhalation, make the sound *Shhhhh,* the sound that's the antidote to anger. Visualize the color *green,* the color that's the antidote for anger. As you do this, think about the emotion that counteracts anger: *joy.* With every inhalation, imagine you are filling yourself up with joy.

To let go of fear: Fear is an emotion that can be buried so deep you may not even know it's there, but at the same time, it can still seem to be just below the surface. Fear is often the emotion beneath anger, or the underlying reason for anger. It often settles into the adrenal glands, which are responsible for the release of adrenalin and noradrenalin. Overstimulation and exhaustion of the adrenal glands can cause chronic fatigue, which is a sign of holding on to fear. Other signs that you're holding on to fear are a decrease in libido, decrease in life force energy, chronic stress (you feel as if you're always in that fight-or-flight state), and anxiety disorders. To help yourself let go of fear, on the exhalation, make the sound *Chooooo,* the sound that's the antidote to fear. Visualize the color *black,* which helps to release fear. As you do this, think about the emotion that counteracts fear: *calm*. With every inhalation, imagine you are filling yourself up with a feeling of calm serenity.

To let go of impatience, anxiousness, and arrogance: These are emotions that settle into the heart. Signs that you are battling these emotions include rash decisions, driven personality, heart palpitations, and high blood pressure. A recent study (heartmath.org) showed that feeling love and appreciation actually had a measurable positive influence on the heart rate. To help yourself let go of impatience, anxiousness, and arrogance, on the exhalation, make the sound *Hawwwww*, the sound that counteracts these emotions. Visualize the color *red*, which helps to release impatience, anxiousness, and arrogance. As you do this, think about the emotions that counteract these: *love, joy, and happiness*. With every inhalation, imagine you are filling yourself up with love and a flood of joy.

To let go of confusion: Confusion stems from what is called the triple warmer or *san jiao* in Chinese medicine. This is what controls temperature and the energy from the brain, lungs, and heart that moves downward to the stomach, spleen, pancreas, liver, kidneys, and adrenals, where it meets the lower energy from the small and large intestines and sexual organs, which moves upward. When this action is balanced, you feel calm and are deeply relaxed. When it gets out of balance, you feel confusion. To help yourself let go of confusion, on the exhalation, make the sound *Heeeeee*, the sound that counteracts confusion. Visualize energy moving in a clockwise motion—*san jiao* doesn't have a color, but instead has this motion. This helps to release confusion. As you do this, think about the emotion that counteracts confusion: *calm*. With every inhalation, imagine you are filling yourself up with calm clarity.

OPEN UP

Finally, the most important thing you can do to emotionally cleanse is to open yourself to the hurt and pain, because if you don't acknowledge it, you cannot process it; and if you cannot process it, it will stay with you, doing its subtle internal damage. This can be incredibly difficult and you may need guidance, but here are some steps to follow:

1. Acknowledge the problem. Speak it out loud to yourself or to someone else.

2. Choose to let go of it. You have to choose this consciously. If you resist, there might be a reason you're holding on. Explore it. Are you gaining something by hanging on to negativity? How would the benefits of letting go outweigh the benefits of hanging on?

3. Be honest about it and others involved. Are others at fault? What role did you play in this? Lay it all out on the table.

4. Acknowledge the pain the problem has really caused. Has holding on to this problem hurt you? Has it hurt others? Are there many casualties, or just you? Look seriously at this. When you realize you're hurting others by holding on to something that no longer serves you, it can make it easier to let go.

5. Give yourself a 12- to 24-hour window to feel sorry for yourself. Cry, scream, mourn, get angry about how unfair it is, pound the pillows, vent to a friend. After that, it's time to move on and focus on solutions.

6. Surround yourself with love, whether from your family, your friends, or even your pets (or all of the above).

7. Learn to love you. This is easy to say and exceptionally hard to do if this is an issue for you, but imagine that you are a young child. You need someone to care for you, nurture you, and protect you. Be that person for yourself. Many people have found healing by becoming their own parent.

8. Fill the empty space with newfound love. Forge new connections, new friends, new bonds. Humans need connection.

9. Remember that you deserve peace and love, no matter what has happened in the past. Don't get stuck in the endless treadmill of self-pity. Jump off and get out there and reclaim your life.

The most important part of all of this advice is to allow yourself to feel, and then to give and receive love. The more you keep an open mind about who you are and what your life is about, the easier it will be to heal past wounds and heartache. Don't let negative emotions become disease in your body. Let that pain and ability to feel it make you more human, more compassionate, and more willing to forgive.

This crisis, whatever it is, will help you to become stronger in the end. You are learning to open up and take risks, and that's a valuable skill. Living in fear is not living. Being afraid of hurt is not living. Burying a failed relationship inside you is not living. Losing a loved one and refusing to let go of the person is not living. To reach your highest potential, you have to take risks and trust that you'll get through to the other side. It may feel like a mighty gamble, but it's the work of this life. As you continue to release, physically, emotionally, mentally, and spiritually, you'll become a greater person than you ever knew you could be. Feed your body with the nutrients it needs, feed your mind with the thoughts that strengthen it, and feed your heart and soul with openness, forgiveness, compassion, and love. *That* is living.

To take your first step toward emotional cleansing, try this next IF Prep Step:

....

INTERNAL PREP STEP #9

IF you are ready to cleanse your emotional life, once a week, perhaps on a Sunday or any day that has a more relaxed pace, sit back and think of something you can let go of. It can be something big, like a harmful relationship, or something little, like a bad habit or an obsessive thought. Spend some time thinking about that thing, and how to let it go so it doesn't hold you back any longer.

....

CHAPTER 10

Taking It to the Next Level with Colonics

COLON HYDROTHERAPY: THE TERM inspires all kinds of emotions. Fear, interest, curiosity. This is my specialty, and the subject that really inspires my passion, but it's also a subject that embarrasses people. It's funny that even though colonics have dramatically improved many lives, unlike other life-changing practices such as diets or exercise programs, nobody wants to get up on a public platform and shout: "Colon hydrotherapy saved me!" Nobody wants to admit he or she has had one, let alone that the person was curious about it.

Yet, every time I attend a swanky New York gala or star-studded Hollywood party, people pull me aside, urgently, furtively, to ask me questions—not about diet, not about cleansing, not about exercise, but about colonics. They have so many questions that are easy to answer, but apparently it must always be done in a whisper. And the number-one comment I get? "I wish you would write a book about this!"

Believe me, I *could* write an entire book on this subject, but since publishers are similarly uncomfortable with the subject, we'll keep it to a chapter—one big, beautiful chapter telling you everything you ever wanted to know about colon hydrotherapy. It's not necessarily an aesthetically pleasing subject, but it's near and dear to my heart; and in my opinion, it's one of the most powerful things you can do to improve your own internal fitness.

LET'S TALK ABOUT POOP

I may be somewhat unusual in that I am perfectly comfortable with the idea of poop talk. I can talk about it all day long. It's the last part of digestion, no less unnatural than the first part, when food goes into the mouth. Poop is simply the parts of food your body can't use mixed with the junk your body has to get rid of in order to stay clean and function properly. It's the end product, so to speak. If you don't poop (and if you don't poop enough, or fully), the stuff that's meant to go out is still in there, and that's not good. When poop sits in your colon for too long, the waste material can leak into your skin, causing acne; your sweat, causing body odor; your saliva, causing bad breath; and your kidneys, causing stinky urine. All of this can also make you look older than you are, and could even contribute to chronic disease. Chronic constipation can also have the following results:

Make you look fatter than you are, because your distended lower abdomen is actually sticking out from the stored poop rather than fat.
Cause lower back pain, from the pressure of backed-up poop.
Give you a stomachache. If you've ever rubbed your stomach and felt tender hard spots, that's often a sign that you are F.O.S. (full of sh*t).

Your digestive tract is really a tube that, aside from capillary action to extract nutrients, is (or should be) completely sealed off from the rest of your body. Food goes from the world into the tube and then out of the tube back into the world. It's when you get a backup in the plumbing that all the trouble begins. This chapter is about how to relieve that trouble and keep the food moving, sweeping up toxic materials and waste and getting them out of your body before they cause any trouble.

And lest you think your particular bathroom situation is anything to be ashamed of, just remember that *everybody poops*. Movie stars, supermodels, professional athletes, high-society ladies, CEOs, and the rest of us, too. And many people have some problems with their poop at some time in life (if not most of the time). So if you still think pooping is weird or gross, get over it—at least for the space of this chapter. Getting on a first-name basis with your own poop can help you monitor your health and digestion (which are one and the same), and can also help you to know what to do to make yourself feel better than you do right now (especially if you haven't been pooping!).

So let's get to your questions—about poop in general, and about colonics in particular. It's everything you didn't even realize you really wanted to know.

POOP FAQS
WHY DOES POOPING FEEL GOOD?

You know how, after a really good poop, you feel light as air, full of energy, and just darned *good?* You've seen those laxative commercials in which people are running and jumping around as if they've never felt so good in their lives. There's a very specific reason for this: Pooping stimulates the vagus nerve. This nerve runs from your brain to your bowels, and when you poop, it gets compressed and results in feelings of euphoria. In some cases and in some people, this vagus nerve stimulation can be too intense, resulting in more extreme reactions, such as nausea, sweating, or even fainting. Ironically, laxatives can have this effect because they make the poop come out so violently (so much for those happy people in the commercials—they should probably be doubled over in the bathroom). When things are operating as they should, it's a great feeling, but chemical laxatives aren't the way to get there. Improving your diet, getting more exercise, and (wait for it) *colon hydrotherapy* are much safer and more pleasant routes to that euphoric feeling.

I'VE HEARD YOU SHOULD SQUAT WHILE POOPING. WHAT'S UP WITH THAT, AND HOW WOULD I DO IT, ANYWAY?

Squatting is an essential part of pooping for any species that has legs. Animals do it, toddlers do it, and people in developing countries do it. You might have even done it while camping. In fact, until the mid-nineteenth century, everyone squatted to have a bowel movement. The only people who used a seated chair-like toilet were royalty and the disabled. But eventually seated toilets became the norm, equipped with increasingly comfortable seats (some even padded and heated) for doing our business. They may be "normal" to us now—but they're not conducive to internal fitness.

People naturally squat to poop because it's the ideal position for complete elimination. During a squat, the thighs come up and press on the left and right sides of the colon, pushing up the cecum on the right and the sigmoid on the left. This allows the colon to completely empty from these two areas. It's no coincidence that polyps and colon cancer are most prevalent in these areas—if you don't eliminate completely, feces can remain lodged in there, spending way too much time in direct contact with the colon wall and causing all kinds of trouble. Sit on a regular toilet and you get no natural pressure on these areas—and we expect them to just clean themselves out? No, we grunt and strain, but the problem is that this causes too much pressure in the wrong direction, forcing feces further into the cecum, even up into the appendix. Pooping shouldn't be so difficult, but it often is, because (1) we started eating food that's more difficult to digest, and (2) we stopped squatting.

Another great thing about squatting is that it protects the pudendal nerve from being overstretched. This is the nerve that carries sensations to the genitals, so let's just say it's in your best interest to keep it functional. Squatting also relaxes the puborectalis muscle, which usually is contracted in order to maintain continence of the bladder and rectum. Short version: You'll be less likely to have little bathroom accidents as you get older. Squatting also helps the ileocecal valve to seal closed while defecating, so the feces do not get pushed into the small intestine by a floppy valve. And, squatting supports the colon and its accompanying muscles, which form a sort of hammock inside your body. It's like supporting a hammock from below so it doesn't get too stretched out or break when a bunch of people pile into it. Without this support, the straining you have to do to dump those "people" out of the hammock can result in injuries like hemorrhoids, hernias, and pelvic organ prolapse.

The problem is that although our ancestors might have been agile and coordinated enough to balance on a toilet seat, most of us probably can't quite manage that level of acrobatic pooping. Fortunately, there are some clever inventions that can help you reclaim your natural right to squat without risking injury. You can use a toddler training potty, but if that's a little too strange for you, check out the Welles Step or the Squatty Potty (I use both of these at the Piper Center: see Resources), or similar inventions that elevate your feet to put you in a more natural position while you're still sitting. It's not exactly like squatting, but at least you'll get the angles right, to simulate squatting. Try it and you'll soon be enjoying a more complete and supported poop experience. Or, book a colonic. Colon hydrotherapists almost always have these in their bathrooms, so this would be a good time to give one a test drive.

MY POOP LOOKS WEIRD. IS IT TRYING TO TELL ME SOMETHING?

Yes! The color, size, consistency, texture, liquidity, solidity, and even the way poop comes out all tell you something about your health and the state of your digestion. Normal feces is made up of

75 percent water and 25 percent solid waste matter from our food and from our body's metabolic processes. This waste consists of dead bacteria, undigested fiber (such as cellulose), cholesterol/fats, inorganic substances (such as calcium and iron phosphates), and protein. Other substances include dead cells, bile pigment, bilirubin, and dead white and red blood cells. This is what gives poop its normal brown color. But poop color and shape can vary widely for many reasons and can tell us about our digestion or indigestion, infections, even cancer.

So what does a healthy poop look like? If you're reading this while eating breakfast, maybe stop and read this later, but here goes. Normal poop should:

Be easy to pass without straining.

Resemble a log or smooth, thick sausage.

Be at least 2 inches wide.

Be long! If you're internally fit, your poop could be 12 or even 18 inches long, with an easy exit and no strain or mess. Championship poop!

Fall into an S-shape in the toilet, which is the shape of the sigmoid region of the lower intestine, where it has been sitting until ready to exit.

Normal poop should not look like clumped-up balls stuck together or little hard pellets that require straining to pass.

Here is a famous chart called the Bristol Stool Chart, widely available on the Internet, that's designed to help doctors gauge health via the stool. It gives some very basic guidance about poop:

BRISTOL STOOL CHART*

Type 1	Separate hard lumps, like nuts (hard to pass)
Type 2	Sausage-shaped but lumpy
Type 3	Like a sausage but with cracks on the surface
Type 4	Like a sausage or snake, smooth and soft
Type 5	Soft blobs with clear-cut edges
Type 6	Fluffy pieces with ragged edges, a mushy stool
Type 7	Watery, no solid pieces. Entirely liquid.

*You can search online for "Bristol Stool Chart" for visuals.

Each of these types is pretty basic—nothing too unusual, but they each let you know certain things about your body. This is my interpretation (which may vary somewhat from the "official" interpretation often published with this chart):

Type 1: You might see type 1 if you are dehydrated. This is a sign of severe constipation. This type of stool has a very slow transit time and is common for people who are only having a bowel movement once a week, or even less often. I often see this type of stool in people with a lot of bad gut bacteria like *Candida*, especially in those who say they don't like to drink water. The person often feels full because a lot of gas is trapped behind the stool and won't come out until the stool is passed. These people tend to say they don't have gas, but really it's just trapped. Too much water is reabsorbed from the stool sitting in the colon for too long a period. During a colonic, this person is often surprised to know he or she has that much gas. This is also the type of stool common to incomplete bowel movements and straining. Some people have been this way for so long that they don't realize that it's not normal and how easy (and frequent) pooping is supposed to be!

Type 2: This type indicates constipation. The person may have a bowel movement every two or three days. This is what we call a stool traffic jam. Water intake is likely low. This type of stool is also frequently associated with moderate to severe malodorous gas, and the person usually has to strain to have a bowel movement. This can eventually lead to hemorrhoids that may or may not bleed, and incomplete bowel movements because of the constant straining. This is not the time to add fiber, which will only make matters worse. More water and probiotics as well as enzymes will do the trick, along with a softer diet.

Type 3: This type indicates mild constipation. You can see there is more stool volume—this is related to a higher fiber intake and more good gut bacteria—but there is still dysbiosis present. However, this type may still be associated with incomplete bowel movements. This type can also be due to a few days' worth of stool backed up and clumping together. Straining is present and can cause hemorrhoids to develop.

Type 4: This is the ideal type. It's a sign that you have adequate fiber and good gut flora. It breaks up when it hits the water. Some may form into a long snake-like shape. It shouldn't contain any mucus. A perfect S-shape comes from the stool having just been in the sigmoid area of the colon.

Type 5: This type of stool may be indicative of too fast of a transit time, which doesn't allow the water to be absorbed from the stool completely and so there are soft blobs of stool present. If a person is having two or three bowel movements a day and eats a relatively clean diet, this type of stool may be normal for the individual.

Type 6: This type is a messy stool. It's hard to get clean afterward by wiping. You might get this kind of stool when eating some kind of irritating food, such as overly spicy food or something that you are allergic to. It's also common after eating dairy products. You could also get this kind of stool when you have a mild case of gastroenteritis or anything else that irritates or inflames the gut lining. Even stress can cause this. Type 6 is also a common kind of stool to get after taking laxatives.

Type 7: Diarrhea. This can actually happen when you are constipated because hard stool impacted in the colon lining may trigger the body to send water to the colon, which flushes out the softer stool but leaves the hard, impacted stool. Being treated with a round or two of antibiotics can also be the culprit behind diarrhea. And I must mention that diarrhea can also be caused by food poisoning or even by parasites—yes, common in the United States! The scenario of having diarrhea while being severely constipated is all too common. You may feel a sense of relief after moving your bowels, even though you still have the problem that caused the diarrhea. I also find that many people immediately take diarrhea medicine because they want the diarrhea to stop (an obvious desire). Instead, I suggest letting it out, hydrating well, and looking at why you got the diarrhea in the first place.

I like the Bristol Stool Chart (page 156), but I also think it doesn't fully cover the complete range of stool I see as a colon hydrotherapist. You can benefit from even more information, especially if you don't recognize your own poop in the types above. I don't have pictures for mine (once you read the descriptions, you might be glad about that!), but I will give you full descriptions so you can have a better idea of what's going on inside. Consider it your special secret poop decoder! I call it the Piper Poop Chart. (Catchy name, right?) My Piper Poop Chart translates all kinds of different poop changes for you, so you can make the necessary lifestyle adjustments. A normal poop can resemble types 3 to 5 in any given adult, as we are all individuals on our own personal health journey.

You're welcome.

PIPER POOP CHART

Yes, you'll need to look in the bowl and smell what's there to understand it, but consider it all in the name of your good health. Here's how to interpret what you see:

COLOR CHANGES

Green poop: Your poop can turn green if you've been drinking a lot of green juice, especially made from vegetables and other things with high chlorophyll content, such as spinach, chlorella, spirulina, liquid chlorophyll, wheatgrass, and E3Live. Food with green dye can also turn your poop green. Did you have green beer on St. Patrick's Day? But poop can also turn green because of an infection from the bacteria *Clostridium difficile* in the GI tract, which can get started after taking a round of antibiotics for some other infection. If you haven't been eating anything green, tell your doctor or, better yet, collect a sample of your green poop.

Yellow poop: Yellow poop is a sign that you're not breaking down fat. Sometimes, yellow poop looks greasy, or you'll even see oil in the toilet water. If you poke the poop, it could move like jelly. This can happen if you are taking Orlistat (brand name Alli), because this drug keeps the body from absorbing some of the fat in your food, for the purpose of weight loss. There are other reasons you might not be absorbing fat, however. Your pancreas releases the enzyme lipase, which breaks down fat. If your poop is yellow and you're not on a diet drug, you might have a lipase deficiency or be having problems with lipase production. Try taking digestive enzymes with a higher amount of lipase to help your body better digest fat. If the problem continues, mention it to your doctor, to be sure it's not a sign of a more serious health issue, like fatty liver. Although yellow poop is most likely due to malabsorption issues, it is (rarely) a sign of a more serious condition, such as Gilbert's syndrome (a mild liver disorder), parasitic infestation, or pancreatic cancer. Hepatitis can also be a cause; when hepatitis is present, then yellow-colored stool may be accompanied by jaundice of the skin and eyes.

Bright red poop: Your poop can turn red from eating red foods like beets or with artificial red food coloring, such as that found in Kool-Aid. If your transit time is slow, your red poop might not show up for a few days after those beets, and you might forget you ate them. However, red poop can also be blood, which means you could have a bleeding hemorrhoid or something more serious, like bleeding in the GI tract or a perforated intestine. If you think you have blood in your poop, talk to your doctor. Hemorrhoids, polyps, and anal fissures can all be causes of bright red colored stool.

Black poop: This is usually from a high dietary intake of iron supplements or Pepto-Bismol, but it could also be caused by bleeding. By the time the blood comes out, it's turned dark because it's no longer fresh. Stool with this dark blood in it is called *melena*. If you're not taking iron or Pepto-Bismol, tell your doctor about black poop. Causes of melena include: bleeding stomach, duodenal ulcers, esophageal variances, peptic ulcers, a gastro-esophageal tear (called a Mallory-Weiss tear), trauma, and gastritis. Some foods can also cause tarry black stool, such as black licorice and beet.

Orange poop: Eating too much food that is high in beta-carotene, such as carrots or sweet potatoes, can turn poop orange. This can also happen with low bile production during digestion, caused by a weak or diseased liver, so if you don't think your orange poop is due to your diet, let your doctor know about it.

Clay poop: When your poop resembles gray clay, it can be due to a blockage in the bile ducts that release bilirubin, which is what gives poop its brown-yellow color. If your poop looks like clay, tell your doctor, or see a gastroenterologist to rule out any liver diseases, hepatitis, or bile duct blockage by gallstones.

White poop: Poop can turn white when you've had to drink that chalky white liquid that preps you for a barium enema, which you might need before an X-ray or CT scan. Otherwise, your poop might look white because of a bile duct blockage. White poop can also be a sign of inflammation. As with clay poop, tell your doctor.

Multi-colored poop: This poop appears in varying colors from dark brown to tan and maybe a hint of green. Multi-colored poop is often a collection of poop from several different meals. All it really means is that you probably aren't pooping often enough.

CONSISTENCY CHANGES

Sticky poop: When there's an abundance of mucus in the gut, especially in the presence of inflammation, poop can get sticky. Here's how it usually comes out: You might feel a sharp cramping pain that seems to take your breath away. You usher yourself to the bathroom and semi-liquid sludge exits. You do your deed and go to wipe. Hmm, feels slippery, so you wipe some more and more and more. Oh my, where are the baby wipes? You can't seem to get clean. This can happen because of too much mucus-forming food in the diet (like gluten and dairy products—especially dairy products!). Lactose-intolerant people also tend to have these types of stools, or this could be due to artificial sweeteners like sorbitol, or low-fat potato chips that can cause diarrhea.

Liquid poop: Oh, diarrhea, how we don't love you! This was in the Bristol Stool Chart (page 156), but permit me to run on (pun intended) a bit longer. In addition to constipation, diarrhea can be caused by many different things, but it is also often due to the body trying to get rid of dangerous bacteria or a virus as quickly as possible. This is why you sometimes have to sprint to the bathroom! I remember going to the movies with friends in St. Thomas years ago. They all ate at a new fast-food restaurant before the movie, and I met them there. During the movie, they all complained of cramping pain, and every one of them had to run out of the theater to the bathroom multiple times. They said the smell was foul and it burned like acid. Food poisoning often results in diarrhea, but so can the consumption of any food to which you're personally allergic or intolerant. Diarrhea is the body's way of saying, "No way, get this food out, and fast!"

Sheep poop or rabbit poop: When your poop comes out in dry little pellets, it's a sign of chronic constipation caused by dehydration. These pellets are hard to pass and you may feel like you didn't pass everything, leaving you feeling unsatisfied or not quite relieved. The colon's job is to absorb water and nutrients from the food you ate. The longer your stool stays in your colon, the more water is absorbed, making the stool drier and harder. By the time you get around to having a bowel movement a day or two or three later, you have sheep pellets. This is a sure sign to drink more alkaline water and eat more alkaline foods.

Oversize chocolate bar poop: When those pelleted poops get all stuck together with mucus, it means you have just enough water to try to form a normal poop but you're still dehydrated. This is often the kind of bowel movement that happens only a few times a week. It means you have a backup of meals in the colon. It's the result of a traffic jam. Drink more water and increase your raw vegetable and fruit intake for a little increase of fiber to sweep things out.

Bubbly poop: When there are air bubbles in your stool, you are experiencing a lot of fermentation in your colon. This means the bad bacteria have taken over and are competing for real estate with the good flora. When this happens, it's time to cut out sugar for a while (including natural sugars like sweet fruits but especially processed sugar) and increase raw vegetables and probiotics supplements or fermented foods!

Pencil poop: This poop is long and very thin—too thin to be the true diameter of the colon. It's smooth, soft, and may leave streaks in the toilet. This stool has some mucus in it. It's evidence that the colon is starting to be impacted because something is blocking the passageway, like old hardened waste, a polyp, or even a cancer-causing tumor (this would be rare, so don't get too worried). If this is not a regular thing for you, it might be from a meal with too much sticky food, especially dairy products such as cheese and ice cream. Pay closer attention to your diet, and add some fiber. If this type of poop persists and it doesn't make sense with your diet, it might be wise to check with a gastroenterologist.

POOP EXPERIENCES

The strainer: If you feel as if you need to poop and even feel the contractions but nothing comes out, you may want to strain to push out your poop. This is a sign that your colon muscles may be weak and the poop is hard and too large. You may get a stream of liquid, but you can tell there is something big in there and you aren't getting it out. You might give up, get up, and try to move on with your day, but just as you leave the bathroom, you get that urge again. Uh-oh! You better go sit back down and try again! This is a sign that you need to try a liquid feast diet to soften things up. You might also make that call to a colon hydrotherapist, or give yourself an enema.

The clogger: Keep the plunger handy! This is what happens when you haven't had a good poop in a few days. Suddenly, you know it's coming. You might break out in a cold sweat. You know you have to get to the bathroom quickly. When it does come out, it can be painful because it is large and in charge. You might have some bleeding. When it's all over, you feel relief but exhausted and empty, with no appetite. Too many of these experiences can cause hemorrhoids.

The anxiety pooper: As a child, you knew you did something wrong when your mom called you by all three names: "Tracy Ayn Piper, you get in here this instant!" Some people poop when they're anxious, and this often starts in childhood, with children who get diarrhea when they are nervous or anxious. It often continues into adulthood in susceptible people. Maybe you've been slacking off at work and then you hear news about potential layoffs. Maybe you are waiting for the loan from the bank that could save your home. Maybe you know you're going to have to have that dreaded conversation with your significant other. Maybe you simply have to give a speech. All these things can set off sudden cramping and the urge to run to the bathroom *now*. Emotions play a big part in bowel movements.

The aha poop: This is that perfect bowel movement—the one that feels satisfying and complete. When you're finished, you feel clear and energetic, as if you can do anything. This is the same feeling you'll get after a great colonic.

The I-need-a-colonic poop: Any kind of abnormal poop—in fact, any kind of poop other than an aha poop—is a sign that you could benefit from a colonic. Colonics make you feel clean and fresh, give you clarity and energy and vitality, increase hydration of the colon, increase muscle tone in the colon, reboot peristalsis to increase the transit time of slow stool, relieve bloat, gas, and abdominal discomfort, and help you to have an easy and complete bowel movement.

Stool odor: The odor of stool can change based on diet, bacteria, fungi, viruses, parasites, and inflammatory diseases such as Crohn's disease and chronic pancreatitis. When there is a foul-smelling odor in the stool, it is probably just something you ate, but it could also be from a more serious health issue, like intestinal obstruction or abdominal abscess. Foul-smelling stool can also be a symptom in patients with cystic fibrosis because of the mucus buildup in the lungs and digestive tract. As you learned earlier, the lungs and large intestines are paired, so one affects the other. Another situation that can also cause smelly stool is undigested food lingering in the colon over an extended period of time from people with leaky gut syndrome and celiac disease.

....

HERBS FOR INTERNAL FITNESS

Skullcap (*Scutellaria baicalensis*) is an herb that nourishes the nerves and muscles, especially in the colon. It's called a nervine because it relaxes and calms the body, making it good for relieving symptoms of IBS, Crohn's disease, leaky gut syndrome, and diverticulitis. There is also some evidence that this herb encourages cancer cell death. It's best taken as a tea or in a tincture form. Have one or two cups of tea. One of them should be right before bed. As a tincture, take 15 to 20 drops in hot water two or three times per day.

....

ABOUT GAS

Call it a fart, flatulence, a toot, a poot, or whatever you like. Whatever you call it, you can't escape it. Passing gas is just one of those things human bodies (and other animal bodies) have to do. It's part of life. People are often embarrassed to pass gas because of the sound it makes, but the silent ones are the real stinkers. You can't win, so you might as well learn to live with it. (And don't blame others for it, either—besides, we all know that "he who smelt it, dealt it.")

The amount of gas any given person emits on a given day varies pretty widely, but averages about 600 cubic centimeters in a healthy person with no gastrointestinal issues. That's a little more than a 20-ounce soda bottle's worth. However, a lot of factors can increase this pretty dramatically. For example, eating beans can increase gas production 175 cubic centimeters every hour! Gases that make up farts are nitrogen, hydrogen, oxygen, carbon dioxide, and methane. The amounts of each varies from person to person, based on the bacteria present in the gut and the diet of the individual. Here's a cute fact: Hydrogen and methane are flammable, so it is possible that you could get a flame going. (If you are a high school boy, you probably already know this.) The gases that give farts their not-so-pleasant scent are indole and skatole (both are the by-products of the digestion of meat), dimethyl sulfide and hydrogen sulfide (responsible for the rotten egg scent), methanethiol, volatile amines, and bacteria. Feces may also contribute to the scent if they are present in the rectum at the time of the fart.

So, do the farts of a raw foodist, vegan, vegetarian, and meat-eater all smell the same? No, because the chemical composition of farts varies based on the types of food eaten and digested.

We can minimize the pressure as well as the odor of gas based on what we eat and how much air we swallow, as well as the amount of good flora in the intestines. Gas-increasing foods include many healthy veggies I hope you won't cross off your list. Just chew them thoroughly to let your digestive enzymes do their work, and take digestive enzymes as well (see Chapter 11). Know your gassy foods, such as:

Asparagus	Chewing gum
Beans of all types	Chickpeas
Beer	Lentils
Broccoli	Milk and other dairy products in people
Brussels sprouts	who are lactose-intolerant
Cabbage	Onions
Carbonated beverages	Prunes
Cauliflower	Unsprouted nuts and seeds

ABOUT PEE

A third of the bodily waste (besides poop and gas) that your body must excrete is urine. Poop and gas are waste products from the colon, while urine is a waste product from the kidneys, but it's similarly affected by what you eat and drink. Pee is yellow because of urobilinogen, a by-product of bilirubin. When you don't drink enough water, this yellow color can get very dark; when you drink enough, your pee will be almost clear. B-vitamin supplements will turn urine a bright fluorescent yellow—but that's nothing to worry about.

Urine has a slight ammonia smell, but if you eat asparagus, you might smell sulfur, and if you have diabetes, your urine might smell like fruit. Urine should be clear, but can become cloudy due to bacteria, blood, or mucus. Severe pain while peeing could indicate a urinary tract infection, or kidney stones. See a doctor if it hurts to pee!

COLON HYDROTHERAPY FAQS

Now that you are well versed in the finer points of poop, let's move on to what to *do* about pooping problems. This, as you already know, is the subject nearest and dearest to my heart. I don't want you to fear colon hydrotherapy. In fact, I hope you'll give it a try, if you can find a good colon hydrotherapist (see Resources). This second half of the chapter should answer all your questions, including the ones you didn't even know you had.

DID YOU DREAM OF GROWING UP TO BE A COLON HYDROTHERAPIST? HOW DID YOU GET INTO THAT FIELD?

Actually, I dreamed of being a doctor, but when a friend of mine died from a burst diverticulum at age thirty-eight, even though he was having a bowel movement every day, I got scared—and curious. The more I learned, the more I realized that this was something people needed help with, and I could be the one to help them.

SO, DOWN TO THE BASICS: WHAT EXACTLY IS A COLONIC? IS IT THE SAME THING AS AN ENEMA, OR DIFFERENT?

Colonics and enemas are similar. They are both safe, effective methods for removing waste matter stored in the large intestine (colon) with the use of water (rather than drugs). Filtered and temperature-regulated water is introduced into the colon via a tube, to soften and loosen up the waste matter and to hydrate the colon in order to stimulate evacuation of waste matter via the action of peristalsis.

The difference between them is that you can do an enema yourself with a tube and a bag, and the enema cleanses the lower part of the colon. You put in the water, hold it, then go to the toilet to let it out (see page 132 for more details). A colonic therapist uses a machine to send the water higher up into the colon and then to evacuate the waste matter through a tube, so you never even have to see it or smell it. It goes through the process of filling and emptying the colon multiple times. It is cleaner and more thorough, but it requires a knowledgeable, trained, and competent colon hydrotherapist to operate the machine and perform the colonic safely.

WHO GETS COLONICS?

Almost anyone could get a colonic (see the next question for contraindications). Some people get them regularly to prevent digestive issues and to maintain or lose weight. Others get them to help with health issues they already have. Anyone suffering from constipation, diarrhea, alternating constipation and diarrhea, acne, bad breath, skin issues, mental fogginess, fatigue, unexplained aches and pain, blurred vision, bloating, excessive gas, recurrent urinary tract infections, yeast infections, body odor, peeling of the skin, dandruff, parasitic infestations, Candida, headaches, colds and flus, multiple sclerosis, rheumatoid arthritis, hemorrhoids, anal itching, rashes, Lyme disease, lupus, or who is preparing for a colonoscopy can benefit from colon hydrotherapy.

WELL, THEN, WHO SHOULDN'T GET A COLONIC?

I think colonics are great for *almost* anybody, but there are a few situations in which colonics are not appropriate. Do not get a colonic if you have any of the following conditions, unless your physician gives you the okay:

Anemia (severe)

Aneurysm

Carcinoma

Cardiac disease

Cirrhosis of the liver

Congestive heart failure

Crohn's disease

Diverticulitis (acute or severe)

Epilepsy/seizures

First or third trimester of pregnancy (if supervised by a doctor, it's okay in the third
    trimester)

Fissures/fistulas

GI hemorrhage/perforation

Hemorrhoids (when excessive bleeding is present)

Hernia (incarcerated abdominal)

Kidney dialysis

Renal failure

Renal insufficiency

Surgery (within 6 months)

Tumors

Ulcerative colitis (severe)

DOES IT HURT? IS IT UNCOMFORTABLE? IS IT EMBARRASSING?

No, colonics should never hurt. If you follow the important preparatory guidelines before the colonic, there should be no need to worry, but if your diet has been filled with not the most stellar of foods—if you ate a lot of gaseous foods, dairy products, or drank alcohol before your session—you might feel a little uncomfortable or there may be some intermittent cramping. It may feel like you have to go to the bathroom, but then you'll get this "ahhh" feeling as gas bubbles and other residue flow out.

As for being embarrassing, different people have different levels of comfort with the process, but in terms of what the colon hydrotherapist does, your dignity is preserved at all times. You're completely covered, and only when the insertion is occurring is any part of your body slightly exposed. You can do the insertion yourself with the aid of the therapist, if you prefer. That is, some clients don't need the therapist to guide them and can insert themselves. A larger-bodied person may need some help. Some other people do not want to deal with doing it at all and may give the therapist permission to insert for them, whether they're able to reach themselves or not. They may simply be uncomfortable inserting the speculum. A good colon hydrotherapist will do everything possible to make you feel at ease and will adjust the process to accommodate you.

HOW DO COLONICS HELP WITH CONSTIPATION, EXACTLY?

Other than jump-starting weight loss, chronic constipation is probably one of the main reasons people seek colonics. Colonics help with constipation in two ways: They ease the immediate problem by softening and hydrating everything so it moves out more easily, and they solve the chronic issue by helping to strengthen, tone, and flex the colon muscles so they get stronger and can do their job more effectively.

I've had many clients come to me with the complaint of chronic constipation. One was Addie, a thirty-year-old woman who was having only about one bowel movement per week.

After she started regular colonics, she began to go on her own more often, but still wasn't having a movement every day. After five colonics in two weeks, she went from every other day to having a daily movement. During her treatments I noticed that she had marks on her ankles from her socks, which is a sign of fluid accumulation, so I began giving her lymphatic massage before her colonics. After just two sessions of massage, Addie's colonic releases became more abundant, and she had a permanent shift. Now she has one to two movements per day. She's drinking more water and having three or four glasses of vegetable juice every day, taking digestive enzymes and probiotics, and making shakes with chia seeds. She continues to have regular lymphatic massages and a weekly colonic, just to keep her system clean and her colon toned. She looks and feels great!

I'VE HEARD COLONICS CAN HELP YOUR SKIN, BUT WHAT DOES ONE HAVE TO DO WITH THE OTHER?

It's true! Toxic buildup in the body has to go somewhere, and the skin is your largest organ of elimination, so when toxins come out through the skin, acne can be the unpleasant result. I had a twenty-five-year-old client with terrible acne that wouldn't resolve with any of the products her dermatologist had prescribed. I suggested she begin a regimen of colonics and that she try the Piper Protocol to improve her diet. Within a month, we saw significant change in her skin. Her acne had almost completely cleared up, and she also said she had a renewed energy and clarity.

ARE COLONICS SAFE? DO I NEED TO SEE MY DOCTOR BEFORE GETTING A COLONIC?

Yes, colonics are safe. Like everything in life, there are some risks, but it's rare that anyone has a problem. As with a colonoscopy, there's a slight risk of a perforated colon, but there are only a few known cases in the history of colonics, and having a knowledgeable and certified colon hydrotherapist greatly decreases the risk.

Some people also worry about cross-contamination. Do not worry! We use disposable speculums and the colonic device filters the water three times before it enters the client. If a filter isn't clean, the device won't work correctly, so you don't have to worry that the practitioner didn't change the filter.

If you have a serious health issue, however, you should definitely tell your colon hydrotherapist about it. If you will feel better asking your doctor if it's okay to get a colonic, please do so. Go over the contraindications and if any apply to you, definitely talk to your doctor. He or she may or may not give you permission to go ahead with it, and may want to monitor you afterward.

BUT WHAT ABOUT DEHYDRATION AND ELECTROLYTE IMBALANCE? IS THAT A RISK?

Many people wonder about loss of electrolytes during a colonic because some websites list this as a "risk." But having a colonic is not the same as having a bout of diarrhea. When a person has diarrhea, the lining of the colon secretes large quantities of water and electrolytes in response to a chemical reaction and/or in response to chronic constipation. When the colon increases in peristalsis action, then the water is forced out of the colon at a high rate in the form of diarrhea. A colonic is a fluid exchange in which the colon is rehydrated. Electrolyte and mineral loss is equivalent to what you would experience during a regular bowel movement. When the colonic is over, the therapist gives the client a probiotic and trace minerals to replace what might have been displaced during the colonic. Do you do that every time you have a bowel movement?

Research supports this practice. A 1989 study, "Effects of Colon Irrigation on Serum Electrolytes," showed no patients experienced any clinically significant symptoms or disturbances from colon hydrotherapy. This study was performed by the National College of Naturopathic Medicine in Portland, Oregon.

Even though the minerals and electrolytes you could lose from a colonic are no more than you would lose from drinking alcohol or coffee, or taking some medications, sweating a lot, or even being stressed, we encourage our clients to eat potassium-rich food after a colonic (such as vegetable broth, green leafy vegetables, or a banana).

WON'T I BE WASHING AWAY ALL MY GOOD GUT BACTERIA WITH A COLONIC?

This is another common worry. I like to compare this scenario to one of my favorite movies, *300*. I look at the ten million bad soldiers as the bad bacteria and the three hundred Spartans as the good microflora. No matter how good the three hundred soldiers are, they cannot beat out the bad soldiers (bacteria) when they're vastly outnumbered. Wiping out almost all the soldiers, including the good guys, evens the odds significantly, so the remaining good guys have more of a chance. Supplementation post-colonic with probiotics and fermented food gives the good microflora a chance to rebuild in a more hospitable environment, with fewer bad guys for competition. In other words, sometimes you have to sacrifice some good guys for the greater good.

CAN I HAVE A COLONIC DURING MY MENSTRUAL CYCLE?

Yes! This is a time when the body is naturally detoxing, so it's actually a great time for a colonic as long as you feel comfortable with your therapist.

CAN I RETURN TO WORK OR BE ACTIVE AFTER MY COLONIC?

Yes. Most of my clients come before work, during their lunch hour, or before or after a long flight (air travel tends to be constipating).

WILL I HAVE ENERGY AFTER MY COLONIC?

This can go both ways. If the majority of the release is gas and mucus, the client usually feels as if he or she has had a massage and wants to relax. If the client releases an abundant amount of stool, that person can have a surge of energy, perhaps wanting to go to a spinning class or on a cleaning spree.

OKAY, YOU'VE CONVINCED ME. IF I WANT TO TRY A COLONIC, HOW DO I FIND A CERTIFIED COLON HYDROTHERAPIST?

Check the list of certified colon hydrotherapists through the International Association for Colon Hydrotherapy, at I-act.org. Click on "Referrals," and that will lead you to a link where you can search by location. If there's no one listed near you, ask your local holistic health practitioners for recommendations. Be sure to get someone who comes well recommended and has a lot of experience. The therapist should never leave the room during a colonic so you always feel safe and supervised. If you can't find someone who is certified and whom you feel comfortable with, stick with enemas for now and keep your ears open for news of a certified and experienced person who might move into your area. Also, be sure to ask any therapists you're considering working with what kind of system he or she uses.

WAIT, THERE ARE DIFFERENT KINDS OF EQUIPMENT? WHAT SHOULD I KNOW?

The equipment used today for colon hydrotherapy is regulated by the FDA (this has been in effect since 1970), which recognizes various types of colon hydrotherapy equipment. Class 1 types include self-administered systems such as an enema bag or bucket (Colema Boards kit). Class 2 types are considered medical devices and can legally be used only by a certified colon hydrotherapist and must be in compliance with manufacturer and country regulations. Class 2 devices include both closed systems (Dotolo, HydroSan, Aquanet) and open systems (Libbe, Angel of Water). The equipment is what doctors prescribe before and/or after colonoscopies, sigmoidoscopies, and certain types of surgery.

Open colonic systems were influenced by the original type of gravity-based methods or the well-known Woods Method. The two most popular open systems are the Libbe and the Angel of Water. The water is temperature-controlled and filtered to be sure it is completely clean. The speculum inserted by the client is the diameter of a pencil and is inserted only 2 to 3 inches. The device has a hole to allow waste matter to exit the body around the tube and flow down into the drain. I find these two devices very helpful for severely constipated clients who may have such large stool that they may need to pass more than can be accommodated by a pencil-size tube. Also, some multiple sclerosis clients may "spill" and the open system may be helpful to them and allow them to push out the stool around the tube, since the stool tends to be very mucus-filled and may clog a regular speculum.

The Gravity System or Woods Method was one of the original methods, and there are many colon hydrotherapists around the world that still use this method. It employs a five-gallon bucket suspended from a shelf. The therapist hooks up filters to it as well as a temperature control on the outside of the bucket, and the water flows down through the tube via the force of gravity.

Closed colonic systems are influenced by the design of a faucet and are the most advanced and precise, in my opinion. This is the type I use in my office. (I use the Dotolo Toxygen). The closed system has three types of filters to be sure the water is thoroughly cleaned, and it has a temperature control and a water control, so the therapist has precise control over the rate at which water flows in and out. I like this method, as I'm able to retrain the colon by doing short fills (like biceps curls for the colon) to strengthen it. I'm not a big fan of pushing the stool out, since most people do that at home rather than allow the peristalsis to move the stool down in a rhythmic fashion. I train the client to not push, because that may lead to hemorrhoids or a hernia, depending on how strong or weak the colon and stomach walls are.

WHAT SHOULD I DO TO PREPARE FOR A COLONIC?

I'm so glad you asked, because this is very important. For two to three days prior to your appointment, you increase your water intake and/or intake of other healthy fluids, such as herbal tea and fresh juice. (Coffee, black tea, energy drinks, soda, and milk don't count.) What you eat is also important for best results. First priority are lots of non-gaseous, colonic-friendly veggies. These include carrots, beets, string beans, arugula, romaine, kale, all leafy green salads, spinach, buckwheat sprouts, and sunflower sprouts. Also eat fruits, especially the less sweet fruits like berries and melons.

What's more important is what you shouldn't eat. The more gaseous the food you eat, the more discomfort you'll have during the colonic, so for two days prior to your colonic, try to avoid gaseous foods (and others that are hard on the digestive system), including the following:

Cabbage, lentils, beans, broccoli, cauliflower, Brussels sprouts, asparagus, bok choy
Dairy products like milk, cheese, yogurt, and ice cream
Soy products like tofu, tempeh, and soy milk
Red meat like beef, pork, and lamb (not gaseous but hard on the digestive system)
Fried food, junk food, fast food (burgers, pizza, fried chicken), and soft drinks
Alcohol
Anything made from refined flour and sugar (such as pastries, crackers, pretzels, white
    bread, bagels, cookies, empanadas, and candy), which can be gaseous for some and
    hard on the digestive system, as well as feeding the bad bacteria in your colon

If you eat some of this stuff, it's no reason to cancel the colonic. You'll still benefit, but there may be a bit more discomfort and a tremendous amount of gas. Colonics are most efficient when the primary need is eliminating waste rather than a bunch of gas. Don't you want to get your money's worth?

WHAT WILL HAPPEN WHEN I GO TO MY APPOINTMENT? CAN YOU WALK ME THROUGH THE PROCESS?

Absolutely. Every colon hydrotherapist does things a little bit differently in the details, but the basic procedure will be the same. This is how I do it in my office:

1. First you'll be greeted and given an extensive intake form to fill out. Your practitioner will go over your form with you, and may have additional questions. This is the time to disclose any health issues and voice any concerns.

2. After all questions on both sides are answered, you'll go to the bathroom and empty your bladder, then return to the treatment room. You disrobe from the waist down, lie face up on the provided sheet or towel with the cover given to you, and wait for the colon hydrotherapist to return.

3. When the practitioner comes back into the room, she'll ask if you're allergic to anything, unless that was already discussed in the intake form. I always begin my sessions by having the client smell an essential oil. Not everyone does this, but many of us do because essential oils are powerful facilitators of the colonic process. The scent activates the olfactory nerve, which sends a signal to the limbic system, which sends a feedback signal to the hypothalamus and then to the enteric nervous system, which signals the colon to release.

    The oil the practitioner chooses for you will depend on whether you are stressed or anxious, or if you noted that you were particularly gaseous. For example, at the beginning of the session, I open the sinuses with eucalyptus oil. If someone is nervous, I may use lavender, which is relaxing. Clove, ginger, and peppermint oil all help to release gas. If the client tends to be cold, I use a warming oil to increase circulation and get things moving. If the person is hot and inflamed, I use a cooling oil, such as peppermint. Further along in the session, if the client has had dairy or other mucus-forming foods, I would use thyme. If we're working on specific emotions, such as anger, I use a blended oil, such as Anger Management blend. If the client is stressed, I use Stress Relief blend and end with lavender or Emotional Rescue blend.

4. The practitioner will have you relax while she massages the area over your colon. This is very important, as it prepares the colon for the session. The massage is in a clockwise direction, going a bit deeper with each circle. To open the colon, I start at the sigmoid area. Most people in demonstrations I see start on the cecum. There's a reason to my madness. If there is hardened stool close to the exit point, it makes sense to me to soften it up and move it down so the other waste to follow can exit the body easily. I start right above the pubic symphysis, massaging in little clockwise circles or in a downward motion,

moving slowly all the way up the left side, turning the corner to go across the navel area, continuing across to the right side corner, and massaging upward, back to where I started. The purpose is to move everything toward the left side, where the exit is.

5. After calming the nervous system and priming the body for the session, the therapist opens the lymphatic ducts. We've already talked about the lymphatic system in Chapter 1, so you know how important it is (you're doing your homework and dry-brushing every day, right?). The culmination of the lymphatic system is in the abdomen, where all the garbage is dumped into the colon, so stimulating the major lymph nodes is essential to wake them up so they can start dumping. To accomplish this, I do a mini-lymphatic massage to get things moving (and during the colonic, I'll work on the abdominal area to stimulate more lymph to be released).

6. Now it's time. Don't stress! The machine regulates the temperature of the water and filters it so it's always clean. The speculum that goes into your body is disposable, so you'll be the only one who will ever use it. You'll turn on your left side, and you can insert the speculum into your rectum yourself, or you can ask the therapist to help you or to do it for you. Don't be embarrassed! Your therapist has done this many times before. Once the speculum is in, some therapists will have you turn on your back immediately, but I prefer keeping you on your side most of the time, at least for the first half of the session. I have performed about 30,000 colonics, and I believe this is the best way, as it gives the therapist a chance to see what works for each individual. As a Licensed Massage Therapist and a Licensed Acupuncturist, I use acupuncture points and massage techniques to help me to help my clients have a better release, so I like to have access to the back.

7. As the therapist works the machine, water will slowly flow into you and back out. There is a back flow valve on the speculum that does not allow the clean water and dirty water to mix, so nothing that comes out will go back in. The client may hold the water in for a few seconds, then it is released. The client tells the practitioner if she feels full or not and of any discomfort, so the practitioner knows when to release.

Everyone is different and every colonic is different every time. If you think something doesn't feel right, just say so. If there's a lot of gas coming out, you may not be able to hold the water in long enough to soften the stool, and that may become uncomfortable. Just try to relax and let it go. A lot of gas tells me that there's some serious fermentation going on in the colon, whether it's from lack of good flora, bad food combining, undigested food particles, excess gas trapped from carbonated drinks or gum chewing, or all the above.

8. At first, the water coming out will be clear with gas and sometimes mucus. You don't have to look, but you can if you want to. Sooner or later the water will begin to turn color, meaning the waste is being released. If you're 15 minutes into the colonic and the water is still clear, no waste matter has been released, then I know there is significant dehydration going on and I need to address fluid intake with you. Don't make the mistake of thinking it means you don't have anything to release in there. Trust me, you do! It's just not letting go yet.

9. When the water does change color, it might stay light or get progressively darker, or change in consistency. This tells me how well the water is softening the stool and it is getting ready to exit. When the stool finally starts coming out, that's when it really gets exciting! I always watch for the consistency and color, because these things tell me a lot. These are some of the things I look for:

- If the stool is long and thin like a pencil, that means the stool is probably blocked against the wall by older hardened stool that doesn't want to come out, or it is a case of spastic colon.

- If the stool comes out like pebbles, I know there has been long-term constipation.

- If the stool releases like diarrhea, unformed and with undigested food, it tells me that you probably have leaky gut syndrome and are not digesting your food properly.

- A lot of mucus tells me that the colonic acid/alkaline balance is out of sorts. You have too much acid and the colon is probably inflamed. The body is trying to protect you by releasing mucus to coat and protect you from the inflammation.

- Intermittent gas leaving in large bubbles and small bubbles on top of the tube can be so plentiful that it looks like foam. This is a sign of excessive fermentation or yeast overgrowth (candida).

- Is the stool too large to pass through the speculum? This may be due to days of constipation or weeks of not going to the bathroom. Some people may be so backed up that no stool is released through the entire session, or only during the last 5 minutes. This happens because it has taken that much time and water to soften things up enough to dislodge them from the colon wall. Large stool is no reason to stop the colonic. On the contrary, the water will soften and break it up so it can be released more easily. (This could take more than one session.)

- If the stool is dark, thick, and sludgy, and moves slowly through the tube as if it doesn't want to go, *ahhh*—this is the deep dark old stuff that's very toxic to the body. When this is releasing, the client usually becomes very quiet or cries, as he may be releasing deep-seated emotional trauma. Sometimes memories come up and stagnant emotional energy releases at the same time. When this happens, I try to keep the client thinking about releasing what no longer serves him. During an emotional release colonic, I have the client talk about an issue that may be bothering him, in order to get this response. Sometimes the client may want to release, but the emotion or trauma is buried deep and it may take a few more colonics to get to the core.

10. When the colonic is over, the therapist will remove the speculum, clean off any excess lubrication, tell you where the bathroom is, and leave the room. You'll go to the bathroom, at which time you'll probably have more release of fluid, poop, and gas. Don't worry about hurrying. Take as much time as you need. Nobody is standing outside the door tapping his or her feet.

    When you sit on the toilet, this is where you apply the squatting technique. There will be a Welles step or Squatty Potty (see Resources) in the bathroom that you'll pull close to the toilet. Put your feet on it so you're in a squatting position. Now you're ready to release the rest. When you're finished, you get dressed and come on out. It's very important, however, to really finish. Sometimes people feel rushed, and they might leave before they have really released everything that is now ready to come out. At the Piper Center, we always urge the client to walk to the elevator after leaving the bathroom, and then come back again. A brisk walk is good. If there is anything lingering in the "corners," the movement can shake it loose. A second trip to the bathroom might be necessary (and is perfectly fine, and common). Better to go back to the bathroom than suddenly have to find a bathroom when you've left our office and you're in the car or on the train.

11. After the first session, the therapist will recommend a schedule for future colonics that is based on what he or she saw and assessed during the first colonic. The therapist might recommend some lifestyle changes based on your colonic, such as increasing your fluid intake, changing your diet, or taking supplements that might help with some of the issues that were noticed. You'll get an after-care sheet that tells you how to continue detoxifying and rebuilding. (If the therapist has a reason to think you might have a health issue based on what was seen, you may be referred to a medical doctor for blood work and testing or a gastroenterologist for an evaluation and/or colonoscopy.)

12. You go home and enjoy the rest of your day feeling lighter and cleaner! And consider going back.

HOW MANY TIMES DO I NEED TO HAVE A COLONIC? AND HOW OFTEN?

Everyone is different, so how many colonics you need will depend on your individual issues and preferences. However, it's customary to have a minimum of three colonics close to each other. If nothing comes out in the first session, or the session is quite minimal in its release, the practitioner might have the client come back the next day, or skip a day and then return. Colonics are not only about releasing waste matter but also about hydrating, strengthening, and toning the colon for better internal fitness. This increases the strength of the peristalsis, speeds the transit time for sluggish colons, and slows it for fast-acting colons, so even if you don't release much, you're still getting benefits.

Once an issue is resolved, it is important that you continue to pay attention to the effect of any dietary changes, such as new efforts to avoid drinking while eating or ways to combine foods for best digestion. It's also important to keep your meals (and life!) as regular as possible and continue to take enzymes and probiotics once or twice a day so you repopulate good gut bacteria and shore up the immune system. When you are feeling like you've got things under control, then it's fine to come in every four to six weeks. Some people like to come in for a colonic every change of season and do three sessions in a row. I understand this impulse, but personally, I'd rather get the grime out more often than wait until it has hardened up and we have to work harder and do multiple sessions to get it all out. This is why I recommend that my clients get on a monthly colonic maintenance schedule. Of course, maintaining your own gut health is your responsibility. The therapist is just there as a guide, to give you a tune-up whenever you decide you need one.

BUT WON'T TOO MANY COLONICS MAKE MY COLON LAZY, SO THAT I WON'T BE ABLE TO POOP WITHOUT THEM?

To the contrary! It's constipation that weakens the colon, because too much waste in the colon weakens and stretches the muscles and impairs the function of the colon. By emptying the colon of impacted waste, we reshape the colon over time so it is healthier, stronger, and more rhythmic in its action. This will assist you with the entire digestive process in the future. The more you tone with colonics, the better your body will work.

WHAT SHOULD I DO AFTER MY COLONIC?

It might surprise you to learn that I don't recommend raw food after a colonic. It takes some time for your body to adjust, so you want to stick to foods that are warming, that increase circulation, and that are easy to digest. You can drink a vegetable juice or a blended juice/smoothie after your colonic with ginger and/or cayenne pepper, for warmth. This will provide the body with quick nutrition and electrolytes. A warm pureed soup that is easy to digest also works, and try to get in as much alkaline water as you possibly can. (Remember not to drink water with your meals—drink it between meals on an empty stomach.) The longer you stay on light liquid or blended foods, the longer you can continue the detoxification of the colon. You can eat salad if you spice it up to give it some warmth, with some hot pepper or ginger dressing. I like to sprinkle some chia seeds or ground flax on my soup or in my blended smoothie for added fiber.

Fiber will give your stools bulk, control your sugar cravings, and also help to keep your cholesterol low. It also acts as food (prebiotics) for the microflora in the colon. Make sure to drink a lot of water, too. Increased fiber should always be paired with increased water. Limit your consumption of refined and processed foods after your colonic (and forever, if you can!).

Just as you're staying away from bad foods, stay away from negative thoughts and reactions. This increases acidity and leads to inflammation. Let your body benefit from its new clean state. Don't cloud it with negativity.

Finally, after a colonic, you're perfectly positioned to begin the Piper Protocol. So how about it? You're clean, you're toned, and you've been practicing your Piper Prep Steps. Are you ready to jump in and change your life? Let's do it together!

Whether you're ready for a colonic or not, I still have an assignment for you this week. Add it to the other nine IF Prep Steps you've been doing so far, and voilà! You have ten awesome new habits that have prepped your body for the Piper Protocol:

....

INTERNAL PREP STEP #10

IF you're serious about your internal fitness, it's time to turn around and face the music. In my world, that's a metaphor for turning around and checking out your poop before you flush. Gross? Maybe, but there's a lot of useful information in that toilet bowl, so take a good look. Consult the Piper Poop Chart (page 158) for clues about your health based on what's coming out. Let this be one more way for you to monitor your health.

....

PREPARE TO BE TRANSFORMED!

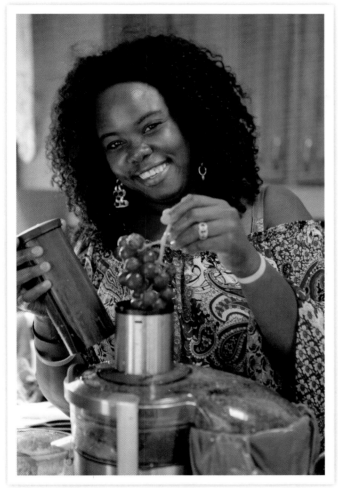

Juicing is easy with a centrifugal juicer like this one.

I've helped movie stars, celebrities, professional athletes, and CEOs achieve optimum health, and now I want to help you. Let's recalibrate your body and rejuvenate your natural beauty using the power of living foods, juicing, and other physical and emotional therapies (from lymphatic massage and deep breathing to letting go of emotional baggage). *The Piper Protocol* includes dozens of techniques and tried-and-true tricks integrated into a step-up plan that starts where you are now and takes you somewhere you've never been before—somewhere beautiful, vibrant, and full of life's energy.

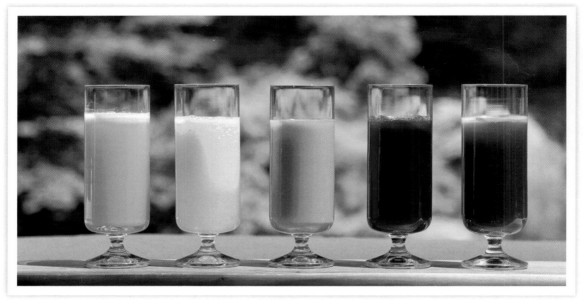

Drink the rainbow! Freshly squeezed juice can be an everyday part of your life.

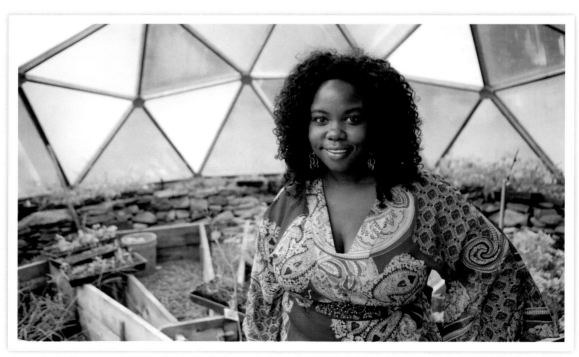

In a greenhouse in upstate New York, we grow many fresh veggies for juicing and herbs and vegetables for meals. Stress relief and concentrated nutrition in one awesome hobby!

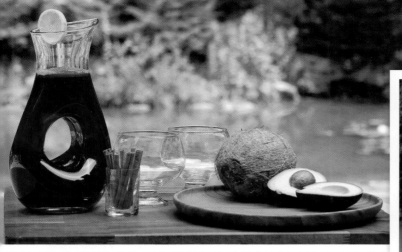

A carafe of juice, a coconut, and an avocado?
Sounds like my kind of happy hour!

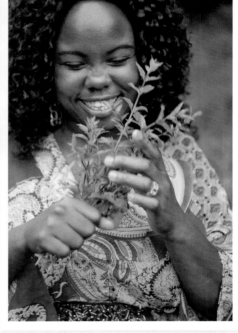

I love the aroma of freshly picked herbs.

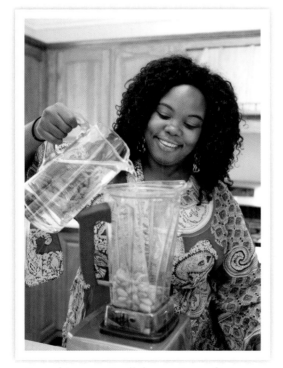

Smoothies contain all the nutrients of juice,
plus all the fiber of veggies and fruits—and
what could be easier than throwing fresh
produce into a blender and pushing a button?

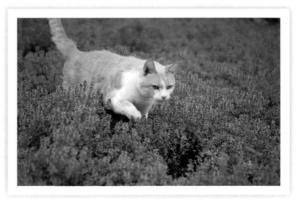

This is Simon, creeping through the flowers on
the farm. He's a mighty hunter!

Are you ready to get started? In the first two weeks, you'll gradually ease into the Piper way of life by improving the quality and gently decreasing the amount of the animal products in your diet. Following the principles of food combining, you'll also be grain-free during these two protein weeks, which will help you slim down and feel energized. You'll enjoy sumptuous dishes like Jamaican Jerk Chicken and Caribbean Beef Stew, and you'll also fill half your plate with bright, delightful, and energizing vegetables in Week 1. By Week 2, you'll be eating 80 percent veggies and just 20 percent animal protein. Don't forget all the amazing freshly squeezed juices and flavorful smoothies you'll also get to indulge in during the first two weeks!

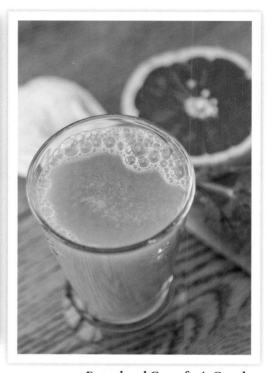

Fennel and Grapefruit Guzzler
A very alkalizing drink first thing in the morning that's cooling and calming on the digestive system.

Jingslinger Jing Jam
This recipe is by my friend in L.A. She makes sure I have a batch as soon as I land. It's divine!

MY GO-TO SUNDAY MEALS . . .

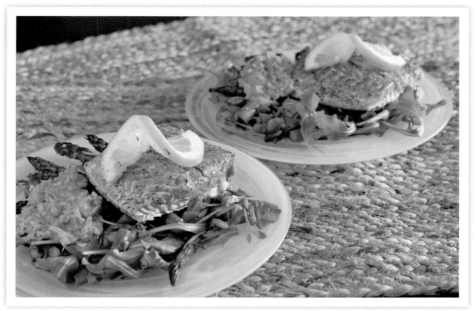

Salmon with Sautéed Asparagus and Arugula Salad

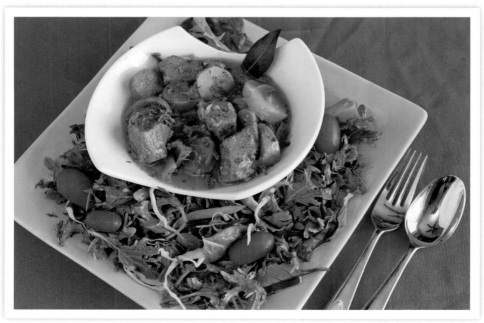

Caribbean Spicy Beef Stew

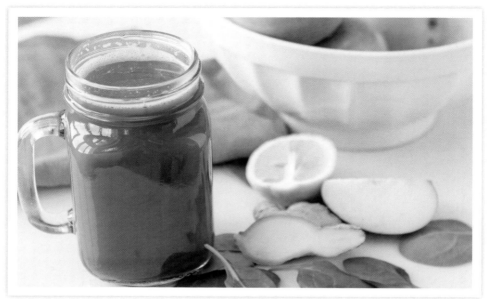

Green Apple Aid *A pick-me-up refresher for any time of day.*

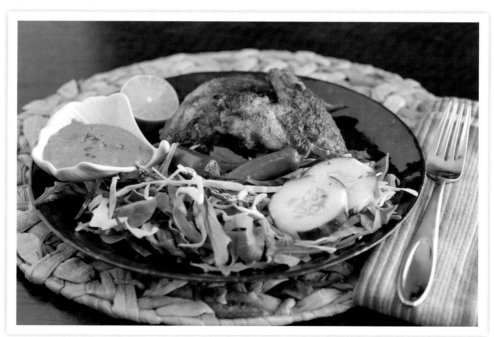

Jamaican Jerk Chicken *My favorite lunch dish! My friends know I jerk almost everything . . .*

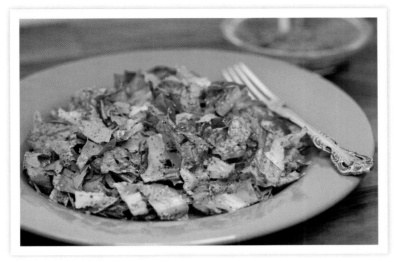

In weeks 1 and 2, always add lots of leafy greens to your meals.

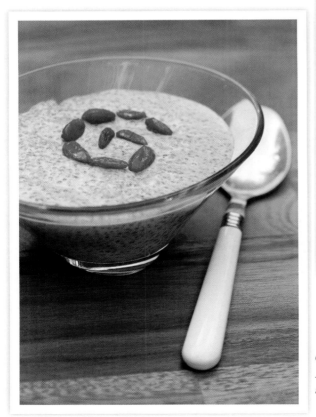

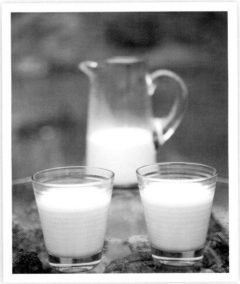

Homemade Almond Mylk
A better way of getting calcium.

Chia Seed Pudding
I'm not a big dessert gal, but this is my midday snack on the weekends.

WEEK 3: 80:20 VEGGIES AND GRAINS

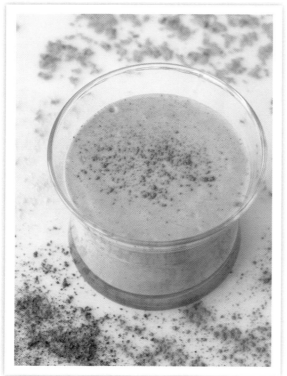

No-Pumpkin Pie Smoothie

Welcome to Week 3! You'll make a fairly dramatic but life-enhancing transition this week, from an 80:20 low-carb diet that can include animal proteins to an 80:20 diet of vegetables and delicious grains. You probably miss grains by now, and this is your chance to get really creative. From homemade Bucky Burgers to Caribbean Wild Rice, you'll indulge in a flavorful plant-based diet that will feel calming and satisfying. And just watch the pounds melt away! This is a good place to settle after *The Piper Protocol*—the gentlest and most nourishing way to eat.

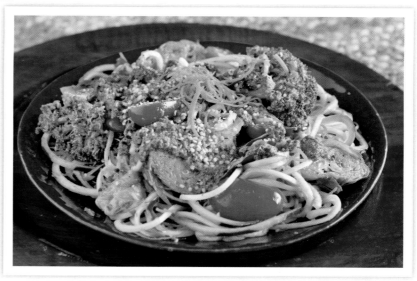

Jingslinger Tuscan Florentine *Veggie Italiano.*

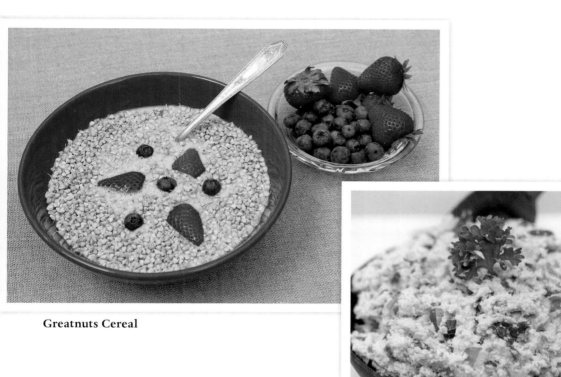

Greatnuts Cereal

Deviled Eggless Salad
*Delicious on a rice cake or
wrapped in baby collard greens.*

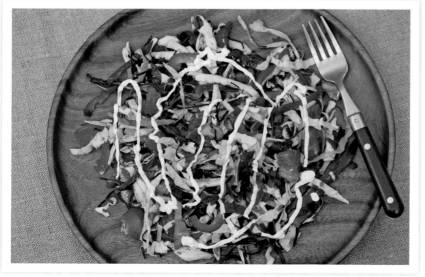

**Rainbow Slaw with
Pinenut Yogurt**

WEEK 3

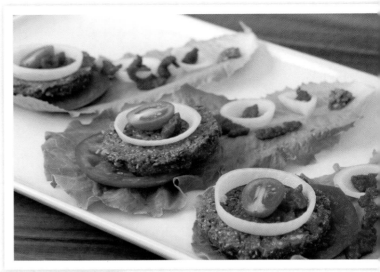

Bucky Burgers
My version of a healthy burger. You can also enjoy on a gluten-free bun.

Caribbean Wild Rice

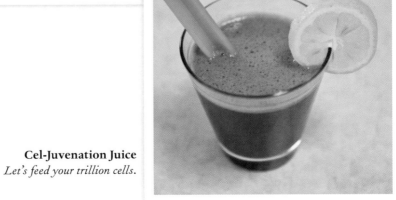

Cel-Juvenation Juice
Let's feed your trillion cells.

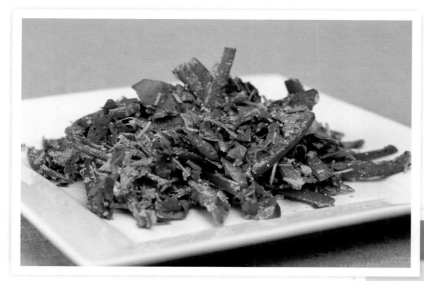

Watercress and Red Bell Pepper Salad

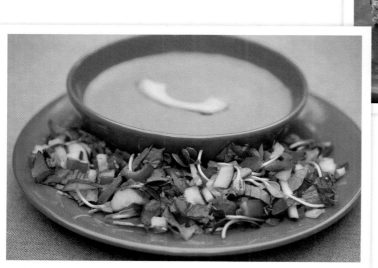

Leigh's Candy *A healthy treat for the kids and you.*

Cream of Vegetable Power Soup

WEEK 4: LIQUID FEAST WEEK

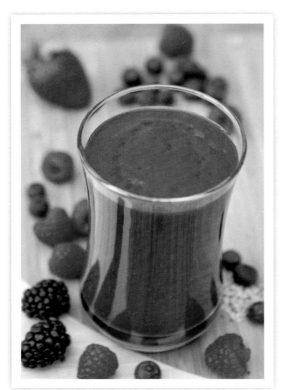

Berry Beauty Smoothie
My version of a Bloody Mary (or Strawberry Daiquiri).

It's time to get a little bit intense, but don't worry—after three weeks on the Piper Protocol, your body has been fully prepped and you're more than ready to try this super-powered weight loss and digestion repair week. Although it's liquids only, you'll get lots of fresh juice, succulent smoothies, and gently warmed or raw soups to keep you full and happy. It might feel like a challenge, but this is a week worth the investment of time and energy because the results are powerful.

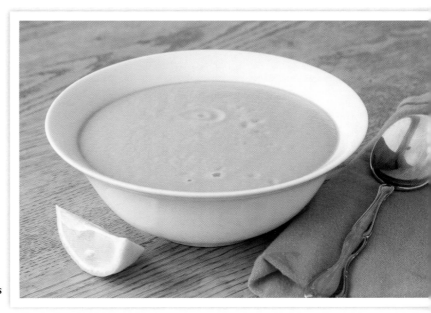

Glorious Greens

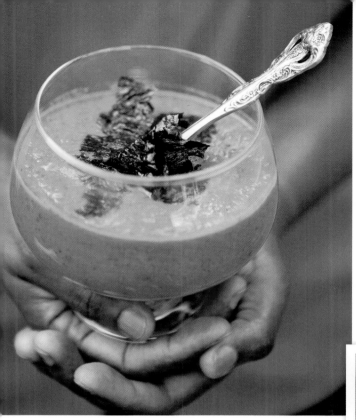

Spicy Veggie Soup
A quick, easy raw soup for the Vitamix or any blender.

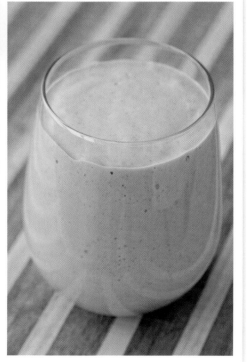

Papayamond
Enzyme-rich and too delicious to save.

WEEK 4: JUICES FOR INTERNAL FITNESS

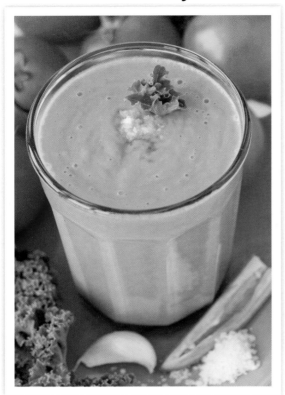

Salty & Spicy Pick-Me-Up

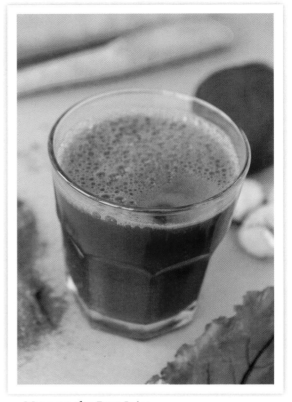

Move-to-the-Beet Juice

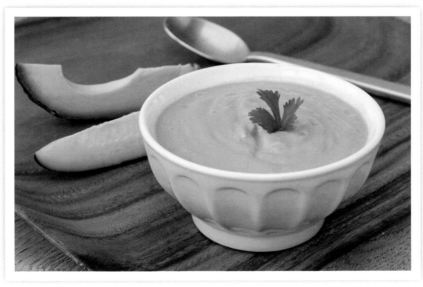

Alkalizing Avocado Gazpacho

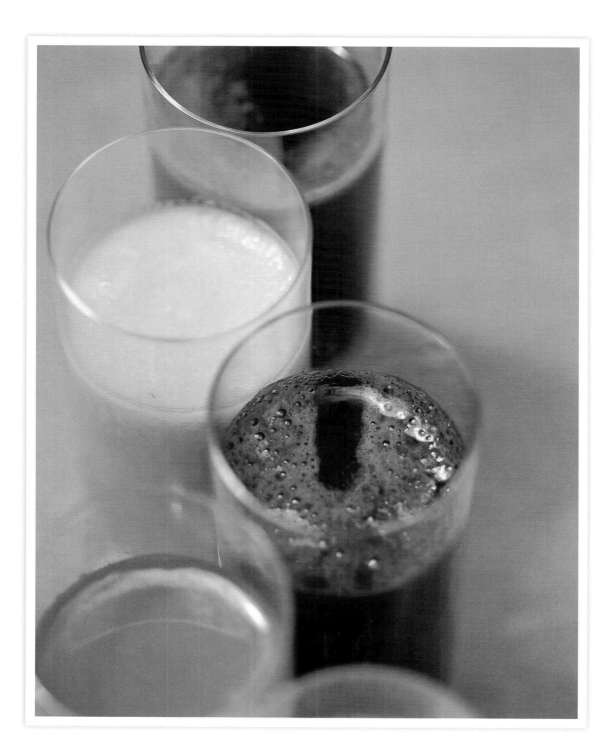

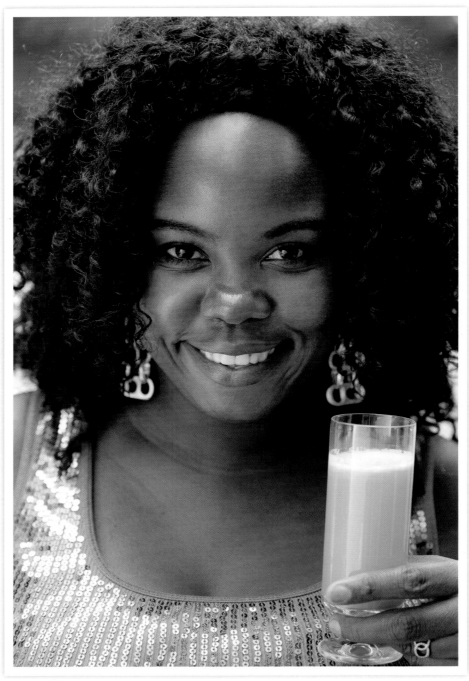

Cooling Cucumber Juice When you face the day fueled by green juice, whole food, self-care strategies, and a positive attitude, you can accomplish anything!

PART THREE

The Piper Protocol

CHAPTER 11

The Piper Protocol in Brief

EVERYTHING YOU'VE READ, TRIED, and practiced in the first two sections of this book has prepared you for this moment. In this chapter, I introduce you to the Piper Protocol and show you how to use it. This is a four-week cleanse, but how you use it depends on what you need, where you are right now with your internal fitness, how quickly you want to move forward, and what you are and are not willing to do. I'll explain it all in this chapter, and I'll also help you get ready. You'll learn the following:

The rules of the cleanse, and why they're important
What equipment you need, and what equipment is nice to have but not required
What herbs, supplements, and other additions can help support your cleanse

The Piper Protocol isn't just a cleanse. It is also a recalibration of your body's internal fitness. And it's ultimately flexible. Think of the Piper Protocol like a carousel—you can jump on at Week One and go all the way around to Week Four before you jump off (taking some new healthy habits and potent nutritional knowledge with you). But you don't have to do it like that.

Maybe you're a meat eater, and you can't imagine giving it up. A lot of my Caribbean people feel this way. Guess what? You don't have to. You can jump into Week One, go to Week Two, and just stay there for a while. You'll notice a significant difference in how you feel. Maybe you'll even make Week Two a new lifestyle most of the time. Or maybe you're a vegetarian and you have no interest in eating *any* percentage of meat in your diet. No problem! Jump in at Week Three, do it for one, two, or even more weeks, and move to Week Four if and when you are ready.

Maybe you'll stay at Week One and never go any further because Week One is enough for you at this time in your life, and it has made a big difference for you. Or maybe you'll love Week Four so much that you decide to do it once a year, or once every few months or even make it your new lifestyle with some maintaining adjustments, working up to it and back out of it each time with a cycle on either side of Week Two and/or Week Three.

The point is that it's *your cleanse*. I want you to find the parts you love, that make an impact on your life and make you feel fantastic, and use them whenever you can. I'm giving you the structure, but you can use it in whatever way you need it. You have freedom on this cleanse, and flexibility, and it's fun, too, because you'll be feeling so good.

This also isn't like typical cleanses, where you don't get to eat anything. On the first three weeks of the cleanse you'll eat a lot of delicious, real food. No starvation! Week Four is a liquid feast, but you'll be taking in so much high-potency nutrition that you'll barely miss chewing. Every single week on this plan can stand on its own, or be a part of a series. You can do a week once, or many times. No matter how much (or how little) you do, you'll be changing your body and improving your internal fitness with new habits that will help you to maintain that awesome after-cleanse feeling. The Piper Protocol isn't a diet—it's the beginning of a better life.

So let's look at what we're going to be doing. Here's a brief summary of each of the weeks, so you can start thinking about where you want to begin, and maybe where you plan to end.

PIPER PROTOCOL SUMMARY
WEEK ONE: 50 PERCENT MEAT, 50 PERCENT VEGETABLES

This is the week that eases you into a more desirable ratio of cooked-to-raw food, and is especially good for those low-carbers, Paleo people, and others who rely on meat as a staple and feel they need it. Instead of filling up your plate with meat *and* grains with a small side of vegetables, we're going to skip the grains and go half meat, half veggies. For most people, this will be an increase in nutrient density, and it's also filling and fulfilling. You'll get plenty of fat, fiber, vitamins, and minerals without the empty calories you might be used to (from sugar and flour, for example).

As you learned in the food-combining chapter, meat and grains do *not* go together, and even though I want you to work toward a mostly raw diet supplemented with cooked gluten-free whole grains or slightly steamed vegetables, many people will find this week the easiest place to begin. This week will help to regulate your blood sugar levels as you're cutting out the grains, which tend to spike sugar levels. This diet will help you lose weight faster, and also will enable your brain to use fat as fuel rather than glucose, which is a beneficial change for better cognitive functioning and some brain abnormalities.

This type of ratio is also great for cardiovascular energy. Some studies have shown that less grain consumption actually reprograms the brain. Eating meat in Weeks One and Two, and omitting grains but keeping lots of non-starchy vegetables, good fats from oils and nuts, and lean quality protein, will be highly beneficial to your internal fitness. You'll still likely be eating a much higher ratio of green vegetables this week than you're used to eating, which will help balance the acidic meat, keeping your body closer to neutral. Note: If you are a vegetarian or vegan, you will start at Week Three.

WEEK TWO: 20 PERCENT MEAT, 80 PERCENT VEGETABLES

This week, you still have your meat, but you'll be cutting it back and phasing it out. This week your meals will consist of 20 percent meat and 80 percent raw vegetables. Meat becomes a condiment rather than a main course. You'll begin to see the impact on your digestion and energy level as you cut back on the meat. If you're carb-sensitive and do not eat any grains, stay at this week until you're used to the larger percentage of vegetables, and then do Week Three using steamed or stir-fried vegetables instead of grains. Or, if you're up for it, skip to Week Four.

....

JUST SAY NO TO WHEAT

Unless you live in a cave, you've probably already heard that gluten, a group of proteins found in wheat, rye, and barley, is bad news. Many people have an autoimmune reaction to gluten, called celiac disease. Others have a non-celiac gluten sensitivity. Still others have an allergic reaction to wheat, but gluten is the trendy protein to blame.

It's true that gluten could negatively affect your immune system, your brain, and your gut. It's also true that more people than ever before are reacting poorly to wheat. Wheat has been hybridized and altered over the years, which makes it more likely to trigger an immune reaction, as well as to contain more gluten than it once did (gluten helps bread rise better). However, gluten isn't the only culprit that makes eating wheat a bad idea for just about everybody.

You could easily react to more than one portion of the gluten protein. Gluten is made of a protein called gliadin, which comes in three different types: alpha, omega, and gamma. Most celiac disease tests only look at alpha gliadin, even if the results say "gliadin antibody." However, you could be fine with alpha gliadin, but have a severe reaction to one of the other gliadins, and never know it from the standard test.

Another element of wheat that is bad for everyone is wheat germ agglutinin (WGA). WGA is most prevalent in the kind of wheat you probably thought was good for you—whole wheat and even sprouted wheat. Many people believe that if they eat sprouted wheat bread, they won't be getting the gluten; however, they'll still be getting WGA, which is a lectin that binds sugar and carbs and can damage the myelin sheath, which coats your nerves. You might never test positive for celiac disease but still have a WGA sensitivity.

I tried sprouted bread, thinking it was gluten-free and therefore just fine. Guess what happened to me? I became so foggy that I could hardly concentrate. I became inflamed and gained 7 pounds in two days, and I developed so much pain in my feet that when I woke up in the morning, it took me 20 minutes before I could walk without limping.

The problem is that WGA passes through the blood-brain barrier and attaches to the myelin sheaths that cover the nerves. When this happens, the nerves are unable to grow because the nerve growth factor is inhibited by the WGA action. This is particularly relevant for people with neurological disorders such as multiple sclerosis, Parkinson's disease, and Alzheimer's disease.

Giving up gluten isn't always easy, especially if you respond to it with the symptoms of an addict. Many people do because gluten has a feel-good effect, working on your opiod receptors. If you give up gluten, you may get withdrawal symptoms similar to when you give up coffee. If you want to know more about your unique reaction to the proteins in wheat, speak to your doctor about getting a Wheat/Gluten Proteome Sensitivity and Autoimmunity Panel, which tests for all antibodies of gluten, not just the basic ones. Or, just give it up. For good. You don't need it, and it very well might be harming you.

WEEK THREE: 20 PERCENT CARBOHYDRATES, 80 PERCENT VEGETABLES

This is where vegetarians will start, and meat eaters should try to continue to here. You might find it really beneficial, and it's only a week! During this week, meat is out and grains are back on the menu, but with a caveat: All grains in this program are gluten-free whole grains.

We're going to keep the 80:20 ratio this week, but this time, 80 percent of your diet will be made of green vegetables and your 20 percent will come from delicious, savory, gluten-free cooked grains.

You might be wondering about putting grain back into your diet after everything I told you in Week Two about how grains increase your sugar level. That's true if you eat a lot of them, but in Week Three, you're only having 20 percent of your meals made up of grains. Most dietary plans keep carbs at 40 percent, but we're going lower specifically because we don't want to increase blood sugar levels.

Why introduce carbs at all? The reason I'm switching you from meat to carbs this week has to do with internal fitness repair. Carbs are less harsh on the digestive system than meat. An 80 percent vegetable to 20 percent grain diet will make digestion easier and put the body into a more alkaline state. This is the case unless you know you are sensitive to carbs and/or don't like to eat any grains. In that case, you should stay at Week Two for a few weeks, then skip to Week Four. Another choice is to have 80 percent of the meal be a raw salad and the 20 percent be steamed or sautéed vegetables. This is great for no-carb people or those sensitive to carbs. For these folks, where you see a gluten-free carb, you substitute slightly steamed veggies or stir-fried veggies. This will allow your gut lining to be healed, as you won't be aggravating it with irritating factors.

Personally, this part of the program with 80 percent raw salad and 20 percent cooked veggies is my favorite, and it's when I feel my best because I'm highly carb-sensitive. Meat is too heavy on my digestive system and leans me more toward acidity, so when I want a treat I do a day or so of Week Two, but try to maintain Week Three without grains. It is *hard*, but I do my best because I truly do feel and see the difference in my body and mind.

....

NO-SOY ZONE

If you are already a vegetarian, chances are you eat soy products—maybe a lot of soy products. Many vegetarians depend on tofu, tempeh, veggie burgers, and other "fake meat" products. These can be useful to help people transition to vegetarianism, but there are issues with soy that make me avoid it, and I don't recommend it for anyone, at least not on a regular basis.

The first problem with soy is over-processing. Many fake meat products are highly processed and are nothing like any real, whole food you would find in nature. I want you to avoid processed foods as much as possible on the Piper Protocol, and that includes many of these fake meat products.

Another problem is that most of the soy available in the United States is from genetically modified soybeans. We don't yet understand or know the effect that genetically modified food will have on the human body because it is such a recent entry in our food supply, but I have not seen enough evidence to trust eating something that did not occur in nature.

Soy is also a phytoestrogen, meaning it mimics some properties of estrogen in the body. When genistein, a compound in soybeans, was isolated and concentrated from the whole soybean, it was linked with an increase in breast cancer. This problem does not seem to exist with whole soy products like edamame and tofu, but soy isolate, a common food additive, is more problematic.

Finally, soy is mucus-forming in the body and many people are allergic to it. For this last reason alone, I keep it out of the Piper Protocol. We are clearing out, not gumming things up, and we are definitely avoiding common allergens. So even if you love soy, give it a break, at least while you are on the Piper Protocol.

WEEK FOUR: 100 PERCENT LIQUID FEAST

This week gets hard core, and not everyone will want to go this far, but if you're up for it, the benefits are extraordinary! This week, you'll have liquids only. I won't take fiber away from you, because I want your bowels to continue to move along, and fiber is a prebiotic to feed your lovely microflora, but you'll be doing minimal to no chewing. This might sound challenging, but your stomach has already gotten used to less food less often, so it won't be as hard as trying to dive into Week Four first (which I do not recommend, as your body probably wouldn't be prepared for it).

We've already tackled your cravings by eliminating processed foods and primed your digestive system to relax, because all your meals will be pre-digested and your system won't have to work as hard. In fact, it can pretty much coast this week, freeing it up for other things your body has been putting on hold, including healing, repairing, and rejuvenation. Week Four won't be without pleasure, however. You'll get to fill up on delicious juices, satisfying smoothies, and comforting soups.

BONUS: CELLULAR CLEANSE

For all you professional cleansers out there, you might want something even stricter and faster-acting. You might want the cleanse I give to my hard-core clients who need miraculous results. This cleanse really works. Many years ago, I was faced with having to do the seemingly impossible: I was asked to get a client to lose 14 pounds in two weeks for a major movie role. I didn't think it was possible, but I said I would give it my best shot. After the first colonic (my famous AcuColonic, which some people call my "Red Carpet Special"), the client called me. "Holy shit!" she said. "I lost four pounds already!" I knew I was on to something. I did another colonic the next day, skipped a day, and did a third colonic that week. Then I put her on this cleanse. Between the cleanse, the colonics, and some regular exercise, she lost 14 pounds in just *one week*—yep, an average of 2 pounds a day. I was so proud of the results when I saw her on screen. Of course, I can't tell you who she is—insider's secret—but then, I was her secret weapon, too.

If you cleanse periodically and you are ready for that kind of intensity, this cleanse might be for you. Beginners who want to try this should do it for three days. Seasoned cleansers can do it for six days.

Like Week Four, this is a liquid cleanse, with the addition of deep detoxifiers to clean out old mucus and old stool.

STEPPING BACK DOWN

Finally, when you finish with the four weeks (or three weeks, or two weeks, or just one week, whatever it is that works for you right now), it's *very important to taper off.* You can undo all the good you did in a cleanse—and do more damage besides—if you gorge on junk food the minute Week Four is over. It's actually dangerous because it's such a shock to your system. The reason I had you work up to the cleanse with your Internal Fitness Prep Steps, and then work gradually toward Week Four, is that this kind of toxin removal is intense and requires a body that's prepared. In the same way, you must step down gradually in order to ease your body back into a mode where it can handle more intense foods.

Fortunately, this is easy to do. You just walk backward. Let's say you did all four weeks in a row. Good for you! After you do Week Four, then I want you to do Week Three again, then Week Two. Then you can ease back into life, keeping your favorite new healthful habits, and ditching your worst habits. If you went only to Week Three, then I want you to step back down through Week Two. If you're already a vegetarian and you started at Week Three and did Week Four, then step back down through Week Three.

Do not skip this step-down! I have seen people get very sick because they broke an intense juice cleanse with a steak and a martini. Respect and love your body, and treat it gently. This is the message throughout this book, so please don't decide to ignore it at the end of the cleanse just because you have a craving.

I also hope you'll hold on to the healthful food choices and the important ratios you learned here. If you keep doing all or at least most of the Internal Fitness Prep Steps, and if you eat 80 percent vegetables, mostly raw, and just 20 percent meat or grains (but never meat *and* grains together, which you learned in the food-combining chapter), then you'll be living the Piper Protocol every day. (For more information on how to do this, see Chapter 17.)

ABOUT JUICING

Starting right away with Week One, you'll be doing a lot of juicing (or buying freshly squeezed juice at a juice bar, if you have access to one and don't want to do it yourself). In fact, the only thing you'll be having between meals is fresh juice, water, or tea. Juicing in particular is excellent for the body and incredibly important for the Piper Protocol. You won't be chewing your snacks, but you will be getting a deep influx of nutrition with every sip.

It's pretty trendy right now, so if you live in a city, you probably have access to a juice bar (or ten), but juicing deserves to be more than a fad. Juicing is the most potent and direct way to deliver live enzymes into your body, as well as concentrated vitamins and minerals. Juicing is the extraction of the liquid part of fruits and vegetables, so you get all the nutrients without the fiber, which slows down absorption and makes you feel full. Fiber is great, in general, but when you want to infuse your body with the nutrients and enzymes from a large amount of veggies and fruit (more than you could eat), juicing allows you to do that without getting too full. I believe it to be an essential practice for optimal health.

When you think about juice, you probably think about fruit juice, but on the Piper Protocol I want to change your mind! Fruits contain many vitamins and antioxidants, but they also contain a lot of natural sugar. For those struggling with inflammation, candida, a slow metabolism, or weight problems, even natural sugars can mess with blood sugar and insulin levels, can stimulate hunger, and can lead to overeating and even bingeing. Instead, I want you to start thinking about vegetable juices.

There are so many vegetables you might not actually eat but that you could gain great benefit from if you juiced them. Leafy greens, root vegetables such as carrots and beets, cucumbers, broccoli, celery—these all make delicious, savory juices. Add some fresh lemon or lime or both, and you have an intensely healing juice that you can also enjoy.

I'm not opposed to ever having fruit in your juice. Fruits with less sweetness, such as green apple and tart berries, make great additions to leafy green juices. I also like orchard fruits such as pears and peaches. But these shouldn't be the main ingredients in your juices. You don't want to start (or continue or end) your day with a glass of what pretty much amounts to pure sugar.

To inspire you, here are some of the great health benefits of juicing:

Optimal absorption of nutrients from the vegetables and fruits

Intense delivery of vitamins, minerals, enzymes, organic salt, and electrolytes

Cleansing effect on the organs, blood, lymph, and cells (juicing is particularly cleansing for the liver)

Palatable way to try a wide variety of vegetables that you may not even look at to cook, including greens like lamb's quarters, sorrel, or bok choy

Significant boost to your immune system

Easy way to balance pH and blood sugar (when the juice contains no fruit)

Instant energy and better mental clarity

Weight loss due to high nutrition in a low-calorie form

Glowing complexion

....

SNACK RESCUE

I would like you to stick to liquids for all your snacks when you're practicing the Piper Protocol. However, I understand that sometimes your caloric needs will be higher when you're under a lot of physical or emotional stress, and sometimes you just have a hungry day. For this reason, I have included some nutrient-dense and delicious snacks in the Recipes chapter (Chapter 18). If you really need something else, or you just want to *chew* something, go to the Snack Rescue options instead of indulging in something crazy that will reverse your efforts. No junk food! Instead, "cheat" in a way that really isn't so bad after all.

....

SUPPLEMENTAL PRACTICES

Now that you have an idea of what's coming your way, let's talk about the supplemental practices that will really give you a boost. I'm not going to load you up with a ton of expensive supplements, but there are a few basics I would like you to take during the entirety of the cleanse, for however long you do it. For each week, I'll tell you exactly when during the day to take which supplements, but here are the types to purchase:

DIGESTIVE ENZYMES

Digestive enzymes are essential on the Piper Protocol to help you digest your food and get their full nutritional impact. Raw food comes packaged with enzymes customized to help you digest those foods, but cooked foods are devoid of enzymes, so you may need some help digesting them. If you aren't used to a lot of raw foods, it could also surprise your digestion a bit, and enzymes can help ease that transition by giving the enzymes already present in raw foods a boost. Look for digestive enzymes with no wheat, soy, gluten, sugar, corn, casein, artificial colors, or preservatives, and eight or ten of the following enzymes (a variety of enzymes will help you to digest a variety of foods):

Alpha-galactosidase	Lactase
Amylase	Lipase
Beta gluconase	Maltase
Cellulase	Pectinase (pectin)
Glucoamylase	Protease
Hemicellulase	Xylanase (non-GMO)
Invertase	

In particular, look for lots of protease during Weeks One and Two to help you break down the protein from the meat you'll be eating, as well as to help you break down the cell walls of bacteria and fungi so your body can eliminate them. If you can find a digestive enzyme with eight to ten of these ingredients, you're doing well. During all four weeks, be sure your enzymes contain plenty of cellulase to help you break down the raw plant food. For more on enzymes, see Chapter 6, and for brands I like and use, see the Resources at the end of the book.

WHEATGRASS OR E3LIVE

These contain super-high-potency nutrition plus chlorophyll, which helps to cleanse your blood. You'll do one shot or dose every morning. If you don't have access to fresh wheatgrass, many stores sell frozen shots that you can defrost the night before. You can also take powdered wheatgrass. Amazing Grass (see Resources) makes a good brand that you can find at most health food stores or Whole Foods Market, or online. Or, try E3Live (see Resources), which is made from freshwater blue-green algae and comes in frozen-liquid form. Defrost and take 1 tablespoon.

COQ10, 100-MG CAPSULES

CoQ10, also known as coenzyme Q10, coenzyme q, or ubiquinone, is an antioxidant supplement that gives you more cellular energy to support you as you heal from a largely cooked diet. Look for 100-mg capsules without any added silicon dioxide or other ingredients, if possible. They should be free of gluten, wheat, corn, soy, dairy, artificial colors, and preservatives. See the Resources section for sources and brands I like.

PROBIOTICS

Probiotics help repopulate your digestive tract with friendly bacteria. If you've been following the prep steps, you should already have these around, but make sure you have enough for the particular recommendations during the weeks you plan to do. (Look for individual recommendations during each week.) Choose probiotics that contain 15 billion organisms per capsule and a variety of different species. Some good ones to look for:

B. bifidum
B. infantis
B. lactis
L. acidophilus
L. plantarum
L. rhamnosus

The Resources at the back of this book will give you some brands I like.

Note: If you find that 15 billion makes you super gaseous, it means they are working too fast, so maybe take half a capsule or start with a lower number of billions and work your way up.

MINERALS

Most of us suffer from mineral deficiency because the soil in which we grow our food is largely depleted of minerals, and because we don't eat enough mineral-rich foods. Look for a good, basic, multi-mineral supplement in liquid or tablet form. The liquid type should say "concentrated trace minerals" and the tablets should have a wide variety of minerals. Liquid minerals are easier to digest and easier for the body to use, especially if you have any digestive issues. If you get a liquid supplement, it should contain no additives. Tablets should contain no wheat, soy, corn, dairy, sugar, or silicon dioxide. Look for a mineral supplement that includes the basics:

Boron
Lithium
Magnesium
Potassium
Trace minerals

THERAPEUTIC OIL

Like the cod liver oil my grandmother used to give me as a child, therapeutic oils lubricate your colon, brain, and joints and reduce inflammation. You'll be taking 2 tablespoons of therapeutic oil every day, which you can add to your smoothie, your salad, or just take by the spoonful. You can also take your oil in capsule form with an enteric coating, if you don't like the taste or tend to feel as if you're "burping" the taste. Remember that fat doesn't make you fat. In fact, ↑ therapeutic oil = ↓ weight. Whenever possible, look for organic, cold-pressed raw oils. Choose from the following:

Coconut oil. Coconut oil is great for increasing the metabolism, killing various types of microbes, and facilitating brain activity as your body shifts from burning sugar to burning fat. It also strengthens the immune system and thyroid function. Coconut oil is a great source of energy and your body tends to burn it instead of storing it as fat.

Extra-virgin olive oil. This oil is not only tasty but also has healthy fats that are good for your body and heart. Be generous with this on your raw veggies because it will help you absorb the nutrients more efficiently, and remember—fat doesn't make you fat (refined carbs and sugar are the real problem).

Fish oil. Fish oil contains high levels of omega-3 fatty acids that your body thrives on, in a form most easily absorbed by humans. If you choose fish oil, you'll probably want to take it in capsule form with an enteric coating so you don't burp up that fishy taste all day.

Flax seed oil. Vegans and vegetarians especially will want to avoid fish oil. To get similar omega-3 fatty acid benefits, try flax seed oil, which also contains lignans. Lignans are phyto-estrogens that act as antioxidants and have cardiovascular as well as cancer-prevention benefits.

Hemp oil. Hemp oil contains the ideal ratio of omega-3, omega-6, and omega-9 fatty acids that the human body needs. It has a nice nutty taste and is excellent alone or on salads.

FIBER

You'll be eating more fiber as you eat more vegetables, but for the sake of spring-cleaning your digestive tract, I also want you to take a fiber supplement to sweep away excess sugars and cholesterol and keep your digestive tract moving everything along. Fiber will slow down your digestion so you feel full longer, keep your blood sugar levels more even, act as a prebiotic to feed the good intestinal microflora, and promote the detoxification of fungus and yeast via the colon. Use the form that's easiest for you to get. You'll be adding 1 teaspoon to a 10-ounce glass of water three times a day. Here are some good options:

Apple pectin
Chia seeds
Ground flax seed
Ground hemp seeds
Psyllium husk

If you want to do the program exactly as I do it with my clients in my office, then you can spend a bit more, add a few more supplements, and look for these brands of supplements (see the Resources at the end of the book). These products are the best of the best, adding intense nutrition to an already-nutritious program. They're especially valuable if you're experiencing a health challenge:

Digestive enzymes. Allegany Nutrition (Digestive Enzymes AL-270) (www.alleganynutrition.com), Digest Gold (enzymedica.com), Transformation Enzymes (www.transformationenzymes.com).

Fish oils. Omega-10 by Metagenics, Dr. Dave's Best Ultra 85 Fish Oil.

MCT (Medium-Chain Triglyceride Oil). Upgraded Octane Oil: coconut oil/palm kernel oil-high in MCT's for increased metabolism. By www.bulletproofexec.com.

Megahydrate. This optional supplement helps the body to absorb water more efficiently and also breaks down oils so you don't get that yucky burping-oil taste. Find it at www.megahydrate.com. I recommend taking two to four capsules daily, or open two capsules and put them in your morning smoothie, then take the other two later in the day.

Minerals. ConcenTrace Trace Mineral Drops (widely available), Quinessentials (www.quinessentialstore.com or www.longevitywarehouse.com).

Orgonosilica. Great for repair and rejuvenation of hair, skin, nails, joints, cartilage.

Prebiotics: Fiber (Beyond Fiber by Garden of Life).

Probiotics. Custom Probiotics (customprobiotics.com) or Renew Life (www.renewlife.com). I also like UltraFlora IB from Metagenics. Soil based probiotics by Prescript-Assist.

Proteolytic enzymes. If you can afford to double up on your enzymes, I recommend adding proteolytic enzymes, which have a higher level of protease enzymes, along with digestive enzymes. Some types I like are Garden of Life Wobenzym N (www.gardenoflife.com), Zymitol (www.life-enthusiast.com), Fibrenza, Phi-zymes (www.jonbarron.com).

DO I REALLY NEED TO BUY ALL THESE SUPPLEMENTS?

I know many of you may wonder why I include so many supplements in the program. With my clients, I actually include even more because my prescriptions are based on their individual needs, but I wanted to make this program both deeply therapeutic and also affordable and accessible to everyone. Still, there are many basics that we should all be taking regularly. Unfortunately, the food we grow is lacking the vitamins and minerals it once contained because of the depletion of vital nutrients in the soil. Increasing supplementation can compensate for this environmental failing. I try to keep supplementation to a minimum, but the ones that I mention are so powerful and so multipurpose that they can fill a lot of gaps.

I remember that, when I was first learning about the raw food and living food lifestyle, I thought it was too expensive. A friend said to me, "But you don't think twice about buying a new pair of jeans or a new handbag or going to a concert. So why are you being so cheap with your health? If you don't have your health, none of that other stuff matters, anyway." I thought about it, and he was right. Somehow I was always able to find the money to do what I wanted to do, but I put my health on the back burner. Do you fall into the same trap?

I'm asking you not to do this to yourself. Put your health first. At the end of the day, being internally fit is the bottom line, and without it, nothing else matters. You want to go through your days feeling good, right? You want to be able to run after your children, or future children, and your grandchildren, or future grandchildren. You want to be able to take a walk, or run out of a building in an emergency. You want to live a strong, productive life, and you want to feel and look as good as you possibly can. For this to happen, you need to feed your trillions of cells the right nutrients, vitamins, minerals, oxygen, amino acids, antioxidants, probiotics, enzymes, and essential fatty acids—and you want your body to be in a state to receive them.

KEEP UP YOUR PREP STEPS

I want you to maintain your Internal Fitness Prep Step schedule throughout the cleanse. As a reminder, this is what you should already be doing. If you haven't been regular with these, it's time to step it up. And you'll continue to do these steps over the course of the cleanse (and beyond!). Here's a reminder:

INTERNAL FITNESS PREP STEPS

1. Once a day, take five minutes to sit, relax, and take five slow, deep breaths. For each breath, inhale for a slow count of 5 and exhale for a slow count of 5 (page 26).

2. Every time you eat, take small bites and chew each bite at least 25 times (page 36).

3. Get into your natural rhythm every morning by drinking a glass of room-temperature water with freshly squeezed lemon juice 30 minutes before breakfast (page 59).

4. Take two probiotics capsules (containing 50 billion bacteria) every morning on an empty stomach. Take the other one with water, then mix one into warm water and swish it around in your mouth (page 76).

5. Test your saliva and urine pH every morning, and drink more alkaline water—8 cups a day for women, 9 cups a day for men minimum—many need more. Test your water source to ensure it has a pH at or above 7, or just add a squeeze of fresh lemon juice to your water (page 95).

6. Drink a raw smoothie every day, from green leafy vegetables, berries, and water or coconut water. During the next four weeks, I'll give you specific recipes to choose from that will feed your body as well as your taste buds (page 105).

7. Never drink and eat at the same time (page 115).

8. Practice oil pulling every morning, right before rinsing with your probiotics (page 140).

9. Once a week, let go of something that is holding you back, large or small (page 151).

10. Pay attention to your poop and what it's telling you about your internal fitness. Check the Bristol Stool Chart (page 156) and the Piper Poop Chart (page 158) every so often to see how you're doing.

ENEMAS, COLONICS, AND LYMPHATIC MASSAGE

I will not require you to get a colonic or do enemas on the Piper Protocol, *but I highly encourage it so you get the full benefits of the program.* Cleansing loosens up toxins and if you don't get them out, they'll be reabsorbed and can cause more harm the second time around. Your body is working hard to purge toxins from the body, and the more you can help with this process, the more effective it will be. An enema or colonic at the end of each week would be wonderful for you, and you'll really get an energy boost as well as a weight-loss bonus if you do this. If you can also schedule a lymphatic massage at least once during the cleanse, you'll reap huge benefits. I'll remind you each week about scheduling these.

PREPARING YOUR LIFE

You're already working on changing your habits, but the cleanse you're about to begin also takes some specific preparation, as does any change to your lifestyle and routine. You can't just decide to cleanse one day and expect your family, your schedule, and your pantry to automatically comply. You need to make space for the Piper Protocol in your life; you need to talk to those who will be affected by these changes; you need to get all the supplies you will need; and you need to get the right food—and get rid of anything that will tempt you away from what you need to do for yourself right now.

The Internal Fitness Prep Steps you have been working on throughout this book are a start. They prepared your body. Now it's time to prepare your life.

SCHEDULE THE PIPER PROTOCOL

The first thing I would like you to do is deliberately schedule the weeks you'll be doing the cleanse. Choose a month (or a few weeks, depending on how much you plan to do) when you don't have unbreakable plans that will interfere, and when your schedule is relatively relaxed. This isn't always possible, but do the best you can. You might always be busy, and that's no reason to put off cleansing, but stress makes cleanses less effective, so you want to be able to relax into this new routine and let the cleanse work on you.

Many people like to cleanse in the spring, and this makes sense because spring is a natural cleansing time. During the winter, people tend to eat heavier foods and be less active. When spring comes, people start to move more and eat lighter foods, as greens begin to sprout and winter stores of heavier foods like animal products, dairy, and root vegetables have become depleted (in traditional cultures). The body naturally wants to let go of its heavy winter layer in the spring, so your natural rhythms will easily cooperate with a spring cleanse. Spring is also an excellent time for juicing and eating raw foods because the weather is getting warmer and all that fresh produce is newly available—especially spring greens and baby vegetables. These foods are cooling and full of juice and water, helping to wash away the accumulated internal residue of winter. So, yes, spring is a great time to do a cleanse.

However, fall is another good time to cleanse. If you've had a decadent summer of cocktails and hot dogs and lying around on the beach, you may want to cleanse to get your body ready for the winter. When cleansing in colder weather, it's important to eat more cooked foods like vegetable soups and to add warming spices to green juices—things like ginger and cayenne pepper. Many of the juice recipes on the Piper Protocol include these warming elements, and are especially good for cooler weather cleansing.

Of course, summer is a fine time to cleanse as well. This is the peak of vegetable and fruit bounty, so you'll have lots of great foods for making your food, juices, and smoothies. Also, good local and/or organic food is cheaper and easier to come by during the summer.

You can even cleanse in the winter, although it's a bit more challenging because this is the time of year when your body wants to hold on to its stores instead of letting them go. As long as you have enough warm and warmly spiced foods, however, you will still benefit from a winter cleanse. New Year's Day is, of course, a popular time to begin a cleanse regimen.

CLEAN OUT YOUR KITCHEN

Next, clear out all the food that you should avoid, especially if you know something will be calling your name. Here's the list of foods that you won't be eating while you're on the program. Get them out of your kitchen if they tempt you, and stop eating these foods *now* so your body can start adjusting to the change:

All grains containing gluten: This includes wheat, barley, rye, spelt, bran, Kamut, couscous, oats, corn, and all products made with wheat flour, including pasta, bread, crackers, bagels, dinner rolls, flour tortillas, pita bread, and pastries like cookies, muffins, doughnuts, pie, and cake.

Soy products: Eliminate tofu, soymilk, tempeh, seitan, and processed soy, including Tofurkey deli "meats," soy "hot dogs," and soy veggie burgers. Most people eat too much soy. It's difficult to digest and usually genetically modified, so even if you love your soy veggie burgers, it's time to take a break from them for a few weeks.

Bad oils: Good oil is great for you, but overly processed oils that are too high in omega-6 fatty acids (polyunsaturated oils) are out! Stick to cold-pressed oils with fats that nourish you, such as extra-virgin olive oil, flax seed oil, hemp oil, coconut oil, sesame oil, and avocados. Cross inflammatory trans fats and other damaging oils off your list. I'm talking to you, Crisco, shortening, margarine, corn oil, and soybean oil!

Mercury-heavy fish: Fresh, wild-caught, cold-water fish such as salmon and shellfish such as shrimp are great for your body, but larger fish, especially from warmer waters, have higher concentrations of mercury and other toxins due to ocean pollution. Avoid tuna, swordfish, and most kinds of sushi for the next few weeks.

Cured and processed meats: These contain carcinogenic nitrites and other nasty additives. Just say no to deli meats, hot dogs, and canned meats, including tuna.

Vinegars: All types of vinegar other than raw apple cider vinegar and raw coconut vinegar.

Bottled dressings: Salad dressing is easy to make—just whisk together extra-virgin olive oil and fresh lemon juice. The bottled stuff is full of sugar and other weird additives.

Caffeinated beverages: This includes coffee, tea, soda (sweetened or diet), and energy drinks. I especially recommend weaning yourself off caffeine a week before the cleanse because it can be difficult. Get the headache and brain fog out of the way so your body can cleanse from other things once you begin the Piper Protocol. For most people, caffeine withdrawal lasts two or three days. By day four, you'll experience a clarity of mind you forgot you could possess! It's totally worth plowing through to the other side of that headache.

Alcohol: Your liver doesn't need to do any extra work. It's going to be busy processing all those fat-soluble toxins from the fat that's going to be melting off your body, so don't make the job any more difficult. You can go for a couple of weeks without a drink, right?

Sweeteners of all types: Corn syrup, high-fructose corn syrup, refined sugar (both white and brown), fruit juice concentrate, cane sugar, beet sugar, and artificial sweeteners (Splenda, Equal, Nutrasweet). These spike your blood sugar, screw up your insulin levels, and can give you some serious mood swings. Plus, sugar feeds the bad gut bacteria and increases inflammation. If you really need to sweeten something in the next few weeks (like your smoothie), use a few drops of pure stevia.

Dairy products: You'll be going dairy-free during the Protocol (I hope forever, especially if we're talking about cow's milk, but this is a start). That means no cow's, goat's, or sheep's milk, or any cheese or cheese substitute, cottage cheese, yogurt, non-dairy creamer, or ice cream. Dairy is incredibly difficult to digest for many people, and while some people seem to be able to handle it all right, it never hurts to take a break from a food you eat too often. Dairy products also tend to cause excess mucus and phlegm, and you don't need that right now (or ever!).

Snacks: Eliminate the chocolates, energy bars, candies, and protein bars. You'll get to have snacks during the cleanse, but they'll be easy to digest, free of sugar and grain, and nutritionally potent. And they won't come in a package! Think freshly squeezed juices and the occasional piece of fresh fruit.

Now's the time to start getting used to taking a break from the foods that don't serve our cleansing purposes. You don't need any of the foods on the above list to be healthy, and we're hyper-focusing on what will super-charge your internal fitness. I'm not saying you can never, ever have a chocolate chip cookie or cheese and crackers again. Just not for the next few weeks, and not the ones laden with gluten and WGA.

EQUIP YOURSELF

The next important step is to get the equipment you need so you can prepare the foods on the cleanse. There are some appliances and tools that will make preparing these foods much easier. You might already have some of them. I highly recommend the following:

Blender: A good-quality blender is by far the best investment you can make. If you splurge on only one small appliance in your life, this should be it! I had a $100 blender and thought it was great until I was introduced to a Vitamix. Oh, my goodness, that Vitamix turned my smoothie into a Smoothie with a capital *S*! The smoothies actually taste better, with fuller, rounder flavors, and I can make them faster. Everything is perfectly, smoothly pureed. The Vitamix is pricey, at between $300 and $600, but it's worth every penny. I still come home, go into my kitchen, look at my Vitamix, and gasp with passion. I tell my clients that the next holiday or birthday they need a gift idea for a loved one, they should pool their resources and buy that person the gift of health.

Blendtec and other options: The Blendtec has been gaining popularity lately for its efficiency and easier cleanup than the Vitamix. If you have one, you are also in great company. In the meantime, if you already have another blender, it should work for the cleanse. You might have to chop things up a bit more to make it easier on the motor. If you don't have any kind of blender, you can start small. A NutriBullet will run you about $75 to just over $125, and it's super-portable, perfect for smoothies at home or on the go.

Cutting board (vegetarian): I prefer that you have one cutting board for meat and another only for vegetables, to avoid any cross-contamination. Bamboo cutting boards are sturdy and resist bacteria. You can use one for Weeks One and Two, and another for Weeks Three and Four. If you already have separate cutting boards, or you don't ever eat meat, you're probably good to go.

Juicers: This seems like a splurge to some—one of those appliances you think you'll use a lot but you only use once. That may be true for some people, but believe me when I tell you that you'll be juicing up a storm over the next few weeks, and you could really use a good juicer. Now, when I say "good" juicer I'm talking about a pretty big range. There are the "best" juicers that cost a lot, and there are the "regular" juicers that cost a lot less. To start, I don't think you need to go crazy and purchase the "best" juicer unless price isn't an issue. Just juicing is a huge step in the right direction, but do look for a juicer that is easy to clean so you'll actually want to use it.

There are two kinds of juicers: those that slowly grind the veggies and fruits, masticating them for the most possible fiber and nutrients (called masticating juicers), and those that quickly grind and spin the veggies using centrifugal force to extract the juice (called centrifugal juicers).

Centrifugal juicers cost less and the juice oxidizes quickly, and they're good if you plan to drink your juice right away. (Here's a trick I use to make my juice last all day long: I put ½ ounce [1 tablespoon] ASAP SilverSol liquid in the juice right after I make it. This kills any bad bacteria so the juice lasts longer and stays fresher. It has no toxins and doesn't change the taste [and it has stem-cell rejuvenating properties].) If you want to go all out, the top-of-the-line in my opinion is the Norwalk juicer. This is a masticating juicer that sounds like a sports car when you rev it up. It's a highly efficient juicer, getting the absolute most out of your produce, and it's a sleek-looking machine, but it costs over $1,000 and up to $3,000!

You can get a high-quality juicer from $200 to $300—good brands include the Hurom, which is a masticating juicer like the Green Star; Omega, which makes a variety of juicers of both types; and Breville, which is one of the most popular brands because it's quick to use and easy to clean (see Resources). The Breville is the one I use most often at home for my own juicing, even though I also have a Green Star, which I use when I'm juicing all day, so there's only one cleanup (it's a bit harder to clean). For those on a budget, there are low-cost juicers for about $50. These won't get as much juice out of your veggies and some can't really handle hard veggies very well, but they're fine for lettuce and cucumbers, and they're an okay place to start. As you get better at juicing, you can upgrade later.

Knives: A set of sharp knives makes all cooking, as well as raw food prep, much easier. They are pretty much essential. Dull knives make food prep more difficult, slower, and more dangerous. Get good knives and keep them sharp!

Salad spinner (optional—but awesome!): I convinced myself this was optional and I could just dab-dry my salads until I invested in this $20 dream machine and I have never looked back. No more watered-down salad dressing because of water on the greens! It's worth every inch of cabinet space, but of course if you're a patient lettuce dabber, then I'm not going to require you to get a salad spinner.

Spiralizer (optional but highly recommended): This is my third favorite tool next to my Vitamix and my Breville juicer. It will allow you to make dinner in five minutes—I kid you not. I've never been a spaghetti girl, but I know it's an easy fix for the nights when you're too tired to make a gourmet meal. This machine turns veggies like zucchini, sweet potatoes, and broccoli stems into pasta noodles—without a smidgen of gluten in sight! It was the best $30 I ever spent. Of course, you can cut your veggies into noodle shapes by hand, but it takes a lot longer and unless you're a raging perfectionist, you're not going to get those beautifully symmetrical and perfectly shaped noodles with a knife.

Dehydrator (optional): This is for the advanced internal fitness cleanser who wants to go the extra mile and make dehydrated foods and snacks. It's a staple for those eating a raw diet because it allows you to make raw snacks by drying them out at a temperature not to exceed 115 degrees F, and the enzymes are not destroyed. However, if your drying needs are minimal and you don't have the budget and/or space for a dehydrator, you can use an oven set to the lowest temperature. Some of the recipes in this book use a dehydrator, but I include alternative directions if you need to use your oven. If you want to invest, Excalibur is a good brand. These run from $125 to $200.

Food processor (optional): You might already have one of these and know how much easier mincing vegetables and grinding nuts are with a food processor. The NutriBullet (see Resources) can do this, too, and it's less expensive. Another option is a Vitamix or Blendtec (see Resources), but be careful not to overblend. A food processor is nice if you want to roughly chop things and don't want to risk pureeing them. They're good for chopping garlic, making salsa, and mincing celery, carrots, sprouted nuts, and onions for soup. (They're also good for making pie crust— but for the next four weeks, pretend I didn't say that!)

That takes care of the major items, but here's some more minor equipment you'll need:

Measuring cups/spoons: You probably already have these, but use them especially when you're first learning to cook and/or you are following a recipe and you want it to come out exactly as intended. Eventually you may begin to recognize amounts, but it never hurts to measure, at least until it becomes second nature and you feel confident. Honestly, I don't usually measure, but I don't usually use recipes, either.

Nut milk bags: For the small price tags on these, I always have two. They're essential for making your own nut milk, which is so much better for you than the store-bought stuff. Just grind up your nuts with water, then squeeze them through these handy bags and voilà!—almond milk, hazelnut milk, hemp milk, or whatever you want to make. (Find a recipe for basic homemade almond milk, plus some delicious variations, on pages 267–271.)

Fine-mesh strainer: This is a must in every household, for rinsing small grains such as quinoa or legumes such as lentils, rinsing berries, and for draining grains and beans after cooking. In a pinch (or in the absence of nut bags), you can also use it for straining nut milk.

Steamer: This is quite handy for lightly steaming your vegetables.

Large salad bowl: Don't you hate trying to toss a salad in a too-small bowl or on a plate and getting lettuce all over the counter? Get a nice, big bowl and make your life easier. You might end up eating a lot more salad.

Garlic press: This isn't entirely essential, but peeling and mincing clove after clove of garlic can get tedious. A good-quality garlic press does the job with one squeeze, and gets more of the juice out of the cloves.

Vegetable peeler: If you're unable to get organic vegetables, a vegetable peeler comes in handy because the skins of non-organic root veggies contain the highest concentration of pesticides. Peel them off and enjoy an almost-organic veggie feast. I also like to use a vegetable peeler for burdock root for my homemade almond milk.

Wheatgrass juicer: Definitely optional but great if you really get into the wheatgrass lifestyle and advanced cleansing. The Omega juicer can juice wheatgrass also.

Mason jars: Great for carrying smoothies, juices, and soups to work with you, or storing leftovers in the refrigerator.

Parchment paper for baking: Do not use aluminum foil to bake, as the aluminum can leach into your food.

Fruit and vegetable wash: I always recommend organic produce, but even organic produce should be washed because it can be covered with contaminants from harvesting and handling. A bottle runs only about $4.

....

WHAT TO COOK WITH

Many types of cookware leach toxic chemicals and heavy metals into food. For the cleanest possible cooked food, I recommend only cooking with:

- Glass

- Porcelain

- Cast iron (although this type of cookware can add some iron to your food if it contains acid like tomatoes, this is usually in amounts that are actually beneficial, especially for the common problem of iron deficiency)

- Stainless steel (do not use if you have a nickel allergy, as stainless steel cookware contains some nickel)

- Copper with stainless-steel lining. This kind of cookware is expensive and requires more care, but it's the safest type of material and it cooks food beautifully and evenly. Never use abrasive scrubbers or cleaners on it!

Note: *Never cook in aluminum*, even if it's coated, and *never use non-stick cookware*, which always eventually flakes into food and also releases toxic fumes into the food and air. You can't see or smell these fumes, but they are there. Teflon, for example, off-gasses toxic particulates at over 400 degrees F, according to a study performed by DuPont. There's even a health problem called "polymer fume fever" associated with this. Do not use it! The one exception is the new green non-toxic, non-stick cookware.

If you have aluminum pans (including anodized aluminum) or non-stick cookware and changing is a hassle or too expensive, slowly change them out, replacing them as they wear out with cast iron, glass, or steel. If your aluminum pots are not scratched and are in good condition, use them, but if they are scratched, please don't use them! Asking for a new set of non-aluminum cookware for a gift is always a great idea.

....

PREPARE YOUR FAMILY

If you don't have support from the people you live with, you'll be much more likely to fail. It's better to tell them what you're doing than to try to do it without anyone noticing. Whether it is conscious or unconscious, the people around you who don't support you are likely to sabotage your progress. You can certainly ask the people around you to join you in your quest for internal fitness, but don't be hurt or discouraged if they aren't up for it. This is something you can only do when you're ready. Instead, just ask that they support what you have chosen to do and not undermine you, even if they don't understand it or wouldn't choose it for themselves. Everyone has his or her own progress and timetable for personal evolution. This is your mission, and as much as it would be great to have your partner doing it with you, living by example is the best teacher. Remember that you're doing this for *you*. This is your time, your health, your body.

KNOW WHY YOU'RE DOING THIS

When the going gets tough, you'll need motivation to stick with the Piper Protocol. Let's define yours. Do you want to lose weight and finally feel good in your own body? Do you want more energy? Does a chronic disease run in your family and you want to avoid it? Do you want to live a longer, healthier life? It might sound great to live into your nineties, but only if you are functioning, vibrant, and alert, right? Nobody wants to be bedridden and a burden, and I have always admired the older women I know who live life fully even into their 80s and 90s.

Decide what your motivation is. Make it specific. I think striving for vitality and longevity is a great reason to do this, but maybe you have other reasons that speak to you more. Maybe you're hoping to start a family. This is a great way of getting your body cleaned and prepared to carry your child. But look further than that. You're building a temple for the future generations. You know the concept of survival of the fittest. Be internally fit, and watch your future generations thrive.

RECORD-KEEPING

Now let's deal with a little bit of paperwork. Or, for that matter, smartphone work. Before my clients begin the Piper Protocol, I like to have them keep a record of the external evidence of their internal fitness, so they can see how these measures of health improve after they change their diets and lifestyles. You can record your progress in an old-school journal, or you can keep it on your phone or on your computer. In your record, before you begin, record the following information:

- **Your measurements:** bust/chest, waist, hips, thighs, calves, upper arms.
- Your weight.
- Any unpleasant symptoms you deal with regularly, such as digestive issues, headaches, or joint pain.
- How your mouth, teeth, and breath feel, look, and smell—do you have a coating on your tongue, does your mouth feel sticky, are your teeth yellow, is your breath not quite as sweet as you wish it was?
- **Ladies:** Describe your cycle. Is it regular or irregular? How long does it last? Do you get PMS, and if so, what kind of symptoms? What color is your flow, and do you have clotting? Record the details.
- **Guys:** Do you wake up with an erection? If not, you may not be getting enough REM sleep, and/or enough circulation through the liver. You should see an improvement on the Piper Protocol.
- What is your libido like lately?
- How is your mood? Good, poor, up, or down?
- Do you find it easy or difficult to fall asleep, and to stay asleep? Are you getting enough sleep?
- When you wake up, are you groggy or alert?
- What is your cholesterol number? LDL to HDL ratio.
- How is your vision? Have you had more trouble seeing lately? Are you getting nearsighted or farsighted? Do you have floaters in front of your eyes? You may notice your vision improving on the Piper Protocol.
- How is your nail health? Hair health? Skin health? Describe.
- What is the typical color of your urine? Does it have an odor?
- Compare your typical stool to the information in the Piper Poop Chart (page 158).
- Do you tend to be cold all the time, or hot all the time?
- Anything else that has been bothering you?

At the end of each week on the Piper Protocol, look over these measures of internal fitness and record how any of them have changed. This will help you to have a more objective view of how the program is helping you, which will be great motivation to keep it up! If you find this is too daunting, then weigh yourself only once a week. Sometimes we plateau and if things don't move it can discourage us. So use what works for you.

So how about it? Do you know which week you want to start with—Week One or Two or maybe Week Three? Do you know how long you want to go? Have you gone shopping? Have you been phasing out the foods you won't be eating for a while, such as sugar, dairy products, and caffeine? Are you excited? Are you inspired? Are you physically, mentally, and emotionally prepared? Do you have the support of friends and family? Then I believe you're ready! Let's jump right into the Piper Protocol and get you internally fit!

CHAPTER 12

Piper Protocol Week One: 50:50 Cleanse Initiation

BEGIN HERE IF:

You eat meat and you're new to cleansing.
You've been on a low-carb diet.
You've been eating a Paleo-style diet.
You eat a standard American diet, high in refined carbohydrates, sugar, and meat.
You want to start out easy.

This first week of the Piper Protocol is the most lenient and the easiest for meat eaters, low-carb people, Paleo people, and anyone who eats a standard American diet. Some of my clients may be surprised that I would include a week that is so lenient, but I know that it's not lenient for many people. My sister, who lives in Texas, often tells me that "normal people" can't just "suddenly eat raw food." She also reminds me frequently that most people can't necessarily afford organic food and a lot of supplements. And *then* she reminds me that many people have emotional attachments to certain foods that may not be the best choices for them, but that they find extremely difficult to give up, and I can't just say, "Don't eat that." Point taken. This is one of the many reasons I value my sister, and also why I created this first week of the Piper Protocol.

I know that not everyone will be interested in becoming a vegetarian or a vegan, and not everyone is interested in embracing a fully raw diet. That's fine, and for those of you who feel that way, or who feel very far away from that kind of diet, start here. (If you still eat meat but not every day and you already eat a very healthy diet, you may start at Week Two or Week Three. If you're a vegetarian or vegan, start at Week Three.)

WELCOME TO WEEK ONE!

Today is the beginning of a new way of life. As you cleanse your body of the things that it doesn't need and fill it with the things that it does need, you'll begin to feel differently. Your clothes will get looser (or are you getting slimmer?). Your shape will become more defined. You'll become less bloated, and the number on the scale will begin to drop rapidly. You'll also feel more energetic, with less brain fog. Your digestion will improve, and you'll notice that you're thinking more clearly and maybe even reacting to the little annoyances in life more calmly. You're going to love how you feel, not to mention how you look. Remember to keep track in your journal of all the changes you notice.

We're gradually lightening the burden on your digestive tract this week as we increase the nutrient-density of your meals. You'll be eating a lot more raw food than you're probably used to eating, and a lot less grain. In fact, you'll be eating *no grains.* You'll drastically decrease your carbohydrate intake this week, and that will make a big difference as you work toward more raw food. Your blood sugar will stabilize, you'll notice less mucus, and your acidity and inflammation will go down, which will make you feel more energetic, lighter, and better. You'll also start burning fat instead of sugar for fuel, which will translate to fast and rewarding weight loss.

You'll also notice that you're doing self-care quite frequently throughout the day—meals, juice breaks, water breaks, supplement breaks, and more. This is why it's good to have a light schedule during the cleanse. You need to be able to stop what you're doing about once every hour to have a juice break or water break, take some supplements, or make a good meal for yourself. You need to be able to take the time each morning to make enough juice for the day, if you don't have time to make it throughout the day (most people don't) or if you don't live in a metropolitan area where you can easily pop out of the office for a few minutes to buy a green juice at a juice bar.

You need to be able to make a good lunch or bring leftovers from your dinner the night before so you aren't tempted by the break-room doughnuts or fast food.

Making time for the cleanse is very important! If you do the cleanse halfway, it won't have nearly the impact as if you do it exactly as I lay it out for you right here. This is the therapeutic process, and if you respect it and honor it, you'll be respecting and honoring your own body. Remember, your body is a temple. Honoring it is the best way to get your body, your weight, and your health to respond.

Be sure to read over the entire day before you start so you know what to expect, and so that you can get everything you need.

WHAT TO BUY

Instead of telling you exactly what to eat this week, I'm going to give you choices. I don't like people telling me what to do, and I bet you don't, either. However, I'll rein in your choices with a variety of recipes. When I say it's time for a juice break, you can choose your juice, but choose something from this book. This is not the time for sweet fruity juices, and the juices on this plan are specifically formulated for Week One purposes. The same goes for the meals, which are formulated to meet the 50 percent meat : 50 percent veggies ratio that we're shooting for this week. Within the parameters of this plan and these recipes, however, you have total freedom. You can eat the same thing every day, or choose something completely different for each meal all week long.

The easiest way to do this is to look over the choices and decide what you'll eat ahead of time, and then go shopping so you have everything you need. However, if you like to decide day by day, just stop by the market after work or whenever it's convenient and get what you need for that day's dinner and the next day's breakfast and lunch.

You'll also need to have enough supplements on hand, and don't forget your pH test kit, so you can monitor your acid/alkaline balance each morning.

SUPPLEMENTS YOU WILL NEED THIS WEEK

In the last chapter, I told you exactly what to look for in these supplements. This is a list of what you will need this week:

Digestive enzymes: You'll be taking two digestive enzyme capsules with each meal and two between meals for a total of 12 per day, so you'll need a bottle at least 84 digestive enzyme capsules in order to get through the week.

Probiotics: 50-billion organism strength (if you're sensitive, start with a lower strength). Continue with your Internal Fitness Prep Step, gargling with one capsule (opened into ¼ cup water) and then taking a second capsule in the morning before breakfast. I'll also have you add one in the evening. You will need a total of 21 capsules this week.

CoQ10 capsules: 100-mg strength. You'll be taking one with breakfast, one with lunch, and one with dinner each day, so you'll need a total of 21 capsules.

Multi-mineral supplement: You'll be taking drops of concentrate in water or a tablet three times per day, between meals. If you use the concentrate, get a bottle. You will take 10 drops of liquid in ¼ to ½ cup water three times per day. If you use the tablets, you'll need 21 tablets this week. If the taste is too strong, add more water.

Therapeutic oil: You'll be taking 2 tablespoons extra-virgin olive oil, fish oil, flax seed oil, coconut oil, or hemp oil per day. Add it to your smoothie, your salad, or if you're taking it in gel-cap form (as you'll probably do if you choose to take fish oil), follow the dosage instructions on the package to determine how much you'll need for the week. Remember coconut oil will rev up your metabolism but you can only have it melted in hot drinks, or you can get upgraded octane oil which can be used hot or cold as it doesn't solidify.

Fiber: You can take any form you prefer: chia seeds, ground flax seed, psyllium husk, apple pectin, or hemp seeds. You'll be taking 1 teaspoon three times per day in 1 cup water or added to your smoothie or juice. You'll be using this throughout the program, so get a large container.

Wheatgrass or E3Live: You'll do one shot of wheatgrass or 1 tablespoon of E3Live every morning before breakfast, so have enough on hand or available for seven shots or 7 tablespoons. Some people can't handle fresh wheatgrass, or they can't find it, but powdered wheatgrass is easier to find and a good option if you can't find or don't want to take fresh.

ABOUT THE SCHEDULE

Ideally, to work in conjunction with your internal clock, you should get up at 5:30 A.M., but I understand that not everybody will be able (or willing) to do this. I've included times on this schedule to help you keep track of when to do each step in the cleanse throughout the day, but if you get up at 7:30 instead of 5:30 (for example), just keep the intervals between the steps the same.

Also, consider scheduling a colonic or a lymphatic massage this week, or doing one of the enemas as described in Chapter 8, to help kick off your cleanse.

DAILY TEMPLATE

Now, let's walk through your day. This is what I want you to do every day for the next seven days. The first few days may seem like a big adjustment, but you'll soon fall into the rhythm. Every meal and snack is pretty light, but you get to eat or drink something often, so you'll continue to feed yourself.

You always have at least two choices about what to eat at each meal and snack, but my suggestion is that you start with heavier meats like red meats at the beginning of the week, then work through the week lightening the load, switching to chicken and turkey midweek, and then to fish and shellfish by the weekend. (Note that I do not recommend eating pork at any time.) This will prepare your system for the lower meat portions in Week Two and will also gradually decrease the burden on your digestive tract.

Also note that whenever I tell you to have any fresh juice, what I mean is to have any freshly squeezed juice in the Recipes chapter (Chapter 18), or a non-fruit-based green juice from a juice bar. These juices should not be mostly fruit and should not be very sweet. This is very important for cleansing on the Piper Protocol.

In the following plan, all recipes in bold type can be found in the Recipes chapter. And if you really need it, flip to the Snack Rescue section on page 307:

5:30 A.M.: Test your pH (saliva and urine) and record the number in your journal.

5:40 A.M.: Do your oil pulling (which you learned how to do on page 127).

6:00 A.M.: Gargle with one probiotics capsule in water, then take your second probiotics capsule with a glass of water with fresh lemon juice squeezed in. This will help to stimulate the first bowel movement of the day. Some morning meditation or light yoga would be good at this time.

6:30 A.M.: Have a shot of wheatgrass or E3Live.

7:00 A.M.: *Breakfast.* Choose from the following:

Breakfast Smoothie (page 265). You can add your daily fiber and/or therapeutic oil to your morning smoothie, if you choose this option.

Asparagus Omelet (page 272).

Along with breakfast, take:

- Two digestive enzymes
- One CoQ10 capsule
- One mineral supplement (1 tablet or 10 drops of liquid in ¼–½ cup water)
- 1 teaspoon fiber supplement in 1 cup water or added to your breakfast smoothie. You will eat less because the fiber fills you up, and also helps cleanse your colon more efficiently as you detox.

8:00 A.M.: *Juice break.* Have any freshly squeezed juice.

9:00 A.M.: *Water break.* Glass of water with juice of ½ lemon.

10:00 A.M.: *Juice break.* Have any freshly squeezed juice. Also take two digestive enzyme capsules.

11:00 A.M.: *Juice break.* Have any freshly squeezed juice. You could finish the rest of either of the juices you've already had today, or try another juice recipe starting on page 258.

12:00 P.M.: *Lunch.* Choose from the following:

Mixed Green Steak Salad (page 282)

Salmon with Sautéed Asparagus and Arugula Salad (page 283)

Jamaican Jerk Chicken (page 285) with green salad

Curry Shrimp Pot (page 286) with sautéed okra or broccoli

Any dinner plate with 50 percent mixed vegetables, raw or cooked, and 50 percent protein, such as beef, chicken, or fish. Remember to start the week with the heavier meats and lighten to fish by the end of the week.

Right before lunch, also take:

- Two digestive enzyme capsules
- One CoQ10 capsule
- One mineral supplement (1 tablet or 10 drops of liquid in ¼–½ cup water)
- 1 teaspoon fiber supplement in 1 cup water

2:00 P.M.: *Juice break.* Have any freshly squeezed juice. Also take two digestive enzymes.

3:00 P.M.: *Tea time.* Choose any of the following herbal teas for your afternoon tea break:

- Pau d'Arco
- Cat's claw
- Uva Ursi
- Matcha green
- Herbal (lemon or chamomile)

Or, have another freshly squeezed juice.

5:00 P.M.: *Juice or water break.* Have either the fresh juice of your choice or water with the juice of ½ a lemon. Note: If you didn't add fiber to your morning smoothie, you can take it now with a glass of water.

5:30 P.M.: *Exercise break.* You can exercise at any time during the day according to your schedule, but this is a convenient time for many people. Take a brisk walk, hit the gym, or try a class. I like Core Fusion from Exhale, with 21 locations in major cities, or SoulCycle, or any gym class in your area. Do whatever you enjoy, so you'll really do it.

6:00 P.M.: *Dinner.* Choose from the following:

Leafy Protein Salad (page 277). You can add your therapeutic oil to this salad if you haven't taken it already.

Chicken Vegetable Stir-Fry (page 278)

50:50 Soup (page 281)

Also take:

- Two digestive enzyme capsules
- One CoQ10 capsule
- One mineral supplement
- 1 teaspoon fiber supplement in 1 cup water

8:00 P.M.: *Enzyme break*. Take two digestive enzymes with 1 glass water.

9:00 P.M.: *Time to slow down*. It's time to get your mind and body ready for sleep. Turn off all the electronics and put your phone away. Meditate, read a book, get your supplements together for the next day. Give thanks. Take one final probiotics capsule before going to sleep.

9:30 to 10:00 P.M.: *Bedtime*. If you can't quite manage going to sleep by 9:30 P.M., at least go to bed by 10:00 P.M. This will help you to get up earlier and stay in sync with your body. It's beneficial to have you in bed sleeping by Gallbladder–Liver Time (11 P.M. to 3 A.M.), so your body can detox.

CHAPTER 13

Piper Protocol Week Two: 80:20 Protein

CONTINUE HERE IF:

You've already done Week One, for as many weeks as you are comfortable.

Begin here if:

You already eat a diet with a lot of raw foods and you want to scale back on your animal
product consumption.

You eat a Paleo diet but with a large proportion of meat.

You want to try being a vegetarian or vegan but you aren't quite ready to go all the way
and you want to ease into it.

Maybe you've just finished Week One. Maybe you did it just once, or maybe you stayed there
for a few weeks to get your body into the swing of this new way of eating. If so, how do you feel
now? Better, lighter, more energetic? In your journal, keep track of any changes you notice and
any problems you had. Now it's time to raise the bar and increase your proportion of raw foods.

Or, maybe you've decided to start here. This week is a good place to begin if you already eat a diet with a lot of raw foods, but you also think you eat too much meat and you want to scale back on animal products. (If you're already a vegetarian, you can skip ahead and start at Week Three.) Either way, get ready to start making some serious and positive changes to the way your body digests food—and to increase the rate of your weight loss even more.

WELCOME TO WEEK TWO!

This week, you'll reduce your meat consumption from 50 percent to 20 percent and increase your complex carbohydrates, in the form of vegetables, to 80 percent. You won't be having any grains or fruit or sweeteners this week, and your body is going to respond by increasing energy, flushing out more toxins, and feeling fantastic. You'll be increasing your body's alkalinity, putting even less stress on your digestive system, and losing more weight, if you're carrying excess weight. You'll also feel less bloated, gassy, or that heavy feeling of being stuffed. By the end of the week you'll be more alert and have more clarity.

As with the first week, you'll be doing something almost every hour during the day, so get ready to be busy cleansing. You'll need lots of breaks throughout your day to make or buy fresh juice, drink water, have tea, or exercise. It's very important to stay on schedule. Even if you don't actually wake up at 5:30 A.M. as I recommend, you still need to keep your intervals going—eating, drinking, and taking your supplements about every hour, as indicated in the day template. This is the best way to achieve exciting and appearance-altering results. By the end of the week you're going to be radiant.

Read over the entire template before you start so you know what to expect, choose your meals, go shopping, and be both physically and mentally prepared.

WHAT TO BUY

Look over the recipes and options for the week and make your grocery list. If you'll be doing your own juicing, plan to go to the store a few times, so your produce is as fresh and enzyme-rich as possible.

All the meals this week are formulated to meet the 80 percent vegetables and 20 percent meat balance or to meet the unique nutritional requirements you have right now, so stick to the recipes for both meals and juices, but introduce as much variety as you please. Maybe you really love only two of the juices and three of the meals. Just stick with those if you prefer, but variety is the spice of life, so I hope you'll try everything at least once.

Also don't forget your supplements and your pH test kit, so you can continue to watch your alkalinity levels rise.

....

CANCER AND WEEK TWO

There's a theory that many people endorse that says sugar feeds cancer. A so-called cancer diet often involves eating large amounts of non-starchy vegetables along with lean protein and no grains or sugars at all. We do know that tumors feed on glucose to grow, so ridding the diet of most carbs lowers the glucose level, and it makes sense that this could starve cancer cells when your body switches to fat burning instead of sugar burning. I'm not promoting Week Two as a cancer diet, but Week Two with leaner meats like fish as the protein source could be part of a lifestyle that can minimize your risk and be beneficial if you do have cancer. When in crisis, Week Four is the best approach to getting the body back in the rhythm of things.

....

SUPPLEMENTS YOU WILL NEED THIS WEEK

Digestive enzymes: You'll be taking three digestive enzyme capsules with each meal this week, as well as three between meals, for a total of 18 per day, so you'll need 126 enzyme supplements this week.

Probiotics: 50-billion organism strength. (Use a lower strength if you are sensitive.) Continue with your Internal Fitness Prep Step practice of swishing the contents of one capsule with ¼ cup water around in your mouth, then taking a second capsule in the morning before breakfast. I'll also have you add one in the evening. You'll need a total of 21 capsules this week.

CoQ10 capsules: 100-mg strength. You'll be taking one with breakfast, one with lunch, and one with dinner each day, so you'll need a total of 21 capsules.

Multi-mineral supplement: You'll be taking drops of concentrate in water or a tablet three times per day, with meals. If you use the concentrate, get a small bottle. You will take 10 drops of liquid in ¼ to ½ cup water three times per day. If you use the tablets, you'll need 21 tablets per week.

Therapeutic oil: You'll be taking 2 tablespoons extra-virgin olive oil, fish oil, flax seed oil, coconut oil, or hemp oil per day, or two capsules of fish oil or other oil. Choose whichever you prefer. Add it to your smoothie, your salad, or if you're taking it in gel-cap form (as you'll probably do if you choose to take fish oil), follow the dosage instructions on the package to determine how much you'll need for the week.

Fiber: You can take any form you prefer: chia seeds, ground flax seed, psyllium husk, apple pectin, or hemp seeds. You'll be taking 1 teaspoon three times per day in 1 cup water or added to your smoothie or juice, so you'll need just a small container.

Wheatgrass or E3Live: You'll do one shot of wheatgrass or 1 tablespoon of E3Live every morning before breakfast, so have enough on hand or available for seven shots or 7 tablespoons. Some people can't handle fresh wheatgrass, or they can't find it, but powdered wheatgrass is easier to find and a good option if you can't find or don't want to use fresh.

ABOUT THE SCHEDULE

Try to get up at 5:30 A.M., to get in sync with your body's natural rhythms, but if that doesn't work in your schedule, just start the day when you get up and keep the intervals consistent. Exercise whenever you can—my exercise time is a suggestion only.

Also consider scheduling a colonic or a lymphatic massage this week, or doing one of the enemas as described in Chapter 8. You're in the thick of detoxing now, and you need all the extra help you can get!

DAILY TEMPLATE

This is your guide for the next seven days. Model each day on the following schedule. If you've already done Week One, this should feel familiar and comfortable. If you're starting here, get ready to make some changes, like spending more time in the bathroom for the first few days, and feeling super-energetic. Weight loss should happen fairly rapidly as well, if you have weight to lose. If weight loss is not your goal, then look for glowing skin, more energy, clarity of the mind, and less bloat.

You'll always have meal choices, but as with last week, when it comes to meat, start with the heavier meats, such as beef, at the beginning of the week (if you want to have them at all). Work toward lighter meats, with chicken and turkey during the middle of the week, and fish and shell-fish at the end of the week. Or, if you've already phased out meat at any level, go ahead and stick to fish and other seafood for your animal protein allowance this week. The lighter your Week Two meat choices, the easier time you'll have transitioning to Week Three.

In the following plan, all recipes in bold type can be found in the Recipes chapter. And don't forget the Snack Rescue section on page 307, in case of emergencies!

5:30 A.M.: Test your pH (saliva and urine) and record the number in your journal.

5:40 A.M.: Do your oil pulling (which you learned how to do on page 127).

6:00 A.M.: Gargle with one probiotics capsule in water, then take your second probiotics capsule with a glass of water with fresh lemon juice squeezed in. This will help to stimulate the first bowel movement of the day.

6:30 A.M.: Have a shot of wheatgrass or E3Live.

7:00 A.M.: *Breakfast.* Choose from the following:

Breakfast Smoothie (page 265)
Spinach Omelet (page 273)
Breakfast Salad (page 274)

You can add your daily fiber and/or therapeutic oil to your morning smoothie or to your porridge.

Along with breakfast, also take:

- Three digestive enzyme capsules
- One CoQ10 capsule
- One mineral supplement (1 tablet or 10 drops of liquid in ¼–½ cup water)
- 1 teaspoon fiber supplement (like unsweetened psyllium or flax seed) in 1 cup water
  or in your breakfast smoothie. You will eat less because the fiber fills you up, and also
  helps cleanse your colon more efficiently as you detox.

8:00 A.M.: *Juice break.* Have any freshly squeezed juice.

9:00 A.M.: *Water break.* Glass of water with the juice of ½ lemon.

10:00 A.M.: *Juice break.* Have any freshly squeezed juice. Also take three digestive enzyme capsules.

11:00 A.M.: *Juice break.* Have any freshly squeezed juice.

12:00 P.M.: *Lunch.* For lunch, choose from the following:

Mixed Green Steak Salad (page 282)
Baked Salmon with Peppers (page 287) and tossed salad
Jamaican Jerk Chicken (page 285), prepared as salad
Curry Shrimp Pot (page 286) with sautéed okra or broccoli
Any dinner plate with 80 percent mixed vegetables, cooked or raw, including salad greens, and 20 percent any protein, such as beef, chicken, or fish.

Add your therapeutic oil to any lunch entrée if you haven't taken it already.
Right before lunch, also take:

- Three digestive enzyme capsules
- One CoQ10 capsule
- One mineral supplement (1 tablet or 10 drops of liquid in ¼–½ cup water)
- 1 teaspoon fiber supplement in 1 cup water

2:00 P.M.: *Juice break.* Have any juice. Also take three digestive enzyme capsules.

3:00 P.M.: *Tea time.* Choose any of the following herbal teas for your afternoon tea break:

- Chamomile
- Lemon
- Pau d'Arco

4:00 P.M.: *Juice break.* Have any freshly squeezed juice.

5:00 P.M.: *Water break.* Have a glass of water with the juice of ½ lemon.

5:30 P.M.: *Exercise break.* If this time works for exercise, try a brisk walk, a yoga class, or anything else that gets your body moving for about 30 minutes.

6:00 P.M.: *Dinner.* Choose from the following:

Vegetable Chicken Stir-Fry (page 278)
Chicken and Asparagus Salad (page 279)
80:20 Soup (page 281)

Also take:

• Three digestive enzyme capsules
• One CoQ10 capsule
• One mineral supplement
• 1 teaspoon fiber supplement in 1 cup water

8:00 P.M.: *Enzyme break.* Take three digestive enzyme capsules with 1 glass water.

9:00 P.M.: *Time to slow down.* It's quiet time! Let your mind and body ease into sleep by turning off the TV and computers, stowing your phone, and getting into calm mode. Do something relaxing, such as taking a bath with Epsom salts to help pull all that stuff you're detoxing out of your skin. Listen to relaxing music, such as classical or meditation music. Or just read a calming book. This is also a great time to meditate and feel gratitude for all that you have.

Also take one probiotics capsule before bed, so it can work while you are sleeping.

10:00 P.M.: *Bedtime.* It's important to get between seven and eight hours of sleep each night, so lights out by 10:00! This will help you stay in sync with your body's natural rhythms, for the most efficient detoxification (and the best-feeling morning!).

CHAPTER 14

Piper Protocol Week Three: 80:20 Carbs

CONTINUE HERE IF:

You've already done Week Two for as many weeks as you are comfortable.

Begin here if:

You're already a vegetarian and have no interest in adding meat to your diet.
You already eat a vegetable-heavy diet and want to jump right in and get quick results.
You're almost a vegetarian and you're ready to go all the way, or even move toward a raw diet.

If you've just come from Week Two, congratulations on making it this far! You'll notice a big change in the diet and in your body this week. Even though we're changing only 20 percent of your plate, you'll feel much different on Week Three than you did on Week Two.

And if you're starting here? Congratulations on already eating a sound and nutritionally dense diet. Now, let's take it to the next level.

Either way, you'll be upping your energy, easing digestion, and losing weight this week.

This is an intense week for some, but most people report feeling a surge of energy and good feeling almost immediately, not to mention the happy buzz you'll get when the number on the scale begins to plummet. If you are carb-sensitive and you still want to try Week Three, you can always substitute any grain for steamed or stir-fried vegetables in an equal amount. That will make this week even more cleansing, so you might want to ease into this.

WELCOME TO WEEK THREE!

This week, we are making a pretty big switch: Meat is out and gluten-free grains are in. (See page 185 for a detailed explanation of why I want you to leave gluten out of your diet.)

If you're a vegetarian, this week will help you reduce your grain consumption and increase your raw food consumption. If you're not a vegetarian, this week will ease you out of the animal protein habit to make digestion easier for you. Animal-based proteins are difficult to digest, so now we're lightening the load even more.

You'll probably notice an increase in bowel movements because of the added fiber this week, which is good because you'll be clearing out your system. You'll have more energy and clarity, and definitely more weight loss. As in the previous weeks, you won't be overloaded with a lot of food in the morning. Your biggest meal will be during the middle of the day, when you're the busiest and need those calories the most. After this meal, you want to start slowing things down with lighter juices and teas and a dinner that's lighter than lunch, with smaller portions. Think of your days like this: light to heavy to light. This trains your body to be more efficient over time at burning food for fuel rather than storing it as fat. You have choices—I'm not militant! I want you to be creative, but within the parameters of the protocol.

You'll be doing a lot of cleansing activity throughout the day, so make room in your schedule for meals, juice and water breaks, and exercise. Although I don't expect you to get up at 5:30 A.M. if that doesn't work for you, keep the intervals between meals and snacks consistent.

The grains and starches that will make up 20 percent of your plate this week will not contain gluten, but will contain dense nutrition. Here's an introduction, in case you haven't met these guys before:

- Quinoa is higher in protein than most other grains and has twice as much fiber. It contains the amino acid lysine, and also contains iron, manganese, and magnesium.

- Millet is the most digestible of the grains, is alkalizing, has a sweet nutty flavor, is a prebiotic, hydrates the colon, decreases c-reactive protein (increases in c-reactive protein signal inflammation) and triglycerides, has a high antioxidant content, contains serotonin, has niacin (which lowers cholesterol and reduces your risk of heart attacks), and has a high protein content.

- Amaranth reduces inflammation due to the peptides in it, reduces cholesterol, lowers blood pressure, is high in protein and the amino acid lysine, has a high fiber content for bulk and prebiotic action, is a rich source of vitamins and minerals, and strengthens the immune system.

- Sweet potatoes are a great source of magnesium, iron, vitamin D, vitamin A, vitamin B6, and vitamin C. They produce collagen, which helps maintain elasticity of the skin.

- Acorn squash, butternut squash, and other deep orange winter squashes reduce high blood pressure, improve the immune system, and aid in reducing the risk of cancer and osteoarthritis.

A SPECIAL NOTE FOR THE GRAIN-FREE AND GRAIN-INTOLERANT

I want you to be able to do the Piper Protocol no matter what your dietary restrictions. Just as some people wouldn't consider eating meat, I know that some of you don't (or can't) eat any grain, even the non-gluten grains I prescribe in this chapter.

You can still stay with us here! You can do Week Three without the grains. Just stick to lots of vegetables, including some starchy vegetables such as sweet potatoes and acorn squash. Even if you normally eat some animal products, it won't hurt you to leave them out for one week, and a vegetable-only diet this week will prep your system perfectly for Week Four. You can even use most of the recipes in this chapter. Just leave out the grain, and be sure to take your weekly fiber.

WHAT TO BUY

This is the time to go over the plan and pick out the recipes you think you'll want to make. Maybe you'll just want to try one or two and repeat them over the week, or maybe you'll want to try them all! I recommend going to the store frequently so your vegetables are always fresh, but make a list and get the basics before you start. Also, remember to get what you need for juicing, unless you're lucky enough to have a great juice bar nearby and plan to get your juice on the outside. And don't forget your supplements and your pH test kit, to keep an eye on your alkalinity.

SUPPLEMENTS YOU WILL NEED THIS WEEK

Digestive enzymes: You'll be taking four digestive enzyme capsules with each meal and four between meals for a total of 24 per day, so you'll need 168 digestive enzyme supplements in order to get through the week. This might sound like a lot, but it's one of the most important supplements you can take on the Piper Protocol!

Probiotics: 50-billion organism strength (use a lower strength if you are sensitive). Continue to gargle with one capsule and then take a second capsule in the morning before breakfast, and I'll also have you add one in the evening. You'll need a total of 21 capsules this week.

CoQ10 capsules: 100-mg strength. You'll be taking one with breakfast, one with lunch, and one with dinner each day, so you'll need a total of 21 capsules.

Multi-mineral supplement: You'll be taking drops of concentrate in water or a tablet three times per day, with meals. If you use the concentrate, get a small bottle. You'll take 10 drops of liquid in ¼ to ½ cup water three times per day. If you use the tablets, you'll need 21 tablets per week.

Therapeutic oil: You'll be taking 2 tablespoons of extra-virgin olive oil, flax seed oil, coconut oil, or hemp oil per day, or two fish oil gel-caps. Add the oil to your smoothie or your salad, or just take a spoonful, if you like it that way.

Fiber: You can take any form you prefer: chia seeds, ground flax seed, psyllium husk, apple pectin, or hemp seeds. You'll be taking 1 teaspoon three times per day in 1 cup water or added to your smoothie or juice, so you'll need just a small container.

Wheatgrass or E3Live: You'll do one shot of wheatgrass or 1 tablespoon of E3Live every morning before breakfast, so have enough on hand or available for seven shots or 7 tablespoons.

ABOUT THE SCHEDULE

If you haven't done so yet, I'd like you to try getting up at 5:30 A.M. (which means getting to bed by 9:30 P.M.—hard at first but totally worth it!), to see what it's like to really work in sync with your internal clock. However, if this isn't possible in your schedule (or in your temperament), then just keep your meals and breaks at the correct intervals based on your wake-up time, and be sure to get in some exercise every day, even if it's just a walk.

Also consider scheduling a colonic or a lymphatic massage this week, or doing one of the enemas as described in Chapter 8. Weekly isn't too often for these cleanse-enhancing practices, and they can really help to get you over the hump if you're having trouble with the meat-to-grain switch. As you detox, you are loosening up things in the colon and stirring up stored toxic material, and cleaning it out before you reabsorb it is key. So be brave and do that enema, or go get a colonic. The ultimate is a lymphatic massage first, followed by a colonic to really get things moving.

DAILY TEMPLATE

Follow this guide for the week. If you've worked up to this point through Weeks One and Two, you already know the drill. Just follow the differing food plans that replace meat with carbs, and load up on your digestive enzymes. If you're starting here, then prepare to drop some weight and add glowing skin, more energy, clarity of mind, and less bloat.

In the following plan, all recipes in bold type can be found in the Recipes chapter. And don't forget the Snack Rescue section (page 307), if you need it!

5:30 A.M.: Test your pH (saliva and urine) and record the number in your journal.

5:40 A.M.: Do your oil pulling (which you learned how to do on page 127).

6:00 A.M.: Gargle with one probiotics capsule in ¼ cup water (as you've been doing for your

Internal Fitness Prep Step), then take your second probiotics capsule with a glass of water with fresh lemon juice squeezed in, to stimulate the first bowel movement of the day.

6:30 A.M.: Have a shot of wheatgrass or E3Live.

7:00 A.M.: *Breakfast.* Choose from the following:

Goji Berry Mango Smoothie (page 266)
Cocoa Almond Smoothie (page 266)
Raspberry Coconut Green Smoothie (page 265)
Brain Porridge (page 274)

You can add your daily fiber and/or therapeutic oil to your morning smoothie or to your porridge. Along with breakfast, also take:

• Four digestive enzyme capsules
• One CoQ10 capsule
• One mineral supplement (1 tablet or 10 drops of liquid in ¼–½ cup water)
• 1 teaspoon fiber supplement in 1 cup water or added to your breakfast smoothie or porridge. You will eat less because the fiber fills you up, and also helps cleanse your colon more efficiently as you detox.

8:00 A.M.: *Juice break.* Have 8 ounces of any green juice, such as **Green Juice 1, 2, 3,** or **4** (page 259).

9:00 A.M.: *Water break.* Glass of water with the juice of ½ lemon.

10:00 A.M.: *Juice break.* Have any freshly squeezed juice. Also take four digestive enzyme capsules.

11:00 A.M.: *Juice break.* Have any freshly squeezed juice.

12:00 P.M.: *Lunch.* Choose from the following:

Zucchini Spaghetti (page 302), ½ cup cooked quinoa, and green salad
Rainbow Super Slaw with Pinenut Yogurt (page 291) and 1 baked sweet potato
Watercress and Red Bell Pepper Salad (page 292) with ½ cup cooked amaranth
Deviled Eggless (page 301) with raw veggies for dipping

Spicy Veggie Soup (page 294) with ½ cup black rice (sometimes called "forbidden rice" or "forbidden black rice")

Add your therapeutic oil to any lunch entrée, if you haven't taken it already. Right before lunch, also take:

- Four digestive enzyme capsules
- One CoQ10 capsule
- One mineral supplement (1 tablet or 10 drops of liquid in ¼–½ cup water)
- 1 teaspoon fiber supplement in 1 cup water

2:00 P.M.: *Juice break*. Have any freshly squeezed juice. Also take four digestive enzymes capsules.

3:00 P.M.: *Tea time*. Have a cup of any of the following teas:

- Chamomile
- Lemon
- Red raspberry
- Tulsi Holy Basil Lemon
- Green

5:00 P.M.: *Water break*. Have a glass of water with the juice of ½ lemon.

5:30 P.M.: *Exercise break*. If this time works for exercise, try a brisk walk, a yoga class, or anything else that gets your body moving for about 30 minutes. Otherwise, fit it into your schedule as desired, but be sure to get in 30 minutes a day.

6:00 P.M.: *Dinner*. Choose one of the following:

Spicy Butternut Acorn Squash Soup (page 300) with **Spinach "Caesar" Salad with Pumpkin Seed Dressing** (page 296)

Caribbean Wild Rice (page 297) with **Savory Coconut Cream** (page 297) and a mixed green salad

Amaranth Vegetable Steam (page 293)

Bucky Burgers (page 298) with **Cream of Vegetable Power Soup** (page 299)

Gluten-free Pasta with Green Pesto Sauce (page 295) and a mixed green salad

Sweet Potato Lasagna (page 288) with a green salad

Any dinner plate with 80 percent mixed vegetables, cooked or raw, including green salad, and 20 percent any non-gluten grain, such as quinoa, amaranth, or brown rice pilaf flavored with chopped mixed vegetables, herbs, and spices.

Also take:

- Four digestive enzyme capsules
- One CoQ10 capsule
- One mineral supplement (1 tablet or 10 drops of liquid in ¼–½ cup water)
- 1 teaspoon fiber supplement in 1 cup water

8:00 P.M.: *Enzyme break.* Take four digestive enzymes capsules with 1 glass water.

9:00 P.M.: *Time to slow down.* If you got up at 5:30 this morning, you should be getting drowsy. Wind down by turning off electronics and settling in with a warm bath or a good book. Right before bed, take one probiotics supplement.

9:30 to 10:00 P.M.: *Bedtime.* Now that you've come to the end of Week Three, your digestive system should be well rested, you should be feeling rejuvenated and less bloated, and you've probably already enjoyed a generous weight loss. You can do this week for as many times as you like. If you want to stay here for a while longer, marinate in it and learn more about how you feel with each passing week on 80 percent raw and 20 percent carbs.

When you're ready to go deeper, let's get hardcore with Week Four.

CHAPTER 15

Piper Protocol Week Four: Liquid Feast Week

CONTINUE HERE IF:

You've already done Week Three for as many weeks as you're comfortable.

Begin here if:

You already eat a very nutrient-dense, healthful vegan diet or a raw diet and you want to take it to the next level.

If you've just come from Week Three, congratulations on reaching this far! I'm extremely proud of you. You've probably already dropped a good amount of weight and are feeling more energetic and focused as your body has been purging toxins, tipping into a more alkaline state, and repairing your digestion so everything is working more smoothly and easily.

Now things are going to get a bit more challenging.

WELCOME TO WEEK FOUR!

This week, we go deeper. You enjoy a level of cleansing you just can't get when you eat solid food. This is an intensive cleanse experience, and many of my clients rely on it regularly to reboot their systems and get them feeling great, either before an important event or after an overindulgent one.

But there is a reason this is Week Four, and not Week One. You do not want to jump from a junk food or processed food diet full of meat, dairy, and sugar, straight into a liquid feast week. Your body needs preparation, and that's exactly what you've been doing, as you practiced your Internal Fitness Prep Steps and then the initial weeks of the Piper Protocol. It was all for this! Your body is ready, and now you can get down to business and do some really serious internal fitness work.

But don't fear—you won't be deprived or starving. You might miss *chewing*, just because you're in the habit, but it's only for a few days and you'll have plenty to fill your stomach (and I encourage you to chew your juices, smoothies, and soups anyway!). You'll get to enjoy soups, juices, and greens specifically designed to take the pressure off your digestive system for a deeper, more meaningful toxin purge.

Everything you eat this week will be pre-digested—either blended or juiced. Everything you eat will be from the plant kingdom, and almost everything will be raw. You have already been juicing and having smoothies, so you know what you're doing, but when you take in *only liquids* for a full week, you'll see profound and intense changes in your body as well as in your mind and spirit. Liquid feasting is a difficult but highly rewarding path, and most of the difficulty, frankly, is psychological. It's important to remind yourself that you'll have plenty of time to chew after your body has cleansed itself. If you've made it through the other weeks, perhaps taking your time and spending more than a week on each, you are ready.

WHAT ABOUT LONG-TERM LIQUID FEASTING?

Many of my clients do a week and then they ease back into solid food again, but some of my clients like this way of eating so much that they want to stay on the liquid feast for longer than a week. Once you've prepared your body, this is totally fine, with a few conditions. You need to be getting a lot of variety in the vegetables you are including in your juices, smoothies, and soups, so you get a broader range of nutrients. Lots of different kinds of leafy greens are particularly important—kale, Swiss chard, sorrel, watercress, dandelion leaves—try whatever you can find for your juices. You also need to be including smoothies and pureed soups in addition to juice, so you get enough fiber to keep your digestion moving and initiate peristalsis. In addition, be sure you are not skimping on the ground flax and chia seeds, to sweep the toxins and stools out. Then you can stay on the liquid feast for as long as you are comfortable with it and feeling good. If you've gone longer than a week, however, and you really start feeling like you want or need solid food again, this is the time to ease back out of the liquid diet. You can always do it again later. In fact, many of my clients like to do a liquid feast week once a month, or once each season. Just remember that the more time you spend on the liquid feast, the more slowly you need to come back out, easing gradually out of the cleanse with plenty of gentle veggies and fruit. If you dive straight into a pepperoni pizza, you'll be doubled over with stomach pain from the shock of it.

A WORD ABOUT LIQUID DIETS

You may have received mixed messages as well as heard fantastical claims about liquid diets and juice cleansing. Some people say it can bring you back from the brink of disease. Others say it will destroy your metabolism. I've seen plenty of evidence that juice cleansing can help the body conquer health issues, and no evidence that a well-planned and nutritionally adequate liquid cleanse does any harm to the metabolism or anything else.

Nutritionally supportive liquid feasts give the digestive system a much-needed rest because you won't have to process any solid food. It's easy to process and digest liquid. Because it isn't distracted by digestion, the body can divert all its resources to healing and detoxification. Even a one-day juice fast can increase internal healing, but three days is better. And what's better than three days? Seven days!

What I've noticed in my practice is that by day three on a liquid feast the body is just beginning to make a change. Most people say they start to feel poorly on day three, and then they stop the cleanse. However, it's much more beneficial to stay on a liquid feast beyond that third day when you don't feel so great. That feeling is a sign that your body is purging toxins from a deep level, and if you stop, you won't get everything out. Seven days really gives the body a chance to loosen up toxic waste material from the colon as well as from the cells.

Another complaint I sometimes get is that people get constipated on a juice fast because they aren't getting any fiber, so the bowels have no stimulation to move. Anything still sitting around in there tends to stay in there. People expect miracles from juice fasts, as though the waste will just fall right out of them, but that's not how it works. In these cases, people usually didn't prepare their bodies for what was about to happen, or they have been chronically constipated or have a sluggish colon to begin with and need some help in the form of an enema or colonic. Please give your body what it needs.

I do not expect you to have the problem of constipation during Week Four. You've been preparing your body all along, through the initial weeks, for this week. You haven't been eating junky processed food, or even a whole lot of cooked food. You haven't been eating mucus-forming dairy and gluten, and you've been taking fiber supplements. You've already been purging fat-soluble toxins, so your liquid feast won't be such a shock to you. You've been detoxing for at least a week and possibly even three or more weeks. This eases you into the liquid feast smoothly and comfortably.

Also, I won't be taking away your fiber. I not only want your bowels to continue to get the signal to move toxins through, I also want to keep feeding your good microflora with prebiotics. This will also help you feel full. You'll be amazed at how full you can be on liquids only. If you do get hungry, it will mostly be psychological. You want to chew. You're used to solid food. This is one week only, so it's not going to kill you not to chew for a while. Let your body rest—and that includes your jaw! You're getting plenty of nutrition. Nobody on my cleanse will starve or be even remotely malnourished.

This week, you'll be enjoying delicious juices and smoothies, just as in past weeks. You'll also be getting both cooked and raw soups to nourish you, and you'll be having your supplements, too. Honestly, it's mostly raw soups, but just so you don't hate me I'm putting in a few pureed cooked soups. If you are up for the challenge, however, save these for later and do all raw this week. I promise you the results are out of this world. It's going to be a great week: Mentally challenging, physically rejuvenating, and spiritually enlightening! It's everything you love about the Piper Protocol, culminating in this final powerful week.

WHAT TO BUY

This week, you'll have a lot of fun in the organic produce section of the market, assuming you will be making your own juices. Juice the juices you want to try this week and make yourself a list. And don't forget your supplements and pH test kit! If you're still a bit acidic, you should definitely see your numbers moving in the direction of alkalinity this week.

SUPPLEMENTS YOU WILL NEED THIS WEEK

In the last chapter, I told you exactly what to look for in these supplements. This is a list of what you'll need this week:

Digestive enzymes: You'll be taking five digestive enzyme capsules with each meal and five between meals for a total of 30 per day, so you'll need 210 digestive enzyme supplements to get through the week.

Probiotics: 50-billion organism strength. Continue to gargle with one capsule and then take a second capsule in the morning before breakfast, and I'll also have you add one in the evening. You'll need a total of 21 capsules this week. By now, this amount should be okay with your tummy.

CoQ10 capsules: 100-mg strength. You'll be taking one with breakfast, one with lunch, and one with dinner each day, so you'll need a total of 21 capsules.

Multi-mineral supplement: You'll be taking drops of concentrate in water or a tablet three times per day, with meals. If you use the concentrate, get a small bottle. You'll take 10 drops of liquid in ¼ to ½ cup water three times per day. If you use the tablets, you'll need 21 tablets per week.

Therapeutic oil: You'll be taking 2 tablespoons of extra-virgin olive oil, flax seed oil, coconut oil, or hemp oil per day, or two fish oil gel-caps. Add the oil to your smoothie or your salad, or just take it by the spoonful.

Fiber: You can take any form you prefer: chia seeds, ground flax seed, psyllium husk, apple pectin, or hemp seeds. You'll be taking 1 teaspoon three times per day in 1 to 1¼ cups water or added to your smoothie or juice, so you'll need just a small container.

Wheatgrass or E3Live: You'll do one shot of wheatgrass or 1 tablespoon of E3Live every morning before breakfast, so have enough on hand or available for seven shots or 7 tablespoons.

Optional: Dr. Patrick Flanagan's Crystal Energy (10 drops in 1 cup water). This is optional, but

I love to add it to the routine during this last week because it's a great way to alkalize water and it has a detoxification effect. It adds extra energy to the water, or whatever you are drinking. You can buy it online (see Resources).

ABOUT THE SCHEDULE

This week, you'll be experiencing some intense physical detoxification. Even though you're ready, it will still feel different from the other weeks, when you were eating solid food. You may have more energy, or you may feel as if you need to spend more time relaxing, meditating, taking long baths, and just generally taking it easy. This is a good impulse. The more you can manage stress this week, the more effective the cleanse will be. For that reason, I'd like you to get even more sleep this week, if you can. Shoot for eight to nine hours. I also recommend getting a massage this week and doing gentle, stress-reducing exercise only.

If you haven't done so yet, *I highly recommend* a colonic or enema this week, and a lymphatic massage added would be even more helpful. If you can, do a lymphatic massage first to move the lymph into the colon, and the colonic after to flush it all out.

This is an intense cleansing week, more so than any other week, and the detoxification rate in your body is going to increase. A colonic or enema will really help, especially since you aren't eating solid food. Your body may need just a little coaxing to really clean out the colon at the deepest level, and your lymphatic system could also use some assistance as the cells purge their toxins and send them into the lymph in the colon for removal. Also, be sure to drink a lot of water this week, in addition to your juices and other liquid foods.

DAILY TEMPLATE

This is your plan for the next seven days. As before, you have choices, but these choices are all liquids. As before, you don't have to get up at 5:30 A.M. if you can't, but I encourage it if you can. If you don't, just adjust your meals to the intervals listed.

In the following plan, all recipes in bold type can be found in the Recipes chapter. I'd like you to avoid any solid food snacks this week, even though you may have relied on them in past weeks. It's so important to keep everything that goes into your system liquid this week!

5:30 A.M.: Test your pH (saliva and urine) and record the number in your journal.

5:40 A.M.: Do your oil pulling (which you learned how to do on page 127).

6:00 A.M.: Gargle with one probiotics capsule in water, then take your second probiotics capsule with a glass of water with fresh lemon juice squeezed in. This will help to stimulate the first bowel movement of the day.

6:30 A.M.: Have a shot of wheatgrass or E3Live.

7:00 A.M.: *Breakfast.* **Raspberry Coconut Green Smoothie** (page 265). You could add your morning fiber and/or your therapeutic oil to this smoothie. Also take:

- Five digestive enzyme capsules
- One CoQ10 capsule
- One mineral supplement (1 tablet or 10 drops of liquid in ¼–½ cup water)
- 1 teaspoon fiber supplement in 1 cup water or in your smoothie
- Optional: Dr. Patrick Flanagan's Crystal Energy (10 drops in 1 cup water)

8:00 A.M.: *Juice break.* Have any freshly squeezed juice.

9:00 A.M.: *Water break.* Glass of water with juice of ½ lemon.

10:00 A.M.: *Juice break.* Have any freshly squeezed juice. Also take five digestive enzyme capsules.

11:00 A.M.: *Juice break.* Have any freshly squeezed juice.

12:00 P.M.: *Lunch.* Have both of the following:

Green Juice 4 (page 259)
Potassium Broth (page 304)

Add your therapeutic oil to either your juice or broth, or take it separately, if you haven't already. Right before lunch, also take:

- Five digestive enzyme capsules
- One CoQ10 capsule
- One mineral supplement (1 tablet or 10 drops of liquid in ¼–½ cup water)
- 1 teaspoon fiber supplement in 1 cup water, or in your juice
- Optional: Dr. Patrick Flanagan's Crystal Energy (10 drops in 1 cup water)

2:00 P.M.: *Juice break*. Have any freshly squeezed juice.

3:00 P.M.: *Juice break*. Have any freshly squeezed juice. Also take:

• Five digestive enzyme capsules
• Optional: Dr. Patrick Flanagan's Crystal Energy (10 drops in 1 cup water)

5:00 P.M.: *Juice or water break*. Have either the freshly squeezed juice of your choice or water with the juice of ½ lemon. Note: If you didn't add fiber to your morning smoothie, you can take it now with a glass of water.

5:30 P.M. or 6:00 P.M.: *Exercise break*. Take it easy this week. A gentle walk in the fresh air, a gentle yoga class, or just some relaxed stretching is plenty. You could also do an easy yoga DVD.

6:00 P.M.: *Dinner*. Choose one of the following:

Spicy Butternut Acorn Squash Soup (page 300) topped with ground flax or hemp seeds
Any homemade vegetable soup made into a puree
Any pure-vegetable smoothie or juice

Also take:

• Five digestive enzyme capsules
• One CoQ10 capsule
• One mineral supplement
• 1 teaspoon fiber supplement in 1 cup water or in your juice
• Optional: Dr. Patrick Flanagan's Crystal Energy (10 drops in 1 cup water)

8:00 P.M.: *Tea break*. Have a cup of Pau d'Arco tea. Also take five digestive enzyme capsules with a glass of water.

8:30 P.M.: *Time to slow down*. It's time to get your mind and body ready for sleep—the earlier the better. Even if you didn't do a lot today, you might still feel tired because of all the hard detoxification work your body is doing. Turn off all the electronics, put your phone away, and meditate to cleanse your mind and spirit while you're cleansing your body. Also take your final probiotic supplement with a glass of water.

9:00 P.M.: *Bedtime.* It may seem early, but try going to bed at 9:00 this week. If you can sleep from 9:00 to 5:30 or 6:00 A.M., you're doing great things for your detoxification. Your body can really use that extra time right now.

At the end of the week, if you're not doing another round of Week Four or moving to the optional bonus cleanse in the next chapter, and have chosen to end your cleanse, it's *extremely important* for you to read Chapter 17. *Do not immediately return to solid food* after doing Week Four. You must step back down and ease back into eating solid food.

In the meantime, you did it! I know you're feeling fantastic and looking glorious right now. You should also be on an energy high. This is living! And you did it for yourself.

CHAPTER 16

Bonus Three- to Six-Day Cellular Cleanse

FOR THE ULTIMATE INTERNAL fitness experience, here's a bonus cleanse experience. You can do it after Week Four, or you don't have to do it at all. Many of my readers and some of my clients won't take cleansing to this level, and it's completely up to you whether you want to get this intense, but this is the program I give to my celebrity clients who have to look dramatically different in a few days, for a *Sports Illustrated* Swimsuit Issue photo shoot or for presenting at the Academy Awards or for a movie shoot.

This is a total body overhaul, like a deep scrubbing of your oven after a Thanksgiving dinner. But here you're scrubbing out your cells, instead. It's not necessarily meant to be done in the four-week cycle, although you should always at least do Week Three attempting this, so you can prepare your body for this level of intense cleansing. You'll begin to pull toxins from a very deep level, even from outside the colon wall, to travel in the colon to be eliminated. The therapeutic ingredients in this cleanse can absorb up to 30 times their weight in toxins. The fiber gathers it and makes the elimination easier.

WHY CLEANSE SO INTENSELY?

The world has changed dramatically, even since my childhood. Our air, water, and soil are full of industrial chemicals. We put chemicals on our skin and we eat them in our food, and it has become a real burden on our body's detoxification pathways. I believe this toxicity is behind the epidemic of autoimmune disease that we've seen in recent years, along with increases in the incidence of childhood leukemia and autism.

The food we eat is nothing like what it once was, and we've largely forgotten the ancient practice of cleansing the body on a regular basis. This is very important at several key stages in life—especially before becoming pregnant, so the body doesn't pass as many toxins to the unborn child, but also following times of toxin exposure, great stress, hormonal changes, and life transitions. Cleansing used to be a seasonal ritual, too, especially in the spring. We can reclaim this ancient practice and bring its benefits into the modern world, where we need them more than ever. Not only will deep cleansing help to prevent chronic disease and improve physical health and mental clarity, but it will also allow the body to absorb and assimilate more nutrients from food, increase the oxygen in the blood, and even increase longevity.

If you're new to intense cleansing, just do three days the first time. If you're a veteran cleanser, you can try the six days, or anywhere in between. The main difference between this week and Week Four is in the supplements that scrub the walls of the colon clean.

SPECIAL FEATURES OF THE BONUS CLEANSE

This cleanse is powerful. So powerful, in fact, that I require you do a colonic or two or an enema daily this week. In particular, I recommend a coffee enema every other day during the cleanse (I explain how to do this on page 137), followed by a wheatgrass implant later that day if you can. If you do a three-day cleanse, do the enema and implant on the first and third day. If you do a six-day cleanse, do it on days one, three, and five or two, four, and six. Or, get a colonic at the beginning and end of your cleanse. As you release at this intense level, you'll be amazed at how much comes out of you. I've seen even very tiny people release huge amounts of waste during this week. Where were they keeping it, I wonder? The average weight loss I see on this cleanse is 2 pounds per day, so in three days, you could lose 6 pounds. That's a lot of weight in a very short amount of time, and you will feel it. You will feel lighter, emptier, and more buoyant, and you'll look brand-new.

This week is similar to Week Four, but we'll be adding more supplements and more detox elements for greater intensity. Let's go over some of the special ingredients we're going to utilize this week:

Zeolite: This is a mineral with a honeycomb-shaped structure that traps toxins within it. Zeolite comes from a mixture of volcanic ash and sea salt. Most volcanoes are on islands surrounded by water, so when they erupt, the lava runs into the ocean and mixes with the salt, forming this unusual mineral. I wonder if they ever searched for zeolite off the island of Montserrat, where my father is from, since they've had volcanic activity in recent years.

Zeolite is a very safe way to remove toxins from the body. Its structure isolates toxins and delivers them out of the body safely. Six to eight hours after taking it, it moves through the system and out. It's a smart detoxifier because it removes the heavy metals and not the good minerals you want. You add it to water or juice, and it has no bad taste. It's a bit expensive—it's about $52 for a 14-ounce jar—but if you choose to do this bonus cleanse, it's an essential purchase.

Ground flax seeds and psyllium husks: You've already been taking fiber supplements, but now I want you to get your fiber from either of these two specific and highly effective fiber sources, and you'll be taking more than you were before. These are both easy to find, but look for gluten-free varieties. Some people get bloated with psyllium, so if you're one of those people, choose ground flax seed. It's important to use ground flax seed, which has a rough surface that can scrape debris from the colon, rather than whole flax seeds, which are smooth. Ground flax is also a rich source of fiber and micronutrients such as vitamin B1, manganese, and alpha-linolenic acid (ALA), which the body converts to omega-3 fatty acid. Omega-3 is very useful for reducing inflammation in the body. Studies suggest flax seed could lower your risk of heart disease, diabetes, and cancer, and that it also has benefits for breast and prostate health because of the omega-3 fatty acids. Flax seeds are also rich in lignans, also called phytoestrogens, which help to eliminate free radicals in the body, lower cholesterol, improve blood sugar levels, and protect against skin radiation through their anti-inflammatory and antioxidant properties.

Wheatgrass: You've had the option to take wheatgrass or E3Live in the past weeks, but this week I want you to buddy up to wheatgrass for real. (If you cannot find wheatgrass, E3Live is still an acceptable substitute.) There are many ways to take wheatgrass. You can buy it in powdered form, you can buy frozen shots at the health food store (just defrost and drink), or you can even grow your own and juice it yourself in a masticating juicer. If you're not in an area where you can buy wheatgrass patches and growing it seems daunting, then go with one of the easier options. Do what's possible.

Wheatgrass is an amazing health tonic. Some people find its intense grassy taste hard to take, but it does great things for your body. Do the shot quickly and it will all be over in a flash. Personally, I have to chew it in my mouth until it becomes like water and has no taste, then I swallow it and take a deep breath through my open mouth to get the leftover taste out. It works. I don't get nauseous or queasy. Wheatgrass increases your red blood cell count while it lowers blood pressure. It's a purifier of the blood, organs, and the digestive tract. It encourages the metabolism by stimulating the thyroid gland. This aids weight management and other related digestive issues, including indigestion and constipation. Wheatgrass also alkalizes the blood because it's filled with alkalizing minerals. Because of this function, it has been used to aid in the healing of peptic ulcers, IBS, and ulcerative colitis.

Freshly squeezed wheatgrass is filled with abundant living enzymes that are used for every function in the body. Because wheatgrass has a high percentage of chlorophyll, which is chemically similar to our own blood (only the center molecule differs—for blood it's iron and for chlorophyll it's magnesium), it has an affect similar to a transfusion. It increases energy in the body, rejuvenates skin, and has anti-aging properties. It also helps to neutralize the toxic effects of heavy metals and other dangerous substances such as cadmium, mercury, nicotine, polyvinyl chloride, and strontium. You may also remember that I like to use wheatgrass in enemas because it feeds the body with minerals via the sigmoidal vein, which goes right into the liver. It can also help to heal a damaged intestinal lining of the lower gastrointestinal tract.

Astragalus tea: This immune-boosting herb is excellent during this cleanse because it helps protect you as you release potent toxins. It has a sweet, pleasant taste, and it also encourages you to flush out excess water your body is holding.

WHAT TO BUY

This week, you'll focus on liquids but you'll still be preparing things for yourself, so look over the schedule and the recipes and make yourself a list. You'll have more supplements to buy this week as well, and of course, your trusty old pH strips!

SUPPLEMENTS YOU WILL NEED DURING THE BONUS CLEANSE

Digestive enzymes: You'll be taking five digestive enzyme capsules with each meal and five between meals for a total of 30 per day, so take that times the number of days you'll be doing this cleanse. If you're doing it for three days, you'll need 90 digestive enzyme supplements.

Probiotics: 50-billion organism strength. Continue to gargle with one capsule and then take a second capsule in the morning before breakfast, and I'll also have you add one in the evening. You would need nine capsules for three days.

CoQ10 capsules: 100-mg strength. You'll be taking one with breakfast, one with lunch, and one with dinner each day, so you'll need a total of nine capsules for three days.

Multi-mineral supplement: You'll be taking drops of concentrate in water or a tablet three times per day, with meals. If you use the concentrate, get a small bottle. You will take 10 drops of liquid in ¼ to ½ cup water three times per day. If you use the tablets, you'll need nine tablets per week.

Therapeutic oil: You'll be taking 4 tablespoons extra-virgin olive oil, flax seed oil, coconut oil, or hemp oil per day, or two fish oil gel-caps. Add the oil to your smoothie or your salad, or just take it by the spoonful.

Zeolite: You'll be taking a total of 6 tablespoons per day, so you'll need enough for 18 tablespoons for a three-day cleanse. A standard-size jar should be fine.

Fiber: This week, you'll be taking 1 tablespoon psyllium husk or ground flax seed three times per day along with your zeolite, which comes to 9 tablespoons for a three-day cleanse. A small container should be plenty. You should have some left over from previous weeks.

Wheatgrass: You'll do one shot of fresh wheatgrass or 1 tablespoon powdered wheatgrass in 1½ cups water every morning before breakfast, and again every evening, so have enough on hand or available for six shots or 6 tablespoons.

Dr. Patrick Flanagan's Crystal Energy (10 drops in 1 cup water): This was optional last week, but required this week, for an intensely alkalizing experience and to increase detoxification.

Astragalus tea: As described on page 246. You'll be having 2 cups per day, so you'll need six tea bags for three days.

S. A. Wilson Gold Roast Enema Coffee: Available online (see Resources). This is for the coffee enema I want you to be doing every other day, if you are doing this instead of getting a professional colonic.

Enema bag and necessary equipment: As described in Chapter 8.

ABOUT THE SCHEDULE

This cleanse is pretty simple. You will do exactly the same thing each day for three days (four to six days, if you are an experienced cleanser). However, it's intense and takes a lot of concentration. If you can do this cleanse during a three-day period when you don't have any other significant obligations, that is ideal. Then you can precisely follow the schedule, including rising at 5:30 A.M. and doing everything at the exact times I specify. This is a *strict* cleanse, and I want you to do it exactly right for the maximum benefit. A long weekend with no work or social engagements is perfect.

You will notice a dramatic difference in your body and skin. Your stomach will be flatter, your facial features will become more defined, and you'll see more muscle definition. You'll feel energetic and light as air.

In previous weeks I recommended a colonic or enema, but this week, I *require* you do at least one of these. For the best results, take a coffee enema every other day to help you remove all the toxins that are coming out at a higher rate than normal from your liver. As you learned in Chapter 8, the coffee enema is an intensive liver detoxifier, and that's just what you need right now. Coffee enemas will get the toxins out quickly to keep your body from reabsorbing them. At the end of the cleanse, a colonic with a professional will be the icing on the cake. (Much better than actual icing or cake!)

Note:

Do not do this cleanse for more than six days.

Do not do this cleanse if you haven't prepared your body by first doing at least Week Three and preferably Weeks Three and Four.

Come off this cleanse carefully, according to the directions in the next chapter.

Do not do this cleanse if you are pregnant or think you might be pregnant.

DAILY TEMPLATE

For the next three to six days, follow this plan. Do everything in order. Do your best to follow the actual times. If you can get time off work to do this cleanse, or do it on a long weekend, that is ideal and allows for following the schedule as precisely as possible.

5:30 A.M.: Test your pH (saliva and urine) and record the number in your journal.

5:40 A.M.: Do your oil pulling (which you learned how to do on page 127).

6:00 A.M.: Take your probiotics capsule with a glass of water with fresh lemon juice squeezed in, then gargle with one probiotics capsule in water. This will help to stimulate the first bowel movement of the day.

6:30 A.M.: Have a shot of fresh wheatgrass, or 1 tablespoon powdered wheatgrass in 1½ cups water.

7:00 A.M.: *Zeolite blend*. Mix 2 tablespoons zeolite blend and 1 tablespoon ground flax seed or psyllium husk in 3 cups water. This will fill you up and serve as breakfast. Also take:

- Five digestive enzyme capsules
- One CoQ10 capsule
- One mineral supplement (1 tablet or 10 drops of liquid in ¼–½ cup water)
- 4 tablespoons therapeutic oil (or mix it into your juice at 10:00 A.M.)
- Dr. Patrick Flanagan's Crystal Energy (10 drops in 1 cup water)

8:00 A.M.: *Juice break*. Have any freshly squeezed vegetable juice. Add 10 drops Dr. Patrick Flanagan's Crystal Energy to your juice.

9:00 A.M.: *Water break*. Have a glass of water with the juice of ½ lemon.

10:00 A.M.: *Juice break*. Have 2 cups of any **Green Juice** (page 259), no fruit other than lemon. Add 10 drops Dr. Patrick Flanagan's Crystal Energy. Also take five digestive enzyme capsules.

11:00 A.M.: *Juice break*. Have any freshly squeezed vegetable juice. Add 10 drops Dr. Patrick Flanagan's Crystal Energy.

12:00 P.M.: *Zeolite blend*. Mix 2 tablespoons zeolite blend and 1 tablespoon ground flax seed or psyllium husk in 3 cups water. This is your lunch and it will fill you up. Also take:

- Five digestive enzyme capsules
- One CoQ10 capsule
- One mineral supplement (1 tablet or 10 drops of liquid in ¼–½ cup water)
- 4 tablespoons therapeutic oil (or mix it into your juice at 10:00 A.M.)
- Dr. Patrick Flanagan's Crystal Energy (10 drops in 1 cup water)

2:00 P.M.: *Juice break*. Have 2 cups of any **Green Juice** (page 259), no fruit other than lemon. Add 10 drops Dr. Patrick Flanagan's Crystal Energy.

3:00 P.M.: *Juice break*. Have any vegetable juice. Add 10 drops Dr. Patrick Flanagan's Crystal Energy. Also take five digestive enzyme capsules.

4:00 P.M.: Have a hot cup of Astragalus tea.

5:00 P.M.: *Juice or water break*. Have either the freshly squeezed juice of your choice or water with the juice of ½ lemon. Add 10 drops Dr. Patrick Flanagan's Crystal Energy.

5:30 P.M.: *Exercise break*. This is no time for anything strenuous. Take a meditative walk outside or do some gentle yoga stretches to get your lymphatic system moving.

6:00 P.M.: *Zeolite blend*. Mix 2 tablespoons zeolite blend and 1 tablespoon ground flax seed or psyllium husk into 3 cups water. This is your dinner. Also take:

- Five digestive enzyme capsules
- One CoQ10 capsule
- One mineral supplement (1 tablet or 10 drops of liquid in ¼–½ cup water)
- 4 tablespoons therapeutic oil (or mix it into your juice at 10:00 A.M.)
- Dr. Patrick Flanagan's Crystal Energy (10 drops in 1 cup water)

7:00 P.M.: *Wheatgrass break.* Have another shot of fresh wheatgrass, or 1 tablespoon powdered wheatgrass in 1½ cups water.

8:00 P.M.: *Juice or water break.* If you are hungry and need some more nutrients, here you can add another **Green Juice** (page 259). Otherwise, just have a glass of water with fresh lemon juice. Add 10 drops Dr. Patrick Flanagan's Crystal Energy. Also take five digestive enzyme capsules.

8:30 P.M.: *Time to slow down.* Start winding down now. Although you haven't been externally taxing yourself, your body has had a very active internal fitness day, so begin calming your mind. This is an excellent time to meditate and work on your emotional cleansing, letting go of baggage and thoughts and ideas that no longer serve you.

9:00 P.M.: *Tea break.* Have another hot cup of Astragalus tea, then turn in and get a good, long detoxifying sleep.

9:30 P.M.: Lights out—it's bedtime!

....

TOO HARD, TOO FAST?

This cleanse is intense. You are pulling toxins from very deep inside, and some people may find that they are detoxing too quickly, which can result in some unpleasant symptoms, especially if you aren't drinking enough water to help your body flush everything out so that the toxins don't get ahead of your natural detoxification system. Some signs that you are detoxing deeply and/or quickly include:

Severe headache
Cystic acne
Nausea
Body odor
Really stinky, weird-looking stool and/or urine
Brain fog
Weakness

If you notice any of these symptoms, first try drinking more water. If your symptoms go away, hydration was the issue. If they don't, check if you need an enema or if it's time for a colonic. This usually solves the problem. If it doesn't then it's time to back off the cleanse. Go back to Week Four, then Week Three. You can always work back up to the cellular cleanse as your body gets a little more detoxed and accustomed to the process.

....

After this cleanse, you'll notice that you have more energy, you're absorbing nutrients from your food more efficiently, you have better digestion, and you even look younger. Many of my clients also tell me they get a surge in their libido—and that's always nice!

Now that you've come to the end of the cleanse cycle, it's time to decide how to live your life, post-Piper. In the next chapter, I'll walk you through your new life and show you the sights. You're going to love it here.

CHAPTER 17

Living the Piper Protocol

NOW THAT YOU'VE REACHED the end of the four-week plan, you've dissolved and flushed away the cellular toxins within you that negatively affect your internal terrain and, by extension, your internal fitness. So why go back to all your bad habits that made you feel so much heavier, more sluggish, and less beautiful than you feel now?

Although I don't intend for you to do anything like Week Four on a daily basis, you can certainly take the essential practices from the Piper Protocol with you into your everyday life. In this chapter, I'll show you how.

KEEP YOUR INTERNAL FITNESS PREP STEP HABITS

If you're practicing all the Internal Fitness Prep Steps as you learned them, and maintained them through the cleanse, then they should be good, established habits. Why ditch a good habit? These are all easy things you can do every day to keep your body, mind, and spirit thriving and to encourage and maintain internal fitness. You are internally fitter today than you were when you first picked up this book, so let the Prep Steps help you stay that way. Here they are one more time, so you can love them and live them every day, for as long as you want to stay internally fit:

INTERNAL FITNESS PREP STEPS

1. Once a day, take five minutes to sit, relax, and take five slow deep breaths. For each breath, inhale for a slow count of 5 and exhale for a slow count of 5.

2. Every time you eat, take small bites and chew each bite at least 25 times.

3. Establish a more regular body rhythm by going to bed at the same time on most nights and getting up at the same time on most mornings (and sleep for seven to eight hours in between!).

4. Take two probiotics capsules (containing 50 billion bacteria) every morning on an empty stomach. Mix one into warm water and gargle it, and then take the other one with water.

5. Test your saliva and urine pH every morning, and drink more alkaline water—8 cups a day for women, 9 cups a day for men. Also, test your water source to ensure that it has a pH at or above 7, or just add a squeeze of fresh lemon juice to your water to make it more alkaline.

6. Drink a raw smoothie every day, from green leafy vegetables, berries, and water or coconut water.

7. Never drink and eat at the same time.

8. Practice oil pulling every morning, right before rinsing with your probiotics (see page 127).

9. Once a week (or more often, as needed), let go of something that is holding you back, large or small.

10. Pay attention to your poop and what it's telling you about your internal fitness. Check the Bristol Stool Chart (page 156) and the Piper Poop Chart (page 158) every so often to see how you're doing.

And here's one more I just can't help adding:

11. Whenever you're willing and able, visit a certified and experienced colon
    hydrotherapist, and/or give yourself a therapeutic enema. It's one of the best things you
    can do for your internal fitness!

REMEMBER YOUR FOOD-COMBINING RULES

Just because you're done cleansing doesn't mean you should start messing up your digestion all
over again. Food combining is powerful, and I hope you'll continue to remember what *never* to
eat together. Here's a summary:

Always eat fruit alone, or before a meal, never after.
Don't mix protein and starchy carbohydrates. (In other words, when you are eating 80:20,
the 20 percent should be *either* protein *or* carbohydrates, such as meat or gluten-free
grains.)
Don't mix beans with meat or eggs with meat or dairy with meat. In fact, the only thing
you should ever mix with meat is vegetables.
Eat grains only with vegetables/salad.

MAINTAIN YOUR RATIOS . . . MOST OF THE TIME

Whether you're a meat-eater or a vegetarian, a cooked-food aficionado or a raw foodist, you can
always maintain, for the most part, a healthful 80:20 ratio. When you eat a meal, make 80 percent of it vegetables, preferably raw. The other 20 percent can be cooked—meat *or* grain or even
starchy vegetables such as sweet potatoes. Just don't mix the meat and grain (as per sound food-
combining principles).

If you eat like this at most meals, then the occasional indulgence won't affect your weight or
internal fitness. It might affect your digestion, but this will be temporary, as long as you get back
to your food-combining rules and your 80:20 ratio.

STAY BROKEN-UP WITH GLUTEN, DAIRY, AND SUGAR

You might still want them because they have an addictive effect in your body, but gluten, dairy, and sugar all work against your internal fitness, add toxic elements to your body, are difficult to digest, and/or contain useless, nutrient-void calories. I'm not saying you can never have another piece of birthday cake or wedge of good cheese, but I *am* saying that you'll be better off without those things, and if you never, ever eat gluten, dairy, or sugar again, you'll be better than fine. Think of them as that bad boyfriend or girlfriend your friends warned you about but you just wouldn't listen. Yep, all three of them are no good!

Listen to me, now! Many companies make excellent gluten-free food products (but still read the labels), and there are also many great gluten-free cookbooks, so you can start playing around with recipes on your own. As for dairy, that's easy. Almond milk, coconut milk, hazelnut milk, hemp milk—the alternatives are out there and delicious (see the Recipes for homemade almond milk and variations on pages 268–271).

KEEP THE PIPER PROTOCOL WEEKS IN PLAY

You can always do the cleanse in this book again, whenever you feel your internal fitness lagging. You can also jump in anywhere again—start at Week Three, or go back and forth between Weeks Two and Three for a month, or do Weeks Three and Four, and then back to Week Three. There are so many options because the Piper Protocol is ultimately customizable for you and how you want to use it.

For many of my clients, I recommend they eat like this all the time, alternating Weeks Two and Three. For vegetarians, I recommend they stick with Week Three most of the time. And when you need to get a little more intense, you can always throw in another round of Week Four, with or without the subsequent bonus cleanse afterward. Just remember to step up and step back down through the weeks whenever you do a liquid feast.

Some of my clients get even more fancy in mixing the weeks into their daily lives. They might do Week Two for the first half of the week, and Week Three for the remainder, or Week Three for half a week, and then end the week with Week Four, using the Week Two ratio for special occasions. This second option is a staple at the Piper Center, and it can be your new way of eating, too.

DON'T FORGET EMOTIONAL CLEANSING

When you don't deal with your emotional issues, they'll surface as physical issues. I guarantee it. Repressing emotional issues causes stress in the body, and the chronic release of stress hormones acidifies tissue, contributes to inflammation, and eventually causes a cascade of imbalances that can lead to chronic disease. Whatever it takes for you to handle your emotional issues, know that this is just as important as your physical issues for achieving true internal fitness. Keep up with your healthy habits, but practice stress relief such as meditation, yoga, and exercise, and have someone to talk to. Whether it's a group of supportive friends or a good therapist (or both!), you need to get the toxins out—toxic feelings included!

That's it. It's simple. Because the Piper Protocol, at its heart, really *is* simple. It's about living in harmony with your body, mind, and spirit. It's about living in sync with your internal rhythms, and the rhythms of the natural world around you. This is how you take care of yourself. Don't you think you deserve it? I *know* you do.

Finally, I haven't talked about God in this book until now, but having a connection to something greater than yourself can give you not only a sense of purpose but also a sense of balance and calm. It can help you let go of things that don't really support you anymore, and it can aid you in knowing how supported, loved, and guided you are. It might not be God for you, but if you can find something to turn to when life gets a little too much for you (or even when everything is wonderful), you'll discover greater strength in your efforts to take care of and cherish yourself.

> *"Do you not know that your body is a temple of the Holy Spirit within you?"*
> —*1 Corinthians 6:19*

> *"Whether you eat or drink, or whatever you do, do in the glory of God."*
> —*1 Corinthians 10:31*

Cleansing and rebuilding will unveil the true extent of what health can feel like for you. It is an ancient practice, a whole-life practice, and now it is *your* practice, helping you to grow into and fully flourish as yourself. Now that you know how to be internally fit, let it become your way, your path, your life. And what a life you'll have to look forward to!

Yours in Cleanliness and Godliness,
Tracy Piper

CHAPTER 18

Recipes

JUICES

For all juice recipes, simply put all the listed ingredients in a juicer and process. The order doesn't matter. It's difficult to say how much each juice recipe makes because this will vary depending on the size and juiciness of your vegetables and fruit and the type of juicer you have chosen. In general, however, have about 8 to 12 ounces (1 to 1½ cups) of juice per serving, and save any remaining juice in an airtight container in the refrigerator to drink throughout the day. Finish it within 12 hours, for best enzyme retention. If you have leftover juice you can't finish within 12 hours, freeze it in an ice cube tray and add the concentrated veggie nutrition to anything you are preparing later, like soup or a smoothie.

CARROT JUICE

4 to 6 medium carrots

CARROT/APPLE JUICE

4 to 6 medium carrots
1 apple

GREEN JUICE, SIX WAYS

All of these versions of Green Juice are packed with nutrition, but they get less sweet as you go down the list, so start with Green Juice 1, and as you get used to juices with a greater proportion of vegetables, move through the numbers until you're enjoying Green Juice 6. Also note that juices that include ginger (like Green Juice 2) are especially helpful when the weather is colder. Raw vegetables make you cold, but ginger and cayenne warm everything up without requiring any heat or cooking. Juices with cucumbers and lemons or limes (like Green Juices 1 and 4) are particularly cooling in hot weather.

GREEN JUICE 1

½ bunch of leafy kale

1 apple

1 small cucumber

1 lime, peeled

GREEN JUICE 2

1 small head or ½ large head of romaine lettuce

1 apple

1 medium cucumber

2 celery stalks

¼-inch piece of fresh ginger

GREEN JUICE 3

1 bunch of dandelion leaves

1 bunch of fresh parsley

1 apple

½ bunch of leafy kale

1 lemon, peeled

GREEN JUICE 4

1 bunch of spinach or 2 cups packed leaves

1 medium cucumber

½ lemon, peeled

1 apple (optional)

GREEN JUICE 5

1 small head or ½ large head of romaine lettuce

1 medium cucumber

2 celery stalks

1 lemon, peeled

GREEN JUICE 6

2 bunches of leafy kale

1 large head of romaine lettuce

1 medium cucumber

2 celery stalks

1 to 1½ lemons, peeled

LIV4EVER JUICE

This juice is a great liver cleanser.

1 large beet, trimmed

1 apple

1 lemon, peeled

1/3 medium cucumber

4 to 6 dandelion leaves

SNACK JUICE

1 bunch of leafy kale

1 small head of romaine lettuce

2 apples

3 to 4 stalks fennel

1 medium cucumber

1 lime, peeled

3 to 4 mint leaves

RUBY JUICE

2 medium carrots

1 beet, trimmed

1/2 bunch of fresh parsley

1 bunch of fresh spinach (or 2 packed cups of leaves)

1/4-inch piece of fresh ginger

1 lemon, peeled

SWEET KALE JUICE

1 bunch of leafy kale

1 or 2 green apples

1 lemon or lime with rind (only if organic)

1 tablespoon powdered wheatgrass

2 medium cucumbers (organic)

1 teaspoon moringa powder

CEL-JUVENATION JUICE

6 celery stalks

1 large cucumber

2 cups alfalfa, sunflower, or other sprouts

1 apple

1/2 lemon or lime, peeled

FENNEL AND GRAPEFRUIT GUZZLER

1 grapefruit, peeled, seeded, and segmented

1 small fennel bulb

2 green apples

1/2 lemon, peeled

Put the ingredients through your juicer, alternating the apples with the grapefruit and fennel in order to get the most juice out of everything. Consume unstrained or strain with a fine mesh sieve.

GREEN APPLE AID

2 organic green apples

2 lemons, peeled

4 cups organic spinach, loosely packed

1-inch piece fresh ginger, plus more to taste

3 drops alcohol-free liquid stevia, plus more to taste

Alternate the apple and lemon with the spinach through your juicer to get the most juice out of the leafy greens. Consume unstrained for the maximum benefit, or strain if preferred. Stir in the desired amount of liquid stevia.

. . . .

MOVE-TO-THE-BEET JUICE

2 beets, peeled

4 carrots

1-inch ginger knob

½ peeled lemon

1-inch piece fresh turmeric or ¼ teaspoon ground turmeric

Tiny pinch cayenne pepper

Place the beets, carrots, ginger, lemon, and fresh turmeric (if using) through your juicer. Consume unstrained or strain. Stir in the dried turmeric (if using) and the cayenne pepper.

SMOOTHIES

For all smoothies, just put all the ingredients in a high-speed blender and process until smooth. All smoothies serve 1 or 2 people, depending on how hungry you are.

"KEY LIME" GREENY SMOOTHIE

2 limes

½ lemon

2 cups filtered water

2 cups spinach

1 avocado, peeled and pitted (no bruises)

1 cucumber, unpeeled and roughly chopped

1 teaspoon lemon zest

1 teaspoon lime zest

¼ cup fresh coconut meat or ¼ cup unsweetened creamed coconut/coconut butter (not coconut oil)

1 tablespoon hemp oil

10 drops alcohol-free liquid stevia drops, plus more to taste

1 cup ice

1. Zest the limes and the lemon, remove the remaining rind, and set them aside.

2. Add the peeled limes, lemon, zest, and the rest of the ingredients to a blender and blast on high until smooth and creamy. Tweak flavors to taste (you may like more zest and stevia) and enjoy.

SALTY AND SPICY PICK-ME-UP SMOOTHIE

1½ cups filtered water or coconut water

2 cups stemmed, chopped curly kale

2 cups chopped tomato (about 2 tomatoes)

1 cucumber, roughly chopped

1 avocado, peeled and pitted (no bruises)

½ lemon, peeled

½ green chile, seeded, plus more to taste

2 garlic cloves

1 tablespoon coconut oil

1 teaspoon Celtic sea salt or Himalayan salt,
   plus more to taste

2 cups ice cubes

Throw all the ingredients in a blender and blast on high for about 1 minute, until smooth and creamy. Tweak the flavors to taste (you may want more chile, salt, or garlic).

. . . .

BERRY BEAUTY SMOOTHIE

1½ cups water (more if using frozen berries)

1 cup ice cubes (if using fresh berries)

2 cups radish greens (from the tops of 1 bunch of red
   radishes)

2 cup mixed berries, fresh or frozen

1 green apple, cored and roughly chopped

2 teaspoons minced fresh ginger

Pinch lime zest, plus more to taste

¾ teaspoon ground cinnamon

1 teaspoon chia seeds

1 teaspoon flax meal

1 teaspoon hemp seeds

1 teaspoon maqui powder (optional)

20 drops alcohol-free liquid stevia, plus more to taste

Throw all the ingredients in a blender and blast on high for about 1 minute, until smooth and creamy. Tweak the flavors to taste (you may like more ginger, lime zest, and stevia).

NO-PUMPKIN PIE SMOOTHIE

1 cup strained raw carrot juice (about 8 large carrots)

1 cup raw unsweetened almond milk, strained

1 cup raw coconut meat

¼ cup raw almond butter

½ teaspoon alcohol-free vanilla extract

¾ teaspoon ground cinnamon

¼ teaspoon ground nutmeg

Pinch ground ginger

30 to 40 drops SweetLeaf English toffee alcohol-free liquid stevia

1 cup ice or more to your preference

Place all the ingredients in a blender and blast on high for about 1 minute, until smooth and creamy. Tweak the stevia to taste. For the best flavor, chill in the fridge for a couple of hours to allow the stevia to settle and the flavors to mesh.

. . . .

ENERGY SMOOTHIE

This is a high-protein breakfast that will get you through the morning having tons of energy and feeling full. The optional L-Glutamine powder also helps to heal your intestinal lining.

2 cups unsweetened (or homemade) almond milk

Handful of ice cubes

1 scoop (or 1 tablespoon) protein powder (dairy-free and sugar-free)

1 teaspoon moringa powder (optional)

1 tablespoon flax seed oil

1 heaping teaspoon hemp seeds

1 teaspoon L-Glutamine powder (optional)

¼ teaspoon chlorella

¼ teaspoon spirulina

10 drops Dr. Patrick Flanagan's Crystal Energy (optional)

Add a small amount of water if the smoothie is too thick for your taste.

BREAKFAST SMOOTHIE

1 cup unsweetened (or homemade) almond milk

½ cup cold filtered water

4 or 5 ice cubes

1 scoop (or 1 tablespoon) protein powder

1 tablespoon flax seed oil

½ medium banana, peeled

½ teaspoon chlorella

½ teaspoon maca

½ teaspoon moringa (or Ormus Supergreens by Sunwarrior)

½ teaspoon spirulina

. . . .

RASPBERRY COCONUT GREEN SMOOTHIE

1 cup raw unsweetened coconut water (direct from the coconut, or packaged)

1 handful of fresh spinach

½ cup fresh raspberries

¼ cup goji berries, rehydrated in a little water for about 10 minutes

1 tablespoon chocolate protein powder (naturally sweetened or unsweetened, no cane sugar) or Sunwarrior Protein
  Powder

1 tablespoon chia seeds or hemp seeds

½ teaspoon spirulina

1 dropperful of stevia (optional)

GOJI BERRY MANGO SMOOTHIE

1 to 1½ cups raw unsweetened coconut water (direct from the coconut, or packaged)

1 cup mango slices

1 tablespoon soaked chia or ground flax seeds (see Note)

1 tablespoon flax seed oil

1 probiotics capsule, opened

½ avocado, peeled and pitted

¼ cup goji berries, rehydrated in a little water for about 10 minutes

Note: Soak the chia and flax seeds for 5 to 10 minutes before using them in this smoothie.

COCOA ALMOND SMOOTHIE

1½ cups unsweetened (or homemade) almond milk

2 pitted dates

2 tablespoons almond butter

1 probiotics capsule, opened

½ medium banana, peeled

½ tablespoon raw cacao powder

½ tablespoon maca

ELIXIRS

Elixirs are medicinal "milks" containing super-powered healing ingredients. Enjoy them as a snack.

GREEN BANANA MYLK

SERVES 1 OR 2

Green banana skins are high in iron, so they are great for anemia. They are also high in antioxidants, they lower cholesterol, are full of antihistamines, they reduce weight, and are great for mood stability because of the amino acid tryptophan. In the Caribbean, we use green banana skins along with green papaya to soften meat while cooking.

4 green banana skins (reserve the bananas for another use)
1 cup unsweetened (or homemade) almond milk
Stevia (optional)

1. Clean the skins of the green bananas thoroughly of any pesticides and dirt, using a vegetable wash. Place them in enough water to cover and bring to a boil. Boil until the water is reduced to 1 cup. Discard the skins. Add the almond milk to the water to give the drink a thicker consistency as well as to add protein. Blend to mix well. Sweeten with stevia to taste and enjoy warm or cold.

2. Green Banana Mylk keeps for 3 days in the refrigerator. If you can't finish it all by then, freeze it in ice cube trays. When you get a craving for something sweet, throw the frozen cubes in a blender with some strawberries, and blend for a perfectly healthful and delicious Strawberry "Ice Cream."

HOMEMADE ALMOND MYLK

SERVES 2 TO 4

You can buy unsweetened almond milk in the store, but this homemade version is simple and you know exactly what's in it: almonds and water. Period. Use this as a base for any kind of flavoring. Add a pinch of sea salt and some vanilla stevia, or any pureed fruit. (See pages 269–271 for some delicious and therapeutic variations.) Use it in smoothies, on cereal, with a gluten-free cookie, or just to drink. Make sure to buy your almonds from a reputable online company. "Raw" almonds from the grocery store are actually pasteurized, which destroys the natural enzymes in this most nutritious of tree nuts.

1 cup raw almonds
6 cups filtered water

1. Place the almonds in a large bowl and cover them with 3 cups of the filtered water. Let them soak for at least 8 hours or up to overnight. Drain and rinse the nuts twice to make sure the enzyme inhibitors, tannic acid, and phytic acid are washed away.

2. In a heavy-duty blender, combine the soaked almonds and the remaining 3 cups filtered water. Blend on high for 1 to 2 minutes. Pour the mixture into a nut milk bag over a large bowl and squeeze the milk from the solids. At this step, you now have unsweetened Homemade Almond Mylk that you can flavor or enjoy plain. Pour and serve, or store in a glass container in the refrigerator for up to 3 days.

GOJIMOND

This delicious and enzyme-rich plant mylk is low in calories and high in protein. It is an elixir that strengthens the bones and makes the skin glow. It's also full of vitamin E and antioxidants like carotenoids, so it's great for your eyes. In traditional Chinese medicine, this remedy supports the liver and kidneys, builds the blood, stimulates the pituitary gland to release human growth hormone, enhances the libido and fertility, reduces blood pressure, improves fatigue, and has anti-aging properties. Goji berries are available in most health food sections.

½ cup dried goji berries

1 cup filtered water

3 cups Homemade Almond Mylk (see previous recipe)

½ teaspoon ground cinnamon

¼ teaspoon almond extract

¼ teaspoon vanilla bean powder or pure vanilla extract

1 dropperful of vanilla crème stevia

Pinch of sea salt

Rehydrate the goji berries in a small bowl with 1 cup of water for 20 to 30 minutes. In a heavy-duty blender, combine the Homemade Almond Mylk and the goji berries. Blend on high for 1 to 2 minutes. Add the cinnamon, almond extract, vanilla bean powder, stevia, and sea salt. Blend for 30 seconds on high. Pour and serve, or store in a glass container in the refrigerator for up to 3 days.

PAPAYAMOND

SERVES 2 TO 4

This elixir is filled with digestive (proteolytic) enzymes from papaya. People who tend to eat a lot of cooked food can replenish their enzyme supplies with this delicious drink. PapayaMond also increases the libido and enhances male virility, has anti-aging properties, contains a lot of fiber for colon health (my favorite subject!), reduces systemic inflammation, breaks down protein that may have leaked into the blood due to leaky gut syndrome, aids in the oxidation of cholesterol, and is particularly good for the skin, helping to resolve eczema and psoriasis and giving a person a healthy glow. Pumpkin pie spice is optional, but I like it because it makes this elixir taste like pie. Do not overblend medicinal elixirs, which will help them maintain their enzyme activity.

1 ripe papaya
3 cups Homemade Almond Mylk (page 268)
1 dropperful of English toffee stevia
½ teaspoon organic pumpkin pie spice (optional)

1. Cut the papaya in half and scrape out the seeds. Rinse the seeds and set them aside. (You can have them later in plain Homemade Almond Mylk or in the PapayaMond as an additive. In the Caribbean, these seeds are a remedy to kill parasites: Put them out to dry, grind into a powder, and add to salads or smoothies.) Cut half the papaya into chunks (reserve the remaining half for another use).

2. In a heavy-duty blender, combine the papaya chunks with the Homemade Almond Mylk, stevia, and pumpkin pie spice. Blend for 1 to 2 minutes, or until the mixture is smooth. Pour and serve, or store in a glass container in the refrigerator for up to 3 days.

ROOTSMOND

SERVES 2 TO 4

This recipe is almost identical in preparation to GojiMond (page 269), but the burdock root replaces the goji berries, and that makes this a completely different elixir. RootsMond is a powerful blood purifier.

3 cups Homemade Almond Mylk (page 268)
½ piece burdock root, cut into small bits
½ teaspoon ground cinnamon
¼ teaspoon almond extract
¼ teaspoon vanilla bean powder or pure vanilla extract
1 dropperful of vanilla crème stevia
Pinch of sea salt

1. In a heavy-duty blender, combine the Homemade Almond Mylk and the burdock root with the remaining 3 cups filtered water. Blend on high for 1 to 2 minutes. Pour the mixture into a fine mesh strainer or nut milk bag over a large bowl and squeeze the milk from the solids. At this step, you now have unsweetened RootsMond.

2. Discard the solids. To continue with the elixir, place the strained RootsMond back into the blender. Add the cinnamon, almond extract, vanilla bean powder, stevia, and sea salt. Blend for 30 seconds on high. Pour and serve, or store in a glass container in the refrigerator for up to 3 days.

· ·

BREAKFASTS

ASPARAGUS OMELET
(Weeks One and/or Two)

SERVES 1

Note that I use whole eggs, not egg whites, in this recipe. Egg yolks are filled with potent nutrition that the egg whites don't have. The fat in the yolk is not important—sugars are much more detrimental to your cleansing process than fats.

Asparagus is high in glutathione, which helps to detoxify the liver and break down carcinogens. It's also filled with sulfur compounds. (This is why asparagus can make your pee smell stinky!)

2 whole eggs
1 cup chopped fresh asparagus spears
Sea salt and freshly ground black pepper

Lightly coat a glass or cast-iron skillet with ghee (clarified butter) or coconut oil and place over medium heat. In a bowl, lightly whip the eggs with a fork and stir in the asparagus. Pour the mixture into the pan. Cook until firm, lifting the edges periodically to loosen the omelet. Fold the omelet in half and turn it out onto a plate. Season to taste with sea salt and pepper.

SPINACH OMELET
(Week One or Two)

SERVES 1

Here, you get your greens and your eggs and nothing else. You'll feel clean, energized, and mentally sharp all morning long.

2 whole eggs
Handful of washed and dried fresh spinach, finely chopped
A few basil leaves, finely chopped (see Note)
Sea salt and freshly ground black pepper

Lightly brush a skillet with ghee (clarified butter) or coconut oil and heat over medium heat. In a bowl, lightly whip the eggs with a fork and stir in the spinach and basil. Pour the egg mixture into the skillet and cook until firm, lifting the edges periodically to loosen the omelet. Fold the omelet in half and turn it out onto a plate. Season with sea salt and a little pepper to taste.

Note: Fresh basil is great for relieving mental fatigue.

BREAKFAST SALAD
(Week One or Two)

SERVES 1

With this salad, you should choose either turkey bacon or a hard-boiled egg. Having only one protein in a meal makes it easier for your digestive system to do its job.

1 cup chopped romaine lettuce

1 tablespoon flax seed oil

1 or 2 hard-boiled eggs, chopped, or 2 to 4 turkey bacon strips, cooked and diced

Sea salt and freshly ground black pepper

Toss the lettuce with the flax seed oil and place on a plate. Garnish with the egg or bacon pieces. Season to taste with sea salt and pepper, and serve.

. . . .

BRAIN PORRIDGE
(Week Three)

SERVES 1

Keep your brain fueled for hours with this brain-fueling porridge.

½ cup short-grain brown rice

1 cup unsweetened almond milk (or Homemade Almond Mylk; page 268)

¼ teaspoon ground cardamom and/or pumpkin pie spice (use either or both)

1 tablespoon ground flax seeds

Combine the rice and the almond milk in a medium saucepan over low heat and cook for 40 minutes, or until the rice is soft and chewy (the consistency of porridge). Stir in the spices, and serve topped with a sprinkling of flax seed.

GREATNUTS CEREAL
(Week Three)

SERVES 1

For fans of cold cereal who miss their Cheerios, try this crunchy breakfast. It takes a bit of prep time because you have to make the Buckies (page 276) first, but you can make a big batch and keep the Buckies on hand for crunchy cravings. For those with diabetes, candida, or cancer, you should use stevia only and omit the raisins.

½ cup any berries (blueberries, strawberries, raspberries, etc.)
½ cup Buckies (page 276)
1 heaping tablespoon raisins
1 cup unsweetened almond milk (or Homemade Almond Mylk; page 268)
Honey, stevia, or coconut sugar

In a bowl, combine the berries, Buckies, raisins, and almond milk. Add sweetener to taste.

. . . .

BUCKIES
(Week Three)

MAKES ABOUT 6 CUPS

This recipe is a basic preparation you can use in other recipes, like the GreatNuts Cereal (page 275) and Bucky Burgers (page 298). It's basically just dehydrated sprouted buckwheat, and it's easy to make with a dehydrator or in a low oven. If you can't find pre-sprouted buckwheat in your local health food store, sprout your own. To make 6 cups sprouted buckwheat for this recipe, start with 3 cups buckwheat. Put it in a glass jar, cover it with water, and let it sit for 24 hours. The buckwheat will expand, approximately doubling in volume, giving you 6 cups. That being said, you can dehydrate any amount of sprouted buckwheat you like. It all depends on how big a store of Buckies you want to keep on hand. If you eat them every morning, or if Bucky Burgers are a particular fave meal in your household, then you could dehydrate even more.

6 cups sprouted buckwheat

Spread the sprouted buckwheat on mesh dehydrator trays and dehydrate for approximately 4 hours at 95 degrees F, until crunchy. (If you don't have a dehydrator, spread the buckwheat on a rimmed baking sheet and dehydrate in an oven set on the lowest setting, with the door cracked open, for 2 to 3 hours.) Store in a covered glass container at room temperature for up to 2 weeks.

. . . .

LUNCHES AND DINNERS

LEAFY PROTEIN SALAD
(Week One or Two)

SERVES 1

This salad is simple but filling and will keep your blood sugar stable all afternoon. It makes a great lunch with cooked meat left over from dinner the night before.

3 to 4 ounces cooked beef, chicken, turkey, or fish (about half cup shredded or chopped)

2 cups mixed leafy greens

2 cups chopped raw vegetables

1 tablespoon extra-virgin olive oil

1 tablespoon fresh lemon juice (or the juice from half a lemon)

Combine the meat, poultry, or fish with the greens and veggies. Toss with the olive oil and lemon juice, and serve.

VEGETABLE CHICKEN STIR-FRY
(Week One or Two)

SERVES 4

When you have time to whip up something hot, this is a quick and easy meal that makes you feel nourished and will keep you happily humming through the rest of the day. Note that this recipe serves 4, so it is perfect for a family meal. If sharing with one other person or enjoying by yourself, refrigerate the leftovers for another meal.

1 tablespoon coconut oil
1 pound boneless and skinless free-range chicken breasts, cut into bite-size pieces
2 cups chopped broccoli florets
1½ cups sugar snap peas, whole or halved if they are large
1 cup chopped cauliflower florets
1½ cups chopped carrots
1 tablespoon coconut aminos (coconut "soy" sauce)

Heat a wok or large skillet over medium-high heat. Add the coconut oil. When the oil is hot, add the chicken pieces and cook, stirring often, until golden brown, about 4 minutes. Toss in all the veggies and cook, stirring often, until they are brightly colored and crisp-tender, and the chicken is cooked through with no pink in the middle, about 4 more minutes. Stir in the coconut aminos. Toss to coat and serve immediately.

CHICKEN AND ASPARAGUS SALAD
(Week One or Two)

SERVES 2

This is a good meal to make with leftover chicken (or any light meat) and any leftover steamed or grilled vegetables. You don't have to use asparagus—broccoli, Brussels sprouts, bok choy, or green beans would be good, too. This is a quick go-to for me when time is limited.

8 ounces boneless and skinless free range chicken breast, broiled and cooled
2 cups chopped steamed asparagus, cooled or not
Extra-virgin olive oil or toasted sesame oil
Fresh lemon juice

Chop the chicken into small pieces and toss with the asparagus. Drizzle with a little oil and lemon juice to taste. Toss and serve.

GRILLED FISH WITH STEAMED VEGGIES
(Week One or Two)

SERVES 2 OR 3

Lighter than a stir-fry but still filling and satisfying, this is a great option when the grill is fired up. All you have to do is place your steamer basket atop a pot of boiling water, quickly steam, and the dinner is almost ready.

1 cup chopped broccoli florets
1 cup sliced carrots
1 cup snow peas, whole or halved if they are large
2 or 3 skinless white fish fillets (4 to 6 ounces each)
Seasonings of choice
Sea salt and freshly ground black pepper

Combine the broccoli, carrots, and pea pieces in a steamer and steam for 5 minutes, until tender-crisp. Meanwhile, grill or broil the fish fillets for 4 to 5 minutes per side over medium-high heat, or until lightly browned and cooked through. Divide the vegetables and fish fillets on serving plates and sprinkle with your favorite seasonings and salt and pepper to taste.

. . . .

50:50 SOUP (Week One)/80:20 SOUP (Week Two)

SERVES 1

This soup isn't precisely 50 percent veggies and 50 percent meat, but it is balanced enough that it makes a great Week One dinner and is a good way to use leftover meat that you've already cooked (or just sauté the amount of raw meat you need with a teaspoon of coconut oil). Because it has fresh juice as its base, the soup takes a little bit of time but is incredibly nutrient-dense. Warm it over very low heat for maximum enzyme preservation. For Week Two meals, make the same recipe but use just 2 ounces of meat and the same proportion of other ingredients, for 80:20 soup. Again, the proportions won't be exactly 80:20, but you will be reducing the meat, as is the goal with Week Two.

3 medium carrots, cut in chunks

3 medium cucumbers, cut in chunks

1½ lemons

1 beet, trimmed

1 head of romaine lettuce

¼ medium turnip (about 3 inches across), peeled

4 fresh kale leaves, chopped

3 scallions, white and green parts, chopped

2 or 3 garlic cloves

2 jalapeño chile slices

Handful of baby spinach leaves

1 ripe tomato

1 to 2 tablespoons coconut oil (1 teaspoon for 80:20 Soup)

4 to 6 ounces pre-cooked lean beef, chicken, or fish, cut into cubes (2 ounces for 80:20 Soup)

2 tablespoons coconut aminos (coconut "soy" sauce)

Sea salt or other natural salt

1. In a heavy-duty blender, combine the carrots, cucumbers, lemons, and beet. Blend until smooth. Pour into a large bowl. Next, add to the blender the lettuce, turnip, kale, scallions, garlic, jalapeño, spinach, and tomato. Blend until smooth. Add to the bowl and stir to combine the two purees.

2. Heat a skillet with the coconut oil. Add the cubed meat and toss until meat is warmed through, about 15 minutes.

3. Stir the coconut aminos into the raw soup. Stir in the meat, then season to taste with salt and serve.

MIXED GREEN STEAK SALAD
(Week One or Two)

SERVES 1

Think you can't have steak on the Piper Protocol? Think again! For all you beef lovers out there, this is a nourishing meal that lets you have your steak and eat your veggies, too.

Sea salt and freshly ground black pepper

3 to 4 ounces boneless steak

3 cups mixed greens

Extra-virgin olive oil

Fresh lemon juice

1. Season the steak and broil it to your liking. Cool, then slice the steak against the grain.

2. In a bowl, combine the mixed greens with the steak slices, then toss with the olive oil and lemon juice to taste. Add more salt and pepper to taste, and serve.

· ·

SALMON WITH SAUTÉED ASPARAGUS AND ARUGULA SALAD
(Week One or Two)

SERVES 1

You sure get your omega-3 fatty acids and your green vegetables in this interesting and delicious salad. The combination of cool, pleasantly bitter greens and the warm salmon and asparagus makes this a gourmet meal that's very easy to prepare.

One 6-ounce salmon fillet
Sea salt and freshly ground black pepper
1 tablespoon coconut oil
2 cups chopped trimmed asparagus
3 garlic cloves, minced
2 cups arugula
½ avocado, peeled, pitted, and diced
1 tablespoon flax seed oil
1 teaspoon fresh lemon juice

1. Preheat the oven to 400 degrees F. Sprinkle the salmon with salt and pepper. Place the salmon skin side down on a baking sheet lined with parchment paper. Bake for 10 minutes, or until the fish flakes easily with a fork.

2. While the salmon is baking, place the coconut oil in a medium sauté pan and sauté the asparagus and 2 garlic cloves until the asparagus is just tender, about 5 minutes. Let the asparagus cool slightly, then place the asparagus and the arugula in a large salad bowl.

3. In a mixing bowl, combine the avocado, flax seed oil, lemon juice, and remaining garlic. Mash well with a fork (or place in a NutriBullet or other blender to make a smooth dressing). Stir the dressing into the asparagus and arugula mixture. Serve the salmon with the salad.

CARIBBEAN SPICY BEEF STEW
(Week One or Two)

SERVES 6

I couldn't resist throwing in a few of my favorite Caribbean recipes. They may not remind you of your childhood the way they do mine, of course, but I hope you will enjoy the luscious flavors and serve them to your friends and family.

3 tablespoons coconut oil

3 pounds boneless beef chuck roast, cut into 2-inch pieces

2 medium onions, coarsely chopped

5 garlic cloves, minced

¼ cup gluten-free flour (such as almond or quinoa flour)

³/₄ cup water

1 quart low-salt organic beef broth (I like Pacific brand)

5 medium carrots, cut into 1-inch slices

3 parsnips, peeled and cut into 1-inch pieces

2 celery stalks, cut into 1-inch slices

½ teaspoon dried thyme or a pinch of fresh thyme

1 bay leaf

1 tablespoon freshly ground black pepper

2 teaspoons Celtic sea salt

1 teaspoon Grace's Jerk Seasoning (or your favorite all-natural Caribbean-style seasoning)

½ teaspoon natural all-purpose seasoning (I like the one by Simply Organic; see Resources)

TO SERVE

12 cups bite-size kale pieces (or baby kale)

2 tablespoons olive oil

Juice of 1 to 2 lemons or limes

1. Add the coconut oil to a large pot set over medium-high heat. When the oil just begins to smoke, add the beef. Cook for about 3 minutes, then turn the meat over and cook for 2 minutes, so both sides are nicely browned. Add the onions and garlic, and sauté for about 4 minutes more, or until onions become translucent.

2. In a small bowl, combine the gluten-free flour and water. Reduce the heat under the pot to medium, then whisk in the flour and water mixture. Stir continuously until well blended. (Sometimes I use a handheld battery whisk.) Add the broth, carrots, parsnips, celery, thyme, and bay leaf, and stir to combine. Cover, and simmer for 45 minutes.

3. While the stew cooks, gently massage the chopped kale with the olive oil and juice. Spread out on serving plates.

4. Uncover the pot and add the seasonings to taste. Cool slightly, remove the bay leaf, and serve over the kale.

JAMAICAN JERK CHICKEN
(Week One or Two)

SERVES 4 TO 6

Here's another Caribbean favorite. Note that the chicken is marinated overnight for the fullest flavor, so be sure to start this recipe the day before you plan to serve it. This chicken is very good on its own, but my favorite way to eat it is tossed in a green salad. You can find jerk seasoning in most major supermarkets. I like Grace or Miss Lily's brands.

4 garlic cloves

3 jalapeño chiles, chopped

2 medium onions, chopped

Juice of 1 lime

¼ cup apple cider vinegar

¼ cup gluten-free Nama Shoyu

¼ cup olive oil

2 tablespoons jerk seasoning of choice

1 tablespoon fresh thyme leaves

1 teaspoon ground cinnamon

1 free-range chicken, quartered

1. Place the garlic, chiles, onions, lime juice, vinegar, Nama Shoyu, olive oil, jerk seasoning, thyme, and cinnamon in a blender or NutriBullet and blend until smooth. Set some marinade aside to use as a dipping sauce, and rub the chicken thoroughly with the rest of the marinade. Cover and let sit overnight in the refrigerator.

2. Preheat the oven to 350 degrees F. Place the chicken in a baking pan and bake for 30 minutes, basting with the reserved marinade a couple of times. Turn the chicken quarters over and baste again, and bake for 30 minutes more.

3. You can serve a chicken quarter to each of four people and accompany it with a green salad, or you can pull the meat off the bone and chop it into smaller pieces, then toss it with salad greens to serve six persons. (Either preparation should provide 80 percent leafy greens with 20 percent cooked meat.)

Variation: Stewed Jerk Chicken

For variety, start with 2 boneless chicken breasts or 2 skinless boneless chicken thighs, chopped into large chunks. Prepare the marinade as for the master recipe and marinate overnight. The next day, place 2 to 3 tablespoons coconut oil in a large skillet or wok. When the oil is hot, add the marinated chicken chunks and toss continuously until cooked on the outside, about 5 minutes. Add the rest of the ingredients, cover, and simmer on low heat for 40 minutes, continually checking to make sure the chicken doesn't stick.

If you like a thicker sauce, add 1 tablespoon gluten-free flour whisked with ½ cup water and add it to the mixture. Let the chicken cool, then serve it over salad. It's delicious.

CURRY SHRIMP POT
(Week One or Two)

SERVES 1

This dinner is both comfort food and exotic—and it's easy to make, but count on time to marinate the shrimp.

4 scallions, green and white parts, chopped

3 garlic cloves, diced

1 or 2 jalapeño chiles, diced

1 medium onion, diced

6 tablespoons curry powder

1 teaspoon Celtic sea salt

3 ounces shrimp (any size), peeled with tails off

½ cup fresh lemon juice

1½ tablespoons coconut oil

1. In a medium bowl, combine the scallions, garlic, chiles, onion, curry powder, and sea salt. Rinse the shrimp with lemon juice and pat dry. Coat the shrimp with the seasoning mixture and let marinate in the refrigerator for 2 hours.

2. In a saucepan over medium-high heat, heat the coconut oil. When the oil is hot, add the shrimp and sauté until pink and cooked through, about 4 minutes.

3. Serve the shrimp with the scallion salad and some sautéed mixed vegetables of your choice. (Do not overcook the vegetables. They should still be slightly crisp.)

BAKED SALMON WITH PEPPERS
(Week One or Two)

SERVES 2

This is a simple and clean recipe that provides copious amounts of omega-3s, as well as leaving you feeling satisfied. The jalapeño gives it a pleasing zip. (Omit peppers if you have a nightshade allergy.)

4 thyme sprigs
1 jalapeño chile, chopped
1 medium onion, sliced
¼ cup apple cider vinegar
½ red bell pepper, sliced
½ yellow bell pepper, sliced
½ teaspoon Celtic sea salt
¼ teaspoon freshly ground black pepper
Two 6-ounce wild-caught salmon fillets (or other fish of your liking)

1. Preheat the oven to 400 degrees F. Add the thyme, jalapeño, onion, vinegar, bell peppers, salt, and pepper to a large sauté pan set over medium heat. Sauté for 10 minutes, or until the onion is translucent and most of the liquid is gone.

2. Place the salmon skin side down in a baking dish and bake for 10 minutes, or until cooked to your preference.

3. Transfer the fish to serving plates. Pour the sauce over the fish and serve with lightly steamed vegetables and a salad.

SWEET POTATO LASAGNA
(Week One, Two, or Three)

SERVES 4

Veggie comfort food! Although a true lasagna is layered and this is all mixed together, this has the taste and texture of lasagna to me, which is why I call it this. Note that even though this looks vegetarian, this is nevertheless a recipe for Week One or Two (because eggs are animal protein).

4 cups peeled and shredded sweet potatoes (about 2 to 4 sweet potatoes, depending on size)
¼ cup clarified butter (ghee), at room temperature
Two 8-ounce packages mozzarella-style Daiya "cheese"
1 cup baby spinach
6 whole eggs
½ cup gluten-free bread crumbs

1. Preheat the oven to 375 degrees F and grease a 9 x 13-inch baking pan lightly with some coconut oil.

2. In a large bowl, combine the sweet potatoes and butter. In a medium bowl, combine the Daiya "cheese," spinach, and eggs. Gently mix the "cheese" and spinach mixture into the sweet potatoes. Spread the mixture evenly in the baking pan and bake for 45 minutes. Sprinkle the bread crumbs evenly on top and bake for 15 minutes more, or until the bread crumbs are golden brown.

Butter is a dairy product, which I usually don't support, but pastured organic butter doesn't have a lot of the issues of milk, so it's okay in this recipe if you tolerate it. Otherwise, you could use vegan butter, like Earth Balance.

If you can't find gluten-free bread crumbs, toast and crumble a slice of gluten-free bread, or you could also use ground flax seeds or just skip this step.

. . . .

MOCK TUNA
(Week Three)

SERVES 4

This recipe resembles tuna salad, but it is much more alkaline and fiber-rich. Note that you must allow the seeds to soak overnight before preparing the recipe. Measurements for seeds are before soaking.

1 cup sunflower seeds, soaked overnight, drained, and rinsed (see pages 101–102)
1 cup pumpkin seeds, soaked overnight, drained, and rinsed (see pages 101–102)
1 garlic clove
2 tablespoons lemon juice
1 to 2 tablespoons powdered dulse or kelp, or to taste
1 celery stalk, minced
1 small onion, minced
¼ red bell pepper, minced (omit if you have nightshade allergies)
Sea salt

Put the soaked seeds, garlic, lemon juice, and dulse in a blender and pulse until the mixture is combined and roughly chopped; it should have the texture of tuna. Put the seed mixture in a bowl, and add the celery, onion, red pepper, and sea salt to taste. Mix thoroughly and serve with Flax Seed Crackers (page 290) or crudités or with a salad.

FLAX SEED CRACKERS
(Week Three)

MAKES 1 SHEET OF CRACKERS (ABOUT 12 CRACKERS, BROKEN INTO PIECES)

This recipe works best if you have a dehydrator, but you can also try it in the oven. Allow time overnight to soak the seeds before you start the recipe.

½ cup flax seeds, soaked overnight and drained (see pages 101–102)
1 tablespoon fresh lemon juice
1 teaspoon celery salt
1 teaspoon onion powder
½ cup water
2 tablespoons scallions, green and white parts, trimmed and finely minced
1 tablespoon chopped fresh parsley

1. Combine the soaked flax seeds, lemon juice, celery salt, onion powder, and water in a blender. Blend until smooth. Add the scallions and parsley, and mix well.

2. Spoon the seed mixture onto a dehydrator sheet and spread to the thickness of your preference. Dehydrate for 36 to 48 hours at 110 degrees F, until crisp. (If you don't have a dehydrator, spread the mixture on a rimmed baking sheet lined with parchment paper or a silicone baking mat and bake at 100 degrees F or the lowest possible temperature on your oven; this could take anywhere from 4 to 12 hours, depending on your oven, so keep an eye on it.)

3. Allow the cracker to cool completely, then break into pieces. Store in an airtight container at room temperature for up to a week.

. . . .

RAINBOW SUPER SLAW WITH PINENUT YOGURT
(Week Three)

SERVES 8

This is another recipe you can have with or without added grain on the side during Week Three. Note that the pinenut yogurt is time-intensive, but if you do it beforehand and have it ready to go, this recipe is super quick. This is a somewhat advanced raw-food-lifestyle kind of recipe, so if you love cooking and want to get into that, give it a try.

PINENUT YOGURT

2 cups pinenuts (pignoli)
Filtered water

RAINBOW SUPER SLAW

1 large handful arame kelp

Filtered water

1 head of green cabbage, cored and grated or very thinly sliced

⅓ head of red cabbage, cored and grated or very thinly sliced

2 ripe tomatoes, chopped

½ medium carrot, grated

1 red bell pepper, seeded, cored, and julienned

Juice of ½ lime or lemon

Gluten-free Nama Shoyu or Celtic sea salt

1. To make the pinenut yogurt, soak the pinenuts overnight in a bowl of filtered water. Drain, rinse, and let sprout at room temperature for 8 hours. Rinse again. Put the nuts in a blender with ¾ to 1 cup filtered water and blend until you have a creamy mixture. Pour the nut cream into a muslin or nut milk bag and squeeze the liquid out. You should have about 1½ cups liquid.

2. Put the pinenut liquid into a wide-mouth glass jar, cover with a muslin cloth, and let sit at room temperature for 5 to 7 hours in hot weather or 8 to 12 hours in cooler weather. The whey should separate from the "cream," which will rise to the top.

3. Place the jar in the refrigerator for 3 hours, or until the "cream" solidifies. The "yogurt" is ready to serve at this point, and will last for 5 days.

4. To make the slaw, soak the arame in filtered water for 5 to 10 minutes, then drain. In a large bowl, combine the arame, cabbages, tomatoes, carrot, and bell pepper with the yogurt (serving as a substitute for mayonnaise). Add the lemon or lime juice and season to taste. Serve at once. (The slaw will keep for 3 days in the refrigerator.)

WATERCRESS AND RED BELL PEPPER SALAD
(Week Three)

SERVES 4

For a grain-free Week Three, enjoy this as a complete lunch. Otherwise, have it with any gluten-free grain on the side or mixed in.

3 red bell peppers, cored, seeded, and julienned

2 bunches of watercress, trimmed and chopped

½ cup pumpkin seeds, ground to a powder

3 tablespoons dehydrated, flaked, or powdered onion (or minced fresh onion)

1 tablespoon flax seed oil (or ½ tablespoon flax seed oil and ½ tablespoon toasted sesame oil)

1 or 2 garlic cloves, put through a press

Juice of ½ lemon

A small piece of fresh ginger, put through a garlic press

Gluten-free Nama Shoyu or Celtic sea salt (optional)

Clover or alfalfa sprouts, for garnish

1. In a large bowl, combine the peppers, watercress, ground pumpkin seeds, and onion. Set aside.

2. In a small bowl, blend the oil, garlic, lemon juice, ginger, and Nama Shoyu or salt to taste. Pour the dressing over the salad and toss well. Transfer to serving bowls and garnish with the sprouts around the edges. (This salad will keep for 1 day in the refrigerator.)

· ·

AMARANTH VEGETABLE STEAM
(Week Three)

THE SERVING SIZE HERE DEPENDS ON THE AMOUNTS OF VEGETABLES AND AMARANTH YOU USE

Toss any steamed vegetables you have on hand (such as broccoli florets, carrots, kale, snow peas) with some cooked amaranth. Serve with a green salad with Sweet Lime Dressing (recipe follows) on the side.

SWEET LIME DRESSING

MAKES ABOUT 1½ CUPS

2 garlic cloves, put through a press
Small handful of fresh basil leaves, minced
1 cup cold-pressed extra-virgin olive oil
Juice of 2 limes
2 tablespoons honey

In a bowl, whisk the garlic and basil with the olive oil. Add the lime juice and honey. This dressing will keep for 1 week, refrigerated in a glass jar.

SPICY VEGGIE SOUP
(Week Three, or pureed for Week Four)

SERVES 8

This is another recipe you can enjoy with or without grain. Note that if you're making this soup for Week Four, you'll need to puree it. The soup is high in potassium.

1 medium zucchini, chopped

1 medium yellow summer squash, chopped

1 medium onion, chopped

1 acorn squash, split in half, seeded and peeled, flesh chopped

2 garlic cloves, minced

2 medium carrots, chopped

½ jalapeño chile, chopped

2 fresh kale leaves, thick stems removed and leaves chopped

1 quart gluten-free organic vegetable broth

Sea salt and freshly ground black pepper

Combine all the ingredients in a soup pot. Bring to a boil, then simmer for 2 hours, or until the vegetables are tender. If you need more flavor, season to taste with more sea salt and pepper. For easier digestion, put the soup into a blender and puree.

GLUTEN-FREE PASTA WITH GREEN PESTO SAUCE
(Week Three)

SERVES 2

Soaking the pinenuts for 30 minutes before using them will help to make their nutrients more easily digestible. The amount of pasta you use depends on how hungry you are.

2 tablespoons pinenuts (pignoli), soaked in water for 30 minutes and drained

1 cup fresh basil leaves

1 avocado, pitted and peeled

½ teaspoon Celtic sea salt

1 teaspoon to 1 tablespoon fresh lemon juice

2 garlic cloves

2 to 4 cups cooked gluten-free pasta of your choice

Blend the soaked pinenuts, basil, avocado, sea salt, lemon juice to taste, and garlic. Add water as needed to achieve your desired sauce consistency. Pour over the pasta and serve immediately.

Note: Make gluten-free pasta per instructions on packet or you can make yellow squash and zucchini spaghetti with the spiralizer.

SPINACH "CAESAR" SALAD WITH PUMPKIN SEED DRESSING
(Week Three)

SERVES 4

This salad makes an elegant side dish or a complete light lunch for Week Three.

1 large bunch of fresh spinach, rinsed with filtered water
½ cup pumpkin seeds, soaked for 30 minutes and then ground
2 tablespoons extra-virgin olive oil
1 or 2 garlic cloves, put through a press
Juice of ½ lemon
½ to 1 teaspoon Dijon mustard
Dash of Celtic sea salt
Pinch of freshly ground white pepper

1. Use a salad spinner to remove excess water from the spinach leaves. Place the spinach in a large bowl.

2. Combine the ground pumpkin seeds, olive oil, garlic, lemon juice, and mustard in a NutriBullet, food processor, or blender and process to a puree. Pour onto the spinach and toss. Season with salt and pepper to taste.

· ·

CARIBBEAN WILD RICE
(Week Three)

1 cup wild rice

2 large tomatoes, diced

2 large red bell peppers, diced

2 large yellow peppers, diced

1 medium onion, diced

1 tablespoon fresh grated or dried shredded
(unsweetened) coconut

½ cup Savory Coconut Cream (recipe follows; or use
Pinenut Yogurt, page 291)

2 cloves garlic, pressed or minced

Juice of 1 lime

Zest of 1 to 2 limes, optional

2 teaspoons ground coriander

1 teaspoon ground brown mustard (or 2 teaspoons
prepared brown mustard)

1 teaspoon ground cumin

1 teaspoon chili powder

Gluten-free Nama Shoyu and/or Celtic sea salt, to taste

Soak wild rice for 36 to 48 hours, changing the water twice. In a large bowl, combine the tomatoes, red and yellow peppers, onion, and coconut. Add the soaked wild rice, which will have increased in size (double or more). In a separate bowl, combine the coconut cream or pinenut yogurt, garlic, lime juice, zest, coriander, mustard, cumin, and chili powder. Mix well and pour over the rice mixture. Toss well. Taste and season with Nama Shoyu or sea salt, to taste. Serve immediately, or store for up to 2 days in the refrigerator.

. . . .

SAVORY COCONUT CREAM
(Week Three)

MAKES ABOUT 2 CUPS

Use this cream in Caribbean Wild Rice (above). You can also add it to your smoothies for a rich, creamy, ice-cream taste. I suggest you use a Coco Jack (see Resources) to open the coconut and scrape out the meat.

1 fresh coconut

Open the coconut, draining the coconut water into a blender jar. Scrape out the meat, then add to the blender. Process until creamy. Use immediately or refrigerate the cream, or freeze it in an ice cube tray for later use.

BUCKY BURGERS
(Week Three)

SERVES 4 TO 8

This is a raw-food specialty, but even if you're not eating raw, try it if you want to know what a raw vegan burger tastes like. (Sneak preview: delicious!) You'll have to make them in advance, allowing enough time for dehydration.

1 cup Buckies (page 276)

¾ cup walnuts (see pages 101–102)

½ cup sprouted sunflower seeds (see pages 101–102)

1 cup grated carrot

1 cup finely diced onion

2 to 4 garlic cloves, put through a press

1½ tablespoons mellow white miso, blended with 1 tablespoon filtered water

1½ teaspoons dried basil

1½ teaspoons sweet paprika

¼ to ½ teaspoon ground thyme

Celtic sea salt

Lettuce leaves, for serving

1. Put the Buckies, walnuts, and sunflower seeds in a blender or food processor with the S blade. Blend until the mixture comes together like a grainy dough.

2. Place the buckwheat mixture in a large bowl. Add the carrot, onion, garlic, miso, basil, paprika, thyme, and sea salt to taste. Mix well and form into 8 patties. To check if the burgers are seasoned enough, sample a small bite. You can always add your own seasonings to give these burgers your special touch.

3. Place the burgers on a dehydrator tray and set the dehydrator at 95 degrees F (or place on a baking sheet and put in an oven on the lowest setting). Dehydrate for 4 hours for rare burgers, 10 hours for medium burgers, or 24 to 36 hours for well-done burgers. (If using an oven, dry for 2 hours.)

4. Wrap the burgers in lettuce leaves to serve.

CREAM OF VEGETABLE POWER SOUP
(Week Three, or Week Four if pureed)

SERVES 2 TO 4

Add a grain during Week Three, or not—your choice. You can puree this for Week Four.

3 or 4 large celery stalks, with leaves

2 large cucumbers

1 red or orange bell pepper

2 large ripe tomatoes

1 large handful of fresh parsley, cilantro, or sunflower greens (sprouts)

1 avocado, peeled and pitted

1 small handful of fresh basil

½ teaspoon onion powder (optional)

Gluten-free Nama Shoyu or Celtic sea salt (optional)

Dash of cayenne (optional)

Diced avocado or sunflower greens (optional)

Put the celery, cucumbers, bell pepper, and tomatoes through a juicer. Transfer the liquid to a blender and add the avocado, basil, onion powder, and Nama Shoyu or sea salt to taste. Blend well. If desired, sprinkle cayenne on top and garnish with the diced avocado or sprouts. Serve at room temperature or slightly chilled.

SPICY BUTTERNUT ACORN SQUASH SOUP
(Week Three)

SERVES 2 TO 4

This is another great Week Three dish that can stand as a complete meal without grains because of the starchy squash. Serve with a green salad of your choice.

2 cups grated butternut squash

1 cup grated acorn squash

2 tablespoons finely chopped onion

1 tablespoon fresh lime or lemon juice

1 tablespoon Bragg Liquid Aminos

2 teaspoons ground turmeric

Up to ¼ teaspoon cayenne

2 tablespoons coconut oil

In a large bowl, toss all the ingredients except the coconut oil until well combined. Heat a wok over high heat and add the coconut oil. Stir in the vegetable mixture, and toss quickly—or less than a minute, just to take the chill off the veggies but not long enough to lose the enzymes.

DEVILED EGGLESS
(Week Three)

SERVES 4 TO 6

This is reminiscent of egg salad, but so much better for you. It's one of my personal favorite lunches.

2 cups macadamia nuts, soaked in filtered water overnight and drained (see pages 101–102)

¼ cup fresh lemon juice

1 tablespoon raw honey

2 teaspoons Dijon mustard

2 teaspoons ground turmeric

1 teaspoon ground black pepper

1 teaspoon ground cumin

1 teaspoon garlic powder (optional)

1 teaspoon onion powder (optional)

1 teaspoon Celtic sea salt

1 teaspoon dried thyme

1 cup diced celery

1 red bell pepper, seeded, cored, and diced

½ yellow or green bell pepper, seeded, cored, and diced

½ large onion, diced

Raw crackers or vegetable crudités, for serving

1. Place the macadamia nuts in a blender, and process until smooth. Add a small amount of water, if necessary, but the mixture should not be watery. Add the lemon juice, honey, mustard, turmeric, black pepper, cumin, garlic powder, onion powder, sea salt, and thyme. Blend well.

2. Transfer to a bowl and add the celery, bell peppers, and onion. Mix well and serve with raw crackers or veggie crudités.

ZUCCHINI SPAGHETTI
(Week Three)

SERVES 4

I eat this often—no meat, no grain, but it's filling and satisfying. And it really does make me feel like I'm eating pasta.

1 medium zucchini
1 medium yellow squash
3 ripe tomatoes
3 garlic cloves, chopped
½ cup chopped fresh basil
½ cup cold-pressed extra-virgin olive oil
½ teaspoon celery salt
½ teaspoon cayenne
1 teaspoon Celtic sea salt
½ teaspoon freshly ground black pepper (preferably Tasmanian Black Pepper; see Note)
¼ cup pinenuts (pignoli) or sunflower seeds

1. Put the zucchini and yellow squash through a spiralizer to make "spaghetti." You could also chop it in very long thin noodle-shaped slices with a knife, or with your food processor or mandoline, if you have an attachment that will make your zucchini look like noodles.

2. Put all the remaining ingredients except the pinenuts or sunflower seeds in a food processor, NutriBullet, or blender and blend to make a sauce of your desired consistency.

3. Pulverize the pinenuts or sunflower seeds in a food chopper or food processor until they resemble the texture of grated cheese. Serve the sauce over the "spaghetti," garnished with the crumbled pinenuts or sunflower seeds.

Note: Any other black pepper will work here, but this brand has an enormous amount of flavor—you can find it in high-end grocery stores.

JINGSLINGERS TUSCAN FLORATINA
(Week Three)

SERVES 3 OR 4

This is another zucchini "pasta" recipe, this time from my friends at the raw food recipe company JingSlingers (jingslingers.com). It's full of Italian garden vegetable deliciousness.

2 cups sun-dried tomatoes packed in olive oil

1 medium onion, chopped

6 garlic cloves, 5 minced and 1 left whole

2 cups halved raw Brussels sprouts

2 cups raw broccoli or broccolini florets

2 cups quartered artichoke hearts (from a can or jar, drained)

1 cup sliced baby bella mushrooms

Sea salt

Freshly ground black pepper

1½ tablespoons Italian seasoning

1 cup fire-roasted red bell peppers packed in water

1 cup whole fresh basil leaves

3 large, straight zucchini

Extra-virgin olive oil

1. In a large skillet over medium heat, drain the olive oil from the sun-dried tomatoes until it coats the bottom of the pan. Add the onion and cook until translucent, about 8 minutes. Add the minced garlic, Brussels sprouts, and broccoli or broccolini. Once the veggies are lightly browned and fork-tender (about 5 minutes), add the artichokes and mushrooms. Add the sea salt, pepper, and ½ tablespoon of the Italian seasoning, or to taste. Stir and remove from heat.

2. In a blender, combine the sun-dried tomatoes, red peppers (and their water), remaining 1 garlic clove, and the basil. Blend until smooth. Add the remaining 1 tablespoon Italian seasoning and some sea salt and black pepper to taste. Pour the contents of the blender over the vegetables in the pan. Return the pan to the burner over low heat, stirring occasionally, until everything is heated through.

3. Meanwhile, cut the ends off the zucchini. Using your spiralizer, spiral-cut all three zucchini (we like to leave the skin on). Place in a bowl and season with some sea salt, black pepper, and a touch of olive oil. Mix by hand to combine. (Optional: Warm the noodles in a hot pan, stirring quickly, until slightly tender.)

4. To serve, place the zucchini noodles on serving plates and top generously with the vegetable and tomato sauce. *Mangia!*

POTASSIUM BROTH
(Week Four)

MAKES ABOUT 1 GALLON

This broth is clear but is made with potassium-rich veggies. Make it ahead of time and keep it in the refrigerator in a glass jar for whenever you need a light snack or to add to any meal. It will keep for 5 days. You can also portion it out, freeze it, and thaw it out when you need it.

1 large sweet potato, cut into about 6 pieces
1 beet, trimmed and cut into about 6 pieces
1 bunch of beet greens, roughly chopped
1 bunch of Swiss chard or collard greens
1 bunch of fresh parsley, coarsely chopped
1 medium onion, quartered
4 medium carrots, cut into several pieces
4 celery stalks
8 fresh shiitake mushrooms, cut in half
A 2-inch piece of fresh ginger, roughly chopped
3 garlic cloves, put through a press
1 gallon distilled water (free of minerals)
1 tablespoon sea salt

1. Combine all the ingredients except the salt in a large soup pot over high heat. Bring to a boil, cover, then lower the heat to a simmer and simmer for at least 2 but up to 4 hours. (You can also make this in a slow cooker and leave it on low all day.)

2. Strain the broth, discard the solids, and stir in the salt, or puree the soup to give you extra fiber. Store in a glass jar in the refrigerator until ready to use, or freeze for later use.

ALKALIZING AVOCADO GAZPACHO
(Week Four)

SERVES 4

2 cups filtered water

3 large avocados, peeled and pitted (no bruises)

2 cups peeled, seeded, and cubed cucumber

1 cup fresh cilantro

3 tablespoons chopped red onion

2 fresh garlic cloves

½ small green chile, plus more to taste

3 tablespoons fresh lime juice

1 tablespoon cold-pressed extra-virgin olive oil

1 to 1½ teaspoons Celtic sea salt or Himalayan salt

OPTIONAL GARNISHES

1 avocado, peeled, pitted, and sliced

¼ cup freshly chopped cilantro

1. Throw all the ingredients in a blender and blast on high for about 1 minute, until smooth and creamy. If the soup warms up slightly, add a few ice cubes to chill the blend.

2. Tweak the flavors to your taste (you may like more garlic, onion, lime juice, or salt) and chill before serving.

3. Serve plain or with the optional garnishes.

GLORIOUS GREENS SOUP
(Week Four)

SERVES 8 AS A STARTER OR 6 AS A MEAL (I HAVE MADE THIS GENEROUS FOR FREEZING)

The lemon intensifies as the soup sits, so it's best not to add the lemon juice to the entire pot of soup. This soup freezes really well for those last-minute quick meals. If the soup separates a little or looks a bit woody or lumpy once defrosted, just blend again and heat gently on low.

2 tablespoons olive oil or grapeseed oil

1 medium yellow onion, roughly chopped

2 tablespoons fresh minced garlic (about 4 cloves)

¼ teaspoon Celtic sea salt or Himalayan salt, plus more to taste

1 zucchini, roughly chopped

1 large cauliflower head, cut into florets

1 large broccoli head, cut into florets

8 cups (2 liters) gluten-free vegetable broth (I like the Massel brand)

1 large bunch of asparagus, trimmed and cut into 2-inch pieces

2 cups spinach

¼ cup blanched raw almonds or macadamia nuts

1 to 2 teaspoons fresh squeezed lemon juice, plus more to taste

1. Heat the oil in a large saucepan over medium heat. Add the onion, garlic, and salt and sauté for about 4 minutes, until the onions are just translucent. Add the zucchini and sauté for another 2 minutes, until softened. Add the cauliflower and broccoli and cook for about 2 minutes.

2. Add the vegetable broth, increase the heat to high, and bring the mixture to a boil. Reduce the heat to medium/low and simmer, partially covered, for about 10 minutes, until the vegetables are crisp-tender. Add the asparagus and simmer for about 3 minutes, or until the asparagus is just tender. Throw in the spinach leaves and simmer for 1 minute, allowing the spinach to just wilt.

3. Remove the saucepan from the heat and allow the soup to cool a little. Stir in the almonds. Working in batches, pour the soup into a blender and puree on high for 1 to 2 minutes, until smooth and creamy. Return the soup to the saucepan, add salt to taste, and warm it over medium-low heat.

4. To serve, ladle the soup into bowls and stir a tiny splash of fresh lemon juice into each to bring out the flavors.

SNACK RESCUE

Enjoy these nutrient-dense snacks between meals when you really need them during Weeks One, Two, or Three. Or, if you aren't very hungry, any of these snacks can stand in for a meal.

CHIA SEED PUDDING

SERVES 2

The taste of this delicious pudding is similar to tapioca. It's a wonderful treat when you need something sweet.

1 cup soaked almonds or macadamia nuts (see pages 101–102)

2 cups filtered water

½ cup chia seeds

¾ cup pitted dates

1 tablespoon honey

½ teaspoon ground cinnamon

½ vanilla bean, minced

1 or 2 teaspoons coconut oil

Put all the ingredients into a high-powered blender. Let the mixture sit for 10 minutes to hydrate the chia seeds, then blend until completely smooth. Serve immediately.

APPLE-PEAR SALAD

SERVES 1 OR 2

Adding cinnamon to this simple fruit salad helps to stabilize your blood sugar levels.

1 apple, diced
1 pear, diced
Dash of ground cinnamon

In a bowl, toss together the diced apple and pear. Sprinkle the mixture with cinnamon, and enjoy.

. . . .

ZUCCHINI CHIPS

MAKES ABOUT 4 CUPS

Enjoy as you would enjoy potato chips—but these are so much better for you!

4 medium or 2 large zucchini
1 teaspoon sea salt
1 teaspoon onion powder
½ teaspoon black pepper

1. Slice the zucchini with a mandoline or use the slicing blade on your spiralizer (or cut very thin by hand). Place in a bowl and season with salt, onion powder, and pepper (or just use sea salt, if you prefer). Place on a dehydrator sheet and dehydrate at 110 degrees F for 24 to 36 hours. Check for crispiness.

2. You can also dehydrate the zucchini chips on a baking sheet in a standard oven at the lowest temperature possible, with the door open. Bake until crisp. This could take anywhere from 2 to 4 hours.

TROPICAL ICE CREAM

SERVES 4 TO 6

It's the ultimate summer treat!

1 cup frozen diced mango
1 cup frozen chunked pineapple
1 cup frozen almond milk cubes (almond milk poured into ice tray and frozen)
open 1–2 probiotics and add
2 tsp of Colostrum (optional) for vegan, add Lucuma for creaminess
Stevia (optional)

Put all the ingredients in a blender and puree until the mixture resembles the consistency of ice cream. Add a few drops of stevia if it's really not sweet enough for you (you probably won't need it).

> Note: For a more sorbet-like texture, omit the almond milk cubes and use ice cubes instead.

LEIGH'S CANDY

Many of the raw-foods recipes in this book are from my friend Rhio, who is a raw-food chef and the author of the wonderful book *Hooked on Raw*. Her partner, Leigh, transitioned to a 90 percent raw diet to manage his high blood pressure, and this was one of his favorite things to eat when he craved something sweet. I love this recipe because sometimes we all really want something sweet. This recipe allows you to fulfill that craving without reaching for junk candy. I hope you'll try it—it certainly does the trick for me!

1 cup almonds
1 cup sunflower seeds
1 cup walnuts
8 small dates, pitted
1 tablespoon raw honey
¼-inch vanilla bean, finely sliced
1 teaspoon ground cinnamon
Pinch of Celtic sea salt

Combine all the ingredients in a bowl and form the mixture into 1-inch balls. Set them on a baking sheet lined with waxed paper to firm up, then store in a container in the refrigerator with waxed paper between the layers.

MACAROON CHEWS

MAKES 12 TO 18

This is another sweet that can fill in for junk food when your resolve is wavering.

2 cups coconut pulp (whatever is left over from making Sweet Coconut Cream, page 313, or you could also use
shredded or grated raw coconut, unsweetened)
2 cups filtered water
10 large dates, pitted and halved
A sprinkling of vanilla bean powder

Put the coconut pulp, water, dates, and vanilla powder in a blender. Blend well, or until the mixture is smooth. Drop the mixture by tablespoons onto a dehydrator sheet or a baking sheet and flatten with the back of a spoon so they resemble cookies. Dehydrate at 100 degrees F for 24 to 36 hours, or dry in the oven on the lowest possible setting until firm enough to hold their shape, about 2 hours.

JINGSLINGERS JING JAM

SERVES 4

Here's a snack from my friends at JingSlingers (www.jingslingers.com). This fruity, creamy antioxidant powerhouse is somewhere between a gelatin and a pudding. It uses some special ingredients you will probably have to order unless you live near a well-stocked natural foods store, but the result is well worth it! Eat it for breakfast, lunch, dinner, or dessert. Pair it with a gluten-free muffin, layer it with Sweet Coconut Cream (page 313), or just enjoy it in a pretty glass dish.

2 cups unsweetened pomegranate juice

1 cup chia seeds

1 tablespoon freeze-dried acai powder

1 tablespoon Miracle Reds Powder (a brand of nutrient-dense fruit powder)

1 tablespoon freeze-dried maqui powder (optional—a powder made from maqui berries)

1 tablespoon birch xylitol powder (or your favorite natural sweetener)

One 12-ounce bag frozen organic raspberries

2 dropperfuls of vanilla crème stevia (or to taste)

1. In a bowl or pitcher, combine all the ingredients except the raspberries and stevia. Stir and then set aside to thicken at room temperature for about 15 minutes.

2. Place the frozen raspberries in a blender and pulse a few times to rough-cut the berries. Stir the raspberries and the stevia mixture into the bowl until evenly distributed. Taste for sweetness and add more stevia or xylitol until it is perfect for your palate. Refrigerate until chilled, then enjoy!

SWEET COCONUT CREAM

MAKES 11 OUNCES

Use this ultra-rich cream to garnish your favorite healthful desserts (like Jing Jam—see previous recipe), or swirl a little bit in your alkaline coffee or herbal tea for a special treat.

11 ounces So Delicious Organic Culinary Coconut Milk, original flavor
vanilla créme stevia

In a bowl, combine the coconut milk with the stevia to taste.

. . . .

JINGSLINGERS LIVING WATERS MARGARITA

MAKES 1 LARGE OR 2 SMALL MARGARITAS

Another snack idea from JingSlingers (www.jingslingers.com), here's body-happy hydration in a glass! (No alcohol required.) This delicious potion is mineralizing, alkalizing, and energizing!

½ cup ice cubes
1 cup coconut water kefir
½ cup spring water
¼ cup aloe vera inner fillet (see note below) or aloe vera juice
¼ cup fresh lemon juice
2 to 3 dropperfuls of ginger extract or 1 teaspoon ginger juice
½ tablespoon sunflower lecithin powder

1 tablespoon unsweetened whey protein powder (preferably grass-fed, hormone-free, non-denatured organic whey—you can find this online) One World Whey is best brand
1 tablespoon pumpkin seed oil
1 dropperful of liquid chlorophyll (I like ChlorOxygen brand)
1 dropperful of vanilla crème stevia (or to taste)
Pinch of sea salt

Place all the ingredients in a blender and puree until smooth and frothy. Pour into margarita glasses and serve.

Note: To obtain the inner fillet, cut free the inner gel from an aloe vera leaf.

Acknowledgments

THIS BOOK HAS BEEN a labor of love and I have given birth to my baby. As with every birth, the help of trusted family is crucial. I would like to thank my midwife, Eve Adamson, for her ability to hear my voice, and my two doulas who sat next to me as I wrote this book—Tucan, my cat, and Niko, my dog. I love you guys.

Cassie Jones and the rest of the team at William Morrow, thank you for understanding right from the start that this book was something the world needed. Thank you for believing in me and this book, and for helping me bring it to fruition.

The knowledge this book conveys is knowledge and experience I have acquired over many years and has come from many people. I hoped to have captured everyone, but if you helped me in any way along my path and I haven't mentioned you, please know that you are in my heart and my gratitude is deep.

My fifth-grade teacher, Ms. Smith, opened the door to allow knowledge to enter and encouraged me along the way. Ms. Fleming, you were one of the most beautiful teachers I have ever had, but you were strict like a marshal; you instilled in me from an early age that school was important and there were no do-overs, so I had to put my best foot forward at once and it would carry me through for years to come. Growing up in St. Thomas, going to a university on the beach, seemed like paradise. Okay, yes it was, but the no-nonsense policy at the UVI Science Department kept me focused, and I still use that organized focus and that attitude to get things done.

My dear grandmother, you were the inspiration of my life. Little did you know that you were training me for my life ahead. There is nothing that I do today that isn't in some way a recognition of your love and teachings. Mom, you instilled in me the ability to work hard, and you never gave up on me—you're that tough West Indian mother who has no time for inferiority and you pushed me to be the best I could be. Dad (Pipes), you taught me to love *everyone*. My beloved Aunt Nennen, you taught me that "He will never leave you nor forsake you," and that it does not matter what lies ahead. "God is right there beside you. My sister; you kept it real with me about what real people can really do and eat"—delivered in her Scorpio voice.

Riah, your illustrations helped put what I wanted to say into pictures. Jeff Skerik, "rawtographer," thanks for flying in from L.A. to help me with my baby. Your guidance, calmness, and creative soul brought a lot of life to the photos and me. Thanks for putting our heads together to style our photos, as you knew what I wanted even before I told you. That's true friendship when you know without speaking. I love you.

To Joad, for teaching me that *all* women are Goddesses of Beauty (GOB). Dr. Junger (Ale), I don't know if you realize how much you inspired me with your encouragement and beautiful friendship—I cherish your gentle guidance. And thanks for believing in internal fitness.

JingSlingers—Jay Denman and Joy Coelho—you guys continue to nudge me to strive for ever more greatness. Your passion and commitment to the field of internal fitness is surpassed by none. And the Ann Wigmore Natural Health Institute family taught me about the living foods lifestyle, and how love needs to be in *everything* one eats and does. You opened my mind to a whole new world that changed my life and allowed me to spread that knowledge to others. Leola Brooks and Lalita Salas, thank you for continuing Dr. Ann's work with such passion.

Mera White, my first colon therapist, who truly educated me on the body. Thanks for your guidance.

David (Avocado) Wolfe, wow—words can't say enough about the knowledge you have bestowed on me since 2011. Denise Mari and Doug Evans (Organic Avenue), thanks for giving me my first platform to reach the masses. Tyra Banks, I am so grateful to you for having the vision to produce a show on live colonics for nationwide TV. This move helped so many, as they called and thanked me for bringing the knowledge forward.

Ruth Willis, thanks for putting up with my lateness as I struggled to our appointments in the early mornings after being up all night writing. Thanks for always being there.

A special note to Rachel Kessler, without whom none of this would be happening. Thank you for your post on how I helped you—that was the catalyst for the conception of my child. To my agent, Alex Glass, who read that post and saw this baby before I did, and reached out to me to make it all come true. There are no words to truly say thank you.

To my health teachers, thank you for blessing me with your knowledge: Dr. Derossier, Dr. Richard Hall, Teresa Turner, Dr. Alejandro Junger, Dr. Frank Lipman, Dr. Robert Young, Adam Banning, Dr. Patrick Fratellone, Dr. Jeffrey Bland, David Wolfe, Sandra Duggan at the Edgar Cayce School of Massage.

To all my clients, who not only beyond a doubt challenged and inspired me to keep learning and make colon hydrotherapy fun, but also recognized that being internally fit is more important than just being externally fit. It's a balance of yin and yang. Every client teaches you something; you just have to be open to learning.

Special friends who supported me on this journey are Eileen Short, my first hands-on teacher in the field of medicine who showed passion for my work; Jim Cosares; Jennifer and Andrew Marrus; Terrance White; Marc Herouard; Tess Masters; Brad Roberts; Barbara Bell; Aarti Tandon; Rhio; Leigh Crizoe; Julio Velazquez; and Robert De Rothschild. Also, thank you Scott Brick for being there, sharing our challenge together. And thanks also to Aleta St. James for her Energy Work in keeping me focused when times got really hard. My second family and staff, Joy Santoli, Elanit Cohen, Amy Benton, Dorelle Gibson, and Liz Cuervas, I'm grateful for your keeping The Piper Center running while I took time to gestate my baby.

I extend thanks to my dear friends who contributed recipes: Tess Masters, Rhio and the JingSlingers, Jay and Joy.

When I moved to New York City, it was tough getting acclimated to this new world, so I would love to thank Libby Baker for opening her 200-square-foot apartment in Carroll Gardens and for allowing me to camp out on her futon while I attended massage school.

To Donald, Libby's partner, your passing is what inspired me to change my mind and my world, to cancel my plans for medical school and concentrate on prevention rather than cure. Your passing gave me the courage and insight to help thousands of people learn that "health and death truly begin in the colon."

When I finally got my own place, I had an accident and was left paralyzed for six months due to severe spinal injury. I was able to walk again with the help of Dr. Frank Morgera, the only chiropractor who wasn't afraid to treat me. Thanks also go to the Swedish Institute for sending a massage therapist to my apartment twice a week to help me get better. Dr. Dennis DiGiorgi, thank you for continuing the work of Dr. Morgera and for being the first to say: "Those pain killers are not going to help; you have to get fit from the inside." My gratitude goes also to Jen Owens (Jinabai), for the raw food that helped heal me. It was great being your guinea pig as you learned the raw cuisine.

Special thanks to Jivaro Mordaunt for being an angel, helping me through a tough time when I moved to New York.

"Jay," thank you for just being you and allowing me to fulfill my dreams even though you had no idea. Thank you, Angel and Bobby, for giving me a chance to work with my disability and teaching me everything about running a medical office so I could one day run my own. Dr. Kelly O'Malley, you were the first doctor who believed in me and in what I had to offer the world. Thank you for always being there.

To Gwyneth, thanks for being there wholeheartedly during a life-changing time; also, for showing me that I needed to truly own the energy of my business by changing the name to The Piper Center. Thank you, thank you, thank you.

To all my Scorpio peeps, thanks for that strong Scorpio loyalty, support, and love.

At the birth of this book, I was blessed to meet an enlightened soul who sparked a light in my being that had been dimmed from exhaustion and loss of a little faith as life got hard again. In our short new friendship, he has taught me not to give up and to go for everything I want; in doing that, I need to continue to "exercise big faith in the process." Thank you.

RESOURCES

Here is a comprehensive list of sources for the products I use and those mentioned in the book that I recommend and admire, as well as books and other educational resources I recommend for further reading.

FOOD

Alkaline coffees: Bulletproof Coffee (www.bulletproofexec.com/coffee), Longevity Coffee (www.longevitywarehouse.com)

All-purpose seasoning: Simply Organic (www.simplyorganic.com)

Bragg's Liquid Aminos: www.bragg.com

Broth: Pacific brand organic beef, chicken, and vegetable broth (www.pacificfoods.com)

Coconut aminos: Coconut Secret Coconut Aminos (www.coconutsecret.com)

Coconut water: 100% Raw Coconut water (www.harmlessharvest.com), Vita Coco (www.vitacoco.com), Zico (www.zico.com)

Coffee substitute: Liquid Heaven (www.thepipercenter.com), Dandy Blend (www.dandyblend .com)

Jerk seasoning: Grace (www.gracefoods.ca) and Miss Lily's (www.misslilys.myshopify.com)

Low-glycemic sweeteners (coconut sugar, luo han guo fruit extract, stevia): BioVittoria **Fruit-Sweetness** (www.biovittoria.com/fruit-sweetness), Madhava Natural Sweeteners **Organic Coconut Sugar** (www.madhavasweeteners.com), NuNaturals Sweet Health LoSweet Pure Lo Han Guo Extract Powder (www.nunaturals.com), Swanson Premium

PureLo Lo Han Sweetener (www.swansonvitamins.com), Omica Organics flavored stevia (www.omica.com), SweetLeaf Stevia Sweetener (www.sweetleaf.com)

Maca root powder: Mountain Rose Herbs (www.mountainroseherbs.com)

Ohsawa Nama Shoyu: Gold Mine Natural Foods (www.goldminenaturalfoods.com)

Pepper: Tasmanian Black Pepper from Savory Spice Shop (www.savoryspiceshop.com), World Spice Merchants (www.worldspice.com)

Protein powder: Sunwarrior (www.sunwarrior.com), Longevity Warehouse (www.longevitywarehouse.com)

Superfood Herbs: www.Jingherbs.com, www.dragonherbs.com

Raw nuts: Natural Zing (www.naturalzing.com), Living Intentions (www.LivingIntentions.com)

Tea: Spring Dragon Longevity Tea (www.dragonherbs.com)

Truth Calkins' Chi City, Jing City: Longevity Warehouse (www.longevitywarehouse.com)

SUPPLEMENTS

Aloe vera juice: George's (www.georgesaloe.com)

Clays (bentonite and montmorillonite), Zeoforce: Mountain Rose Herbs (www.mountainroseherbs.com), Sonnes (www.Sonnes.com), Healthforce Nurtitionals (www.HealthforceNutritionals.com)

Liquid chlorophyll: DeSouza's (www.desouzas.com) or World Organic (widely available online)

Coconut oil: organic cold press, upgraded octane oil (www.bulletproofexec.com)

Coenzyme Q10: NOW Foods (www.nowfoods.com), Puritan's Pride (www.puritan.com), Vitamin Shoppe (www.vitaminshoppe.com), Dr. Dave's Best (www.drdavesbest.com-vegetarian source)

Colon cleansers: Colon Detox (www.baselinenutritionals.com), Super 2 (thepipercenter.com)

Digestive enzymes: Allegany Nutrition Digestive Enzymes AL-270 (www.alleganynutrition.com), Digest Gold ATPro (www.enzymedica.com), Pancreatic Enzymes (www.allergyresearchgroup.com, formulated by Dr. Nicholas Gonzalez), Transformation Enzymes (www.transformationenzymes.com), Garden of Life WobenzymN (www.gardenoflife.com), Generation Plus Zymitol (www.life-enthusiast.com), Fibrenza Systemic Enzyme (www.fibrenza.com), Baseline Nutritionals pHi-Zymes (www.baselinenutritionals.com), Transformation (www.Transformation.com, wide variety for specific issues)

Dr. Patrick Flanagan's Crystal Energy, Phi Sciences: www.phisciences.com

E3Live: AFA Fresh Frozen Superfood (www.e3live.com)

Fiber (apple pectin, chia seeds, ground flax seed, hemp seeds, psyllium husk): Bob's Red Mill (www.bobsredmill.com), Organic India Organic Whole Husk Psyllium, (www.organicindia.mercola.com) Beyond, Garden of Life (www.Garden of Life.com), EcoBloom, Body Ecology (www. bodyecology.com)

Fish oil: Metagenics Omega 10 (www.metagenics.com), Dr. Dave's Best Ultra 85 Fish Oil (www.drdavesbest.com), Udo's 369

Mineral supplements: Trace Minerals Research ConcenTrace Trace Mineral Drops (www .traceminerals.com), QuintEssential Marine Plasma (www.quintessentialstore.com)

Probiotic supplements: VSL #3 (www.vsl3.com), Custom Probiotics (www.customprobiotics .com), Renew Life (www.renewlife.com), Metagenics UltraFlora IB (www.metagenics.com)

EQUIPMENT

Blenders: VitaMix (www.vitamix.com)

Coconut tool: Coco Jack (www.coco-jack.com)

Dehydrators: Excalibur (www.excaliburdehydrator.com), Nesco (www.nesco.com), Weston Supply (www.westonsupply.com)

Dry skin brush: Yerba Prima Tampico Skin Brush (www.yerba.com)

Enema supplies: Optimal Health Network (www.optimalhealthnetwork.com)

Food processors: Cuisinart (www.cuisinart.com), KitchenAid (www.kitchenaid.com)

Infrared sauna: Costco (www.costco.com), Momentum (www.Momentum.com)

Juicers: Norwalk (www.norwalkjuicers.com), GreenStar (www.greenstar.com), Omega (www.omegajuicers.com), Breville (www.brevilleusa.com)

Nut milk bags: Vitamix (www.vitamix.com)

NutriBullet: NutriBullet (www.nutribullet.com)

Rebounders: Bellicon (www.bellicon-usa.com), Needak (www.needak-rebounders.com)

pH test strips: CVS (www.cvs.com), Walgreens (www.walgreens.com), pH Miracle Living (phmiracleliving.com.), Phion (www.phion.com)

Spiralizers: Bed Bath & Beyond (www.bedbathandbeyond.com), Williams-Sonoma (www.williams-sonoma.com), Amazon (www.Amazon.com)

Toilet stools: Welles step (www.optimalhealthnetwork.com), Squatty Potty (www.squattypotty.com)

Water alkalizing and filtration systems: Chanson (www.chansonalkalinewater.com), Jupiter Water Filters (www.jupiterwaterfilters.com), Enagic Kangen Water (www.enagic .com), pH Miracle WaterMark (www.phmiracleliving.com), WellBlue Filters (www .wellblue.en.alibaba.com)

SUPPLIES

Carrier oils: Mountain Rose Herbs (www.mountainroseherbs.com)

Castor oil: Baar Products (www.baar.com)

Epsom salts: CVS (www.cvs.com), Mountain Rose Herbs (www.mountainroseherbs.com), Walgreens (www.walgreens.com)

Essential oils: Young Living Essential Oils (www.youngliving.com), (www.Doterra.com)

Herbs: Mountain Rose Herbs (www.mountainroseherbs.com), Organic India Ashwagandha (www.organicindia.mercola.com)

Moringa powder: Organic India Moringa Leaf Powder (www.organicindia.mercola.com), Vitamin Shoppe (www.vitaminshoppe.com)

Nattokinase: NOW Foods (www.nowfoods.com), Puritan's Pride (www.puritan.com)

Salt (Celtic sea salt and Himalayan salt): SaltWorks (www.saltworks.us), Selina Naturally Celtic Sea Salt (www.selinanaturally.com)

S. A. Wilson Gold Roast Coffee: S. A. Wilson (www.sawilsons.com)

Silver liquid: ASAP 365 Silver Liquid, One Silver Solution (www.silversolutionusa.com)

Therapeutic oils (coconut, extra-virgin olive oil, fish oil, flax seed oil): Mountain Rose Herbs (www.mountainroseherbs.com)

Wheatgrass: Amazing Grass Wheat Grass Powder (www.amazinggrass.com)

Zeolite: HealthForce Nutritionals (www.healthforce.com), Vitamin Shoppe (www .vitaminshoppe.com)

ORGANIZATIONS

Holistic dentists: Holistic Dental Association: www.holisticdental.org

Colon therapy: International Association for Colon Hydrotherapy: www.I-act.org

EDUCATIONAL RESOURCES

Acid-Alkaline Diet, Christopher Vasey, trans. Jon Graham (Healing Arts Press, 2006)

Bernard Jensen International, www.bernardjensen.com/nutrition

Chi Nei Tsang: Chi Massage for the Vital Organs, Mantak Chia (Destiny Books, 2006)

The Detox Miracle Sourcebook: Raw Foods and Herbs for Complete Cellular Regeneration, Robert S. Morse, N.D. (Kalindi Press, 2004)

Digestion Connection: Exclusive Expanded Edition, Elizabeth Lipski, Ph.D., and Mark Hyman, M.D. (Rodale, 2013)

Eating For Beauty, David Wolfe (North Atlantic Books, 2003)

Eat Right 4 Your Type, Dr. Peter J. D'Adamo, with Catherine Whitney (Penguin, 1997)

Enzymes: The Fountain of Life, K. Miehlke, R. M. Williams, and D. A. Lopez (Neville Press, 1994)

Enzymes: Go With Your Gut: More Practical Guidelines for Digestive Enzymes, Karen DeFelice (ThunderSnow Interactive, 2006)

Fats That Heal, Fats That Kill: The Complete Guide to Fats, Oils, Cholesterol and Human Health, Udo Erasmus (Alive Books, 1993)

Food Combining and Digestion: 101 Ways to Improve Digestion, Steve Meyerowitz (Sprout House, 2002)

Get the Sugar Out, 2nd ed., Ann Louise Gittleman (Harmony, 2008)

Gut Solutions, Brenda Watson (Renew Life, 2004)

Healthy Mouth, Healthy Body: The Natural Dental Program for Total Wellness, Victor Zeines, FAGD (Xlibris, 2010)

Huangdi Neijing (475 B.C.), various publishers

Longevity Now: A Comprehensive Approach to Healthy Hormones, Detoxification, Super Immunity, Reversing Calcification, and Total Rejuvenation, David Wolfe (North Atlantic Books, 2013)

The pH Miracle: Balance Your Diet, Reclaim Your Health, Robert O. Young and Shelley Redford Young (Grand Central Publishing, 2010)

Probiotics: Nature's Internal Healers, Natasha Trenev (Avery Trade, 1998)

The Raw Food Detox Diet: The Five-Step Plan for Vibrant Health and Maximum Weight Loss, Natalia Rose (William Morrow Paperbacks, 2006)

The Six Healing Sounds: Taoist Techniques for Balancing Chi, Mantak Chia (Destiny Books, 2009)

The Second Brain, Dr. Michael D. Gershon (HarperCollins, 1998)

The Truth About Food—The Good, the Bad and the Downright Dangerous: Revealing the True Nutritional and Vibrational Content of Different Foods and How They Affect Our Health, Gillian Drake (Shank Painter Publishing, 2013)

Index